OXFORD MEDICAL PUBLICATIONS

Managing Alcoholism

Managing Alcoholism

Matching Clients to Treatments

LARS LINDSTRÖM
Department of Educational Research
Stockholm Institute of Education

OXFORD   NEW YORK   TOKYO
OXFORD UNIVERSITY PRESS
1992

Oxford University Press, Walton Street, Oxford OX2 6DP
Oxford   New York   Toronto
Delhi   Bombay   Calcutta   Madras   Karachi
Petaling Jaya   Singapore   Hong Kong   Tokyo
Nairobi   Dar es Salaam   Cape Town
Melbourne   Auckland
and associated companies in
Berlin   Ibadan

Oxford is a trade mark of Oxford University Press

Published in the United States
by Oxford University Press, New York

Original Swedish edition ©1986 Lars Lindström and Liber Förlag
This edition ©Lars Lindström, 1992

A catalogue record for this book is available from the British Library

Library of Congress Cataloging in Publication Data
Lindström, Lars.
[Val av behandling för alkoholism. English]
Managing alcoholism: matching clients to treatments / Lars Lindström.
(Oxford medical publications)
Extensively rev. translation of: Val av behandling för alkoholism.
Includes bibliographical references and indexes.
1. Alcoholism–Treatment.   I. Title.   II. Series.
[DNLM: 1. Alcoholism–therapy. WM 274 L753v]
RC564.7.L5613 1992   616.86'1061–dc20   91-32243
ISBN 0-19-261902-0 (hb)

Typeset by Dobbie Typesetting Ltd.
Printed in Great Britain by Biddles Ltd
Guildford & King's Lynn

For Henning and Ruth,
whose reason and humanity
have inspired my research

Foreword

Dr Griffith Edwards
National Addiction Centre, Institute of Psychiatry, University of London

This book will immediately win its place among the most important reviews of the alcoholism treatment literature to have been published over recent decades. That Dr Lindström is a reviewer of unusual diligence is evident from the broad scope of the issues which he covers, and the immensely comprehensive bibliography which he provides. There are, of course, all too many traps into which the unwary reviewer may haplessly stumble. It is, for instance, possible to be too destructively critical or, on the other hand, too blandly uncritical, or to provide a medley of everyone else's conclusions while coming to no fresh judgement of one's own. Too many reviewers have at a certain juncture simply lost their way in a maze of their own making and into which they duly seek to drag the reader—they leave us lost and baffled, rather than enlightened.

Dr Lindström has fallen into none of these traps, but has, on the contrary, fashioned out of extensive and disparate material an intelligible and original work of scholarship.

If the first point to be made about this book is that it speaks to an unusual mastery of the technical challenge which is always set by the review process when applied to a large and complex field, the second point is that the matter which Dr Lindström tackles is currently of live importance to the alcoholism treatment and research world. Added salience has been given to the issue of treatment matching by the publication of the recent (1990) US Institute of Medicine report on 'Broadening the Base for Treatment of Alcohol Problems'. Lindström's review and the American report might indeed be seen as by happy accident constituting two very complementary approaches to the same large question: how are we to do better in determining the right and person-specific treatment for the individual with a drinking problem, rather than forever employing only the blunderbuss approach? This Swedish book can be seen as giving many of the conclusions drawn in the US report a firm and further scientific underpinning.

Many patients with serious alcohol problems continue to drink unremittingly, and make misery and chaos out of their lives. With equal certainty it can be asserted that even those drinkers who appear to be irrecoverable may at some point escape from their alcoholism, and find recovery, personal growth, and great reward. Recovery never comes about for one reason alone, but always through an amalgam of influences, many of which are quite beyond the therapist's prescription—new hope or new horror, disaster or good fortune, a bad relationship jettisoned or a good one made, the slow process of personal maturity or the cataclysmic event which brings about sudden and radical change. Within that nexus and those mysteries, the formal treatment effort finds its place. With Dr Lindström's generous help we may now be guided more often toward how more accurately to place, time, deliver, and mix the apt treatment interventions.

Preface

The origins of this study can be traced to my experience between 1975 and 1979 as a consultant to a rehabilitation unit in Stockholm, Sweden. The unit provided extensive support to homeless alcoholics who had moved out from a treatment setting to live on their own. Inspired by our 'new' approach to facilitating the social re-entry process, I carried out a survey of evaluations which had compared various approaches to treatment. The implicit purpose was to find justification for what we were doing—whereas the review, in fact, challenged my entire concept of alcoholism, treatment, and human change.

To get perspective and guidance, I felt compelled to take a closer look at the premises, organization, and outcomes of psychosocial treatment of various alcoholic populations. The latter study was started in 1981 and evolved into an interdisciplinary analysis and synthesis of information scattered throughout at least a dozen specialized fields of research. It eventually resulted in the preliminary version of this book, *Val av behandling för alkoholism* (Selection of treatment for alcoholism), which was published by the Liber Förlag (Liber Pub. Co.) in 1986. The book was widely read and quoted, and it was suggested by many colleagues and reviewers that it should be translated into English.

In the process of translation the original book has been extensively revised. It has been updated to integrate literature of relevance to differential treatment appearing up to the end of 1990. As a consequence, 340 new entries have been added to the list of references. Thus, although the main structure is the same, this is in several respects an entirely new book. Among other things, there is a sharper focus on the role of the family, the work environment, and community networks in supporting 'natural processes of healing', and more attention is being paid to the clinical implications of research on treatment of alcoholism.

Along the path that led to this book, I received help, support, and inspiration from numerous colleagues and friends. First, I am indebted to the staff and clients at the 'Krukis' rehabilitation programme in Stockholm for their inspiring optimism and sincere effort.

Next, I owe thanks to my colleagues at the Department of Education at Stockholm University, and especially to Lennart Grosin who was my faculty adviser until 1986, when the dissertation on selection of treatment for alcoholism was examined. I wish to express my gratitude for his patient Socratic guidance, which stimulated me to find and formulate the essentials.

I am grateful also to Hans Bergman, Eckart Kühlhorn, Stig Lindholm, Sten Rönnberg, Ulf Rydberg, and Gunnar Ågren (Stockholm), Lennart

Sjöberg (Gothenburg), Hans Kristenson (Malmö), Torben Arngrim (Århus, Denmark), and Olaf Gjerløw Aasland (Oslo, Norway) for their encouragement and valuable comments on preliminary versions of this book.

The late Nils Bejerot (Stockholm), Griffith Edwards (London), and George Vaillant (Hanover, New Hampshire) provided me with role models for scholarship in the field of addictions.

A visit to the United States and Canada in 1984 gave me an opportunity to meet with several of the researchers and clinicians referred to in the book. Among all those who generously shared their knowledge and experience with me, I especially wish to thank Thomas McLellan, Lester Luborsky, and George Woody (Philadelphia), Frederick Glaser, David Hunt, and Harvey Skinner (Toronto), Alan Ogborne and Brian Rush (London, Canada), and Philip O'Dwyer and Elisabeth Begle (Detroit).

The preliminary study and its publication was supported by grants from The Commission for Social Research at The Swedish Ministry of Health and Social Affairs. The translation and revision of the Swedish treatise was funded jointly by The Swedish Council for Research in the Humanities and Social Sciences, The Commission for Social Research (The Swedish Ministry of Health and Social Affairs), The Swedish Council for Planning and Coordination of Research, and The Swedish Carnegie Institute. Nevertheless, writing this book would not have been possible without the freedom and stimulation provided by my appointment in 1989 as research associate at the Department of Educational Research, Stockholm Institute of Education.

Thanks and appreciation also go to Richard Nord, who helped me translate the original Swedish edition and corrected my extensive revisions.

I wish to thank all the above persons, other colleagues, and friends who have rendered support and assistance, as well as the staff of the library of the Swedish Council for Information on Alcohol and other Drugs, the Karolinska Institute Library, and the National Library for Psychology and Education in Stockholm, who have always given good and prompt service.

Stockholm   L. L.
February 1991

Acknowledgements

The author gratefully acknowledges permission to reprint or adapt the following figures and tables.

Figure 3.1. Schlesinger, Mumford, and Glass 1980, Fig. 5. Copyright by Sage Publications, Inc. Reprinted by permission.
Figure 7.1. Skinner and Allen 1982, Fig. 1. Copyright by the American Psychological Association. Reprinted by permission.
Table 9.1. Marlatt *et al.* 1973, Table 1. Copyright by the American Psychological Association. Adapted by permission.
Figure 10.1. SPRI 1983, Fig. 8.1. Copyright by the Swedish Planning and Rationalization Institute for the Health and Social Services (SPRI). Translated and reprinted by permission.
Table 10.1. Azrin *et al.* (1982), Table 2. Copyright by Pergamon Press. Adapted by permission.
Table 13.1. Sawyer 1966, Table 4. Copyright by the American Psychological Association. Reprinted by permission.
Table 14.1. Pattison 1976, Table 4. Copyright by Pergamon Press. Adapted by permission.
Table 14.2. Pattison 1976, Table 2. Copyright by Pergamon Press. Reprinted by permission.
Figure 15.1. Glaser *et al.* 1984, Vol. 1, p. ii. Copyright by the Addiction Research Foundation of Ontario. Reprinted by permission.
Table 15.1. Glaser 1984*b*, Table 1. Copyright by the Addiction Research Foundation of Ontario. Reprinted by permission.
Table 16.1. McLellan *et al.* 1982, Table 2. Copyright by the American Medical Association. Adapted by permission.
Table 16.2. McLellan *et al.* 1982, Table 3. Copyright by the American Medical Association. Adapted by permission.
Table 16.3. McLellan *et al.* 1981*c*, Table 2. Copyright by Williams and Wilkins. Adapted by permission.
Table 16.4. McLellan *et al.* 1981*c*, Table 4. Copyright by Williams and Wilkins. Adapted by permission.
Table 16.5. McLellan *et al.* 1981*a*, Table 1. Copyright by Elsevier Scientific Publishers Ireland Ltd. Adapted by permission.
Table 16.6. McLellan *et al.* 1983*c*, Table 1. Copyright by Williams and Wilkins. Adapted by permission.
Table 16.7. McLellan *et al.* 1983*a*, Table 3. Copyright by the authors. Adapted by permission.

Table 16.8. McLellan *et al.* 1983*c*, Table 4. Copyright by Williams and Wilkins. Adapted by permission.

Figure 19.1. Annis and Chan 1983, Fig. 1. Copyright by Sage Publications, Inc. Adapted by permission.

Table 19.1. Wallerstein 1957, p. 66. Copyright by Basic Books, Inc. Adapted by permission.

Table 19.2. Wallerstein 1957, p. 137. Copyright by Basic Books, Inc. Adapted by permission.

Figure 21.1. Hunt 1975, Fig. 1. Copyright by the American Educational Research Association. Reprinted by permission.

Figure 21.2. Hunt 1975, Fig. 2. Copyright by the American Educational Research Association. Reprinted by permission.

Figure 21.3. Carr 1970, Fig. 2. Copyright by the American Psychological Association. Reprinted by permission.

Figure 21.4. Witkin *et al.* 1977, Fig. 3. Copyright by the American Psychological Association. Reprinted by permission.

Figure 21.5. Frank 1976, Fig. 1. Copyright by the Johns Hopkins University Press. Reprinted by permission.

Figure 21.6. Skinner 1980, Fig. 3. Copyright by the author. Reprinted by permission.

Table 21.1. McLachlan 1972, Table 1. Copyright by *Psychotherapy*, Cleveland. Reprinted by permission.

Table 21.2. McLachlan 1974, Table 1. Copyright by *Canadian Journal of Psychiatry*. Adapted by permission.

Table 21.3. Frank and Gunderson 1984, Table 1. Copyright by *Psychiatry*. Reprinted by permission.

Table 21.4. Frank and Gunderson 1984, Table 3. Copyright by *Psychiatry*. Reprinted by permission.

Figure 22.1. Orford 1980, Fig. 9.1. Copyright by Croom Helm Ltd. Reprinted by permission.

Table 22.1. Orford *et al.* 1976, Table 1. Copyright by Pergamon Press. Adapted by permission.

Table 22.2. Polich *et al.* 1981, Table 7.8. Copyright by John Wiley and Sons, Inc. Reprinted by permission.

Contents

1. Introduction   1
   Overview   1
   The problem   2
   The integrative review   6

Part I. Research in transition

2. The Hippocratic tradition   13
   Craftsmen and philosophers   13
   Therapy as a cultural phenomenon   16

3. Outcome of alcoholism treatment   20
   Review of outcome research   20
   Are the conclusions plausible?   31

4. New directions in research   34
   Issues in treatment research   34
   Changing notions of treatment   37
   Basic assumptions reconsidered   40

Part II. Conceptions of alcoholism

5. The moral model   47

6. The disease model   49
   The classical model   49
   Scientific critique   51
   Social consequences   55
   Alcoholism—a disease?   57

7. Alcohol dependence   59
   Alcohol-related disabilities   60
   Quantity of consumption   61
   Physical dependence   62
   Dependence as a syndrome   63

8. The symptomatic model   67

Prospective studies   68
Dynamic psychotherapy   74
Alcoholism—a symptom?   77

9. The learning model   79

Conditioning approaches   79
Alcohol expectancies   82
A cognitive-behavioural model   83
Alcoholism—a learned behaviour?   85

10. The social model   88

Symptomatic conceptions   88
Patterns of recovery   93
Environmental resources   96
A social treatment approach   98
Alcoholism—a social career?   101

11. A biopsychosocial perspective   104

The biopsychosocial equation   104
Multivariant and dynamic   107

Part III. Systems of treatment

12. Matching and the systems approach   115

Potentials and criteria   115
Spontaneous remission   117
The non-specific hypothesis   119
The matching hypothesis   120
Monolithic and shotgun approaches   124
The systems approach   126

13. Clinical versus statistical prediction   130

14. Pattison's treatment profiles   137

15. The Core–Shell System   142

The background   142
The core and the shell   143
Primary care   144
Individual assessment   146
Treatment research   147
Implementation   148
Regional systems   149

16. The Penn-VA Project   152

   Is treatment effective?   152
   The Addiction Severity Index   156
   The role of psychiatric severity   161
   Matching—a prospective study   164

Part IV. Studies of interaction

17. Research methodology   173

18. Studies with negative results   177

   Rand Report I   177
   Smart   178
   Finney and Moos   179
   Stinson   181

19. Personality traits   184

   Wallerstein   184
   Annis and Chan   189
   Lyons and Sokolow   192
   Personality typologies   193
   Kadden   195

20. Social and psychological resources   198

   Kissin   198
   Gibbs   201

21. Cognitive styles   204

   McLachlan   204
   Conceptual differentiation   212
   Field dependence and restructuring   214
   Locus of control   221
   Skinner's hypothesis   226
   Therapist–milieu interaction   228

22. Degree of alcohol dependence   233

   Edwards and Orford   233
   Rand Report II   238
   Welte   244
   Foy, Sanchez-Craig   245
   Long-term outcome   247
   Persuasion versus dependence   249

Part V. Selection of treatment

23. Treatment in perspective   255
    Is there a superior method?   255
    Are all alcoholics alike?   256
    Are there effects of interaction?   258
    Conclusion on matching   261

24. Matching clients to treatments   265
    Abstinence versus controlled drinking   266
    Inpatient versus outpatient treatment   269
    Degree of structure and directiveness   273
    Kind of treatment task   279
    Implementing the systems approach   282

25. Strategies of alcoholism treatment   288
    The dynamics of treatment   288
    Supporting the superego   290
    Natural healing processes   293
    Establishing a helping alliance   297

References   305

Name index   357

Subject index   366

1 Introduction

1.1 Overview

Each year about 300 books and 3700 articles are published on alcoholism and its treatment (Mark Keller, cited by Naroll 1983). The scientific production has doubled every seventh year (Moll and Narin 1977). The resulting overload of information has made it impossible for any one person to keep up with the latest developments in the field. This is the case both for those who provide treatment and for the researchers themselves. To an ever increasing extent we have to consult literature reviews as a means of extracting knowledge from the endless flow of information.

Cognizant of the abundance of data, Emrick (1974) noted that: 'adding one more set of findings to an empirical literature can be less helpful than making sense out of and gaining new direction from an existing body of research' (p. 523).

The present review of literature on psychosocial treatment for alcoholism integrates findings drawn from approximately 1000 scientific articles and books. The aim of the project was to study whether the matching of clients to treatments is consistent with current concepts of alcoholism and the body of treatment research, what administrative arrangements it calls for, what consequences it is likely to have for treatment outcome, what client characteristics and treatment dimensions are important, and what conception of effective treatment is thereby implied.

The definition of a problem will influence the way of dealing with it. In this book five concepts of alcoholism are examined: the moral model, the disease model, the symptomatic model, the learning model, and the social model. Alcoholism has traditionally been conceptualized either as a progressive and irreversible disease or as a symptom of social or psychological maladjustment. Recent findings suggest, however, that the view that most alcoholics have been severely disturbed or distressed from the very beginning is based on a retrospective illusion. The disease concept, the learning model, and the social model, on the other hand, all contain elements that are contributing to a biopsychosocial understanding of how alcohol dependence arises, is maintained and can be treated.

This emerging concept of alcoholism draws attention to the differences among alcoholics with respect to both severity of dependence and the social and psychological contingencies that reinforce drinking. The recognition that the population of persons with alcohol problems is multivariant has influenced outcome research and selection of treatment during the past decade. A systems approach has been envisaged as the form towards which the alcoholism treatment enterprise is likely to evolve. This approach is based on the assumption that treatment programmes could maximize their effectiveness by clearly specifying what alcoholic population they can expertly serve, what goals are most feasible for that population, and what methods can be expected to to best achieve those goals. This study examines in depth the rationale and design of three system approaches: Pattison's treatment profiles, the Core–Shell System, and the Penn-VA Project.

In the greater part of the book research on the outcome of alcoholism treatment is examined. This research is reviewed in two stages. Firstly, I try to answer the questions of whether treatment is more effective than no treatment, and whether certain types of treatment are more effective than others. Secondly, the question of whether certain types of clients do better in certain types of treatment is addressed. Thus, I investigate what empirical evidence exists in support of the assumption that a careful matching of clients to treatments will produce outcomes that are superior to those achieved by a unitary approach to treatment. Studies of the effect of client–treatment interaction on outcome are classified according to which types of client variables have been investigated: personality traits, social and psychological resources, cognitive styles, or degree of alcohol dependence. Definitions and research designs are scrutinized. Observed effects of interaction are compared to what is known from the literature on psychotherapy, education, and criminology.

The book concludes with an analysis of what implications this growing body of research has for the design of research and effective clinical practice. The state of the art is summarized with regard to indications for abstinence versus controlled drinking, inpatient versus outpatient treatment, degree of structure and directiveness, and kind of treatment task. Finally, the literature on client–treatment interaction is utilized for an analysis of which healing components characterize successful psychosocial treatment of alcoholics.

This book is intended not only for academics and students but also for practitioners, administrators, and policy makers responsible for the management of alcohol problems. Many of the issues and approaches discussed are applicable to psychosocial treatment in general. They should thus be of interest to those in charge of services for other health problems as well.

1.2   The problem

A doctor seems not even to study health [in the abstract], but the health of man, or perhaps rather the health of a particular man; it is individuals that he is healing.

Thus says Aristotle (1925, p. 1097) in the *Nichomachean Ethics* from the fourth century BC. Himself the son of a doctor, he realized that no two patients, though suffering from the same disease, are quite alike. Hence the idea of matching clients to treatments is by no means new. It is probably as old as the art of healing itself.

Nor is it a recent concept in alcoholism treatment. Already in the late eighteenth century, the British physician Thomas Trotter (1804) noted the variations among alcohol abusers, and suggested that 'very different remedies will be required' (p. 5). The pioneering alcohologists Karl Bowman and Morton Jellinek (1941) maintained in the first major review of alcoholism treatment approaches that probably

the only possibility [for improving the outcome of alcoholism treatment] is to bring greater order into psychotherapeutic procedures. By this we mean that a definite effort has to be made to establish criteria for the suitability of any given method to a given patient; the criteria so far established are definitely superficial. (p. 169–70)

Unfortunately, little attention was given to this problem during the following four decades. Yet a recent initiative by the US National Academy of Sciences has radically changed the situation. From 1986 to 1990, a committee of the Institute of Medicine (IOM) and its study staff, directed by Frederick Glaser, carried out a comprehensive examination of treatment for alcohol problems. Four task forces and more than 200 researchers, practioners, and administrators were asked for reviews and recommendations. In the process a 'vision' of treatment systems or multi-programme networks for people with alcohol problems emerged. Matching was designated 'the central process in the committee's vision' (IOM 1990, p. 287).

However, the fishing expedition strategy, i.e., the strategy of systematically testing out all possible client × therapist × technique × setting interactions, is not feasible. In order for the vision to be implemented, investigators will have to specify a limited number of relevant dimensions across existing modes of therapy.

The IOM committee recommended 'that an expert committee be convened on a regular basis . . . to focus on what is currently known about matching individuals with alcohol problems to appropriate treatments' (IOM 1990, p. 296). In 1989, moreover, the US National Institute on Alcohol Abuse and Alcoholism announced a multi-year effort called the National Collaborative Matching Project (RFA AA-89-02B), which aimed to conduct multisite trials of patient–treatment matching. Studies funded under that project have adhered to the same design and employed a prescribed protocol. As a supplement, separate studies on matching were requested (RFA GR15). Incidentally, such large-scale studies, 'which can be evaluated only after several years', were advocated earlier by Bowman and Jellinek (1941, p. 170).

Thus, although matching is an old concern, there has been a recent renaissance of interest. The assumption that a differential approach characterized by a careful matching of clients to treatments will improve outcome is, indeed, both promising and consistent with common sense. Yet it remains largely unproven and has therefore legitimately been designated 'the matching hypothesis' (Glaser 1980).

The problem investigated in the present study is whether this hypothesis does provide a sound foundation for research and development work in the treatment of alcoholism. Furthermore, new hypotheses are generated on *how* and *why* improvements may be achieved by matching clients to treatments.

The term *matching* was defined by Glaser and Skinner (1981) as 'the deliberate and consistent attempt to select a specific candidate for a specific method of intervention in order to achieve specific goals' (p. 302).

Matching thus refers here to the central process in differential treatment. The requirements for matching are evident from Glaser and Skinner's definition. Any programme will have to specify not only which type of population can be served but also which methods are appropriate and which goals are feasible for that population. Moreover, an efficient procedure for assigning specific clients to specific interventions for the purpose of achieving specific goals must be available.

The IOM committee noted that many programmes exclude applicants by some screening process or provide ancillary services on an individualized basis. Although such practices were commended, the committee were justified in not regarding them as instances of matching. In the committee's view 'matching involves varying the principal treatment approach utilized from one individual to another in accord with a preconceived and explicit plan' (IOM 1990, p. 284). That is, one patient may be assigned to supervised Antabuse, another to relapse prevention training, a third to an approach drawing on the environmental resources available to the alcoholic, and so forth.

The term *hypothesis* is often defined as a theory which has not yet proved its mettle. The 'matching hypothesis' is not a hypothesis in this literal sense. It rather denotes a perspective or a frame of reference. A *theory* is a coherent set of general propositions that are interconnected in such a way that they explain phenomena in reality. Theories are capable of falsification or corroboration (Popper 1959). A *perspective* serves as a tool for organizing or 'framing' information within a field of research. Before theories are formulated, we need a perspective for identifying relevant facts and relationships. The latter must be wide enough to help us view all the important components and their interaction in specific situations.

A given perspective will not in itself explain the phenomena which are the object of investigation. But it may be more or less fruitful as an element in a *research strategy*, or the collection of explicit and implicit views that every researcher holds as to which tasks are most important, how they should be carried out, and which results should be expected.

The matching hypothesis can be regarded as a fruitful perspective for research and development work, if the following conditions are satisfied:

1. *No single treatment has been found superior for all alcoholics.* If, however, a single treatment approach is universally superior to all other approaches, then there should be greater prospects of improving treatment outcome by developing this method than by studying under what conditions less successful ones can best be utilized.

2. *No valid evidence exists for the assumption that alcoholics are essentially alike.* If, however, 'all alcoholics are alike' and have the same needs, we should expect to find one particular treatment approach which is most appropriate to all 'cases'.

3. *Interaction takes place between type of client, form of intervention, and outcome in the treatment of alcoholism.* If different treatment approaches affect different client populations in different ways, improvements can probably be achieved by matching each client with an approach that has been effective for similar individuals.

The question of whether any superior treatment exists is discussed in Part I of the book. Theories on what alcoholics have in common and how they differ are analysed in Part II. Part III elaborates on the usefulness of the matching hypothesis as an element in both a research strategy and a *strategy for intervention*—the systems approach. Empirical studies that attempted to identify effects of client–treatment interaction are classified and reviewed in Part IV.

In Part V, Chapter 23, conclusions are drawn as to whether the matching hypothesis is scientifically and clinically fruitful. Chapter 24 develops a number of hypotheses on how clients and treatments should be matched in order to achieve the most favourable outcome. Chapter 25 formulates a theory on why improved results can be expected from a matching of clients and treatments in the manner suggested.

With well-founded theories about client–treatment interaction, valid definitions of concepts and reliable classification procedures, clients and treatments can be co-ordinated in a 'deliberate' and 'consistent' manner. It will then be possible to test and modify hypotheses on how to match specific clients with specific treatments in order to achieve specific goals.

So far, only one study of alcoholism treatment (McLellan *et al.* 1983*c*) has directly tested a specific matching hypothesis. Furthermore, there are hardly any corroborated theories of interaction, based on valid constructs and reliable classifications of client characteristics and treatment dimensions.

However, these issues are presently high on the agenda of alcoholism treatment research. Matching has been the topic of many scholarly review papers in recent years. Some of these (Matakas, Koester, and Leidner 1978; Ogborne 1978; Glaser 1980; Gibbs 1981; Emrick 1982; Pattison 1982*a*; Miller and Hester 1986*c*; Annis 1987) have summarized empirical findings, while others (McLellan *et al.* 1980*c*; Glaser and Skinner 1981; Skinner 1981*b*; Finney and Moos 1986; Longabaugh 1986; Annis 1988; Marlatt 1988; IOM 1989, Ch. 11; IOM 1990, Ch. 11) have focused on conceptual and methodological issues.

I wish to contribute to this re-orientation in our thinking about alcohol problems and their treatment. The emerging interest in a systems approach to treatment calls for a transformation of the matching hypothesis from a heuristic principle into well-defined hypotheses and ultimately into theories, of increasingly general scope, on the best way to design psychosocial treatment for each particular alcoholic.

Treatment for alcohol problems is defined as 'any activity that is directed toward changing a person's drinking behaviour and reducing [his or her] alcohol consumption' (IOM 1990, p. 46). In general, such treatment involve additional activities aimed at alleviating physical, psychological, and social complications or modifying conditions that are assumed to maintain hazardous drinking. The term intervention is used synonymously with treatment. Client and patient are used as synonyms for a person in treatment.

In order to avoid cumbersome sentence rhythms, I will most often use 'he' instead of 'he or she' as a generic pronoun for alcoholics. It should, however, be remembered that in most industrialized societies today one fourth to one third of all those with alcohol problems and dependence are females. For other persons than alcoholics I will use 'he or she' fairly frequently, in order to remind the reader not to think of men only.

For practical reasons, the topic of this book has been delimited in two important ways. Firstly, I will focus on treatment for alcohol abuse and alcoholism. Thus, preventive measures for problem drinkers having little or no documented physical dependence will be discussed only in passing. Secondly, the focus will be on treatment in voluntary forms. Hence, the conclusions drawn here cannot be generalized to compulsory treatment aimed at protecting the family or preventing severe and permanent damage to the alcoholic himself.

It should be recognized, however, that both of these approaches provide significant remedial opportunities over and above those studied in this book. Alcoholism treatment cannot provide a substitute either for early preventive or for legislative measures. A comprehensive and integrated system of prevention would, however, make it easier for treatment to fulfil its humanitarian mission.

1.3   The integrative review

To test the fruitfulness of the matching hypothesis, I searched literature in primarily three areas:

1. Reviews of outcome research that compared various treatment methods with each other or compared a treatment group with a control group that received no or minimal treatment.

2. Theoretical efforts to describe and explain alcohol abuse and alcoholism.

3. Outcome research that attempted to identify effects of client–treatment interaction.

In addition, I searched studies that indirectly elucidate the question of whether the matching hypothesis is useful in research and clinical practice. The studies of interest were mainly:

4. Analyses of research strategies, i.e. theoretical and methodological approaches, in psychosocial treatment research.

5. Descriptions of administrative arrangements aimed at a deliberate and consistent pairing of clients and interventions in alcoholism treatment.

Cooper (1984) distinguishes between three types of literature reviews. The first type he calls the 'integrative' review. By this is meant 'the synthesis of separate empirical findings into a coherent whole' (Cooper 1982, p. 291). What is typical of this review is the combination of empirical data rather than the goal of integrating material from various sources, which, after all, characterizes any review. I therefore propose that it be called the *empirical review* instead of the integrative review. Empirical reviews summarize past research by drawing overall conclusions from many separate studies that address related or identical hypotheses. The purpose is to present the state of knowledge and to highlight important issues and fruitful directions for future research.

Cooper's (1984) second kind of literature review is called the *theoretical review*. Here, the purpose is to present theories offered to explain a particular phenomenon. These are compared with regard to their empirical support and internal consistency as well as to how convincing they are in explaining the phenomenon. Theoretical reviews will typically contain descriptions of critical studies and promising avenues of research as well as an assessment of which theory is most powerful and consistent with what is known. Sometimes the presentation concludes with an attempt at a new theoretical synthesis.

The third type of review is called the *methodological review*. Its purpose is to examine the research methods and operational definitions that have been applied to a problem area. Methodological reviews are often critical of previous research, arguing that artefacts have distorted the results, that measurement has been misleading or unreliable, or that specific conditions limit the conclusions that can be drawn.

A comprehensive review often addresses more than one of these sets of issues. A review such as the present one, which combines empirical, theoretical, and methodological components, could legitimately be called an *integrative review*. The present study is in the main, or as regards the review of outcome research in alcoholism treatment and related fields, an empirical review. Empirical findings concerning main effects and interaction effects are classified, summarized, and interpreted. The study in Part II of the book, which examines conceptions of alcohol abuse and alcoholism, is a theoretical review. The presentation in Parts I and III of the matching hypothesis and other strategies in research on the outcome of treatment for alcoholism and other health problems may be characterized as a methodological review.

The approach has thus been flexible and adapted to the types of problems dealt with. It can be described as *qualitative*, with a greater emphasis placed on analysis of patterns, agreements, and contradictions within the body of research than is usually the case in quantitative literature reviews, such as meta-analyses. Since the reviewing approach is varied throughout the book, I have chosen to address relevant methodological issues in direct connection with the part or chapter to which they apply. I will confine myself here to making some general comments on the literature search.

My basic bibliographic source has been the library of the Swedish Council for Information on Alcohol and other Drugs in Stockholm, whose literature stock amounts to over 147 000 volumes, of which around 450 are periodicals (Sonja Valverius, personal communication 1990). The library closely monitors developments in its field, which has often enabled me to locate—as catalogued or ordered—alcohol studies identified through other channels. My inter-disciplinary approach and ambition to consult the sources has, however, led me to undertake regular visits to half a dozen research libraries in the Stockholm region, of which the Karolinska Institute Library, the National Library for Psychology and Education, and the Stockholm University Library deserve special mention.

Owing to the scope of the study, limited funds, and the availability of good abstracting services, bibliographies, and citation indexes, I have only occasionally carried out computer searches. There are three kinds of manual literature searching: *unsystematic search*, *chain search*, and *systematic search*. I have combined all of these techniques to track down the about 1000 articles and books referred to in the text.

Examples of unsystematic search are informal communication with Swedish and foreign research colleagues, attendance at professional meetings, contacts with librarians and documentalists at research libraries, looking in directories such as *Books in Print*, browsing in international publisher's catalogues found at libraries or received via subscription (for example, IBIS), utilization of the Esselte literature service, visits to book dealers in Sweden and abroad, reading of book reviews in scientific and professional journals, regular reading of current periodicals and recently acquired literature at the research libraries, etc.

Chain searches start with core references embodying key ideas and basic facts. By citing earlier research on the subject, the authors of these books and articles enabled me to take advantage of their search efforts. Recent literature is particularly useful for such *backward* chain searching. Older titles central to a topic sometimes served as the starting point for *forward* chain search. I made for this purpose use of the *Science* and *Social Sciences Citation Indexes*, which provide a list of fairly recent journal articles (plus certain books) that refer to the title of interest. Combined backward–forward chain searching proved to be a fast and effective method of tracking down literature within a given, limited field of research.

The results of the above techniques are dependent on a number of factors whose influence is difficult to control, for example the interests and qualifications of the persons who are consulted, which books and periodicals the research libraries choose to buy, and which theoretical perspective or empirical research tradition characterizes the studies chosen as a starting point for chain searching. In order to ensure that the selection of information is not overly biased, it must be complemented with some form of systematic literature search.

Given that the topic is relatively narrow, the relevant literature can be sifted out from abstracts, bibliographies, or data bases on the basis of a few descriptors and a specification as to the period and the languages of interest. Crawford and Chalupsky (1977), for example, utilized data bases covering approximately 3000 journals and 1 000 000 technical reports to locate evaluations of psychosocial alcoholism treatment. The literature search was restricted to evaluations which had been published in English during the period 1968–71. By this means, the authors identified 40 evaluations, the majority of which had been published in a few leading journals.

The literature search for the present study, however, could not be restricted to a few years and a handful of descriptors. With my broader problem definition, including empirical, theoretical, and methodological aspects, I repeatedly had to search for relevant titles and authors in the catalogues of research libraries, in the *[Quarterly] Journal of Studies on Alcohol* with its Classified Abstract Archive of Alcohol Literature, the *British Journal of Addiction*, and a dozen other core journals, in handbooks such as *The Biology of Alcoholism* and *Research Advances in Alcohol and Drug Problems*, and in journals publishing reviews, e.g. *Annual Review of Psychology* and *Psychological Bulletin*. In addition, I regularly consulted abstracting services, such as *Psychological Abstracts* and *Drug Abuse* (Stockholm), and bibliographies, notably *Index Medicus* and *Current Contents*. Systematic literature search of this kind is extremely time-consuming, but there is no short cut to locate studies in peripheral sources and to protect the validity of a research review.

Only a few foreign dissertations and unpublished research reports have been procured. Many relevant books were not available in Sweden; but thanks to the extensive contacts between Nordic research libraries, these books could generally be obtained within a few months. Nevertheless, more readily available periodical literature from recent years is probably overrepresented in this study.

The literature search has mainly identified studies reported in English. My survey of untranslated literature in Swedish, Danish, Norwegian, German, and French yielded meagre returns. Studies in English were not only more numerous but generally also of a higher standard, since most of them had been scrutinized by an international network of peer reviewers. It is possible that a more systematic search would have yielded more non-English reports of high quality research. Nevertheless, the result of my survey reflects the dominant position of English as the international language of alcoholism treatment research. However, the research reported in the English-language literature is more distributed among different countries of origin than it was in the pioneering years following World War II, when Ivan Bratt (1953) pointed out that 'writing about alcoholism and leaving out what the Americans have to say on the matter would be like writing about communism and ignoring the lessons from Russia' (p. 131; translated from Swedish).

Finally, it should be remembered that even if the identified studies were representative of all published and unpublished studies, the elements contained might differ from all elements of interest. For example, Miller and colleagues (1970) observed that conclusions from alcoholism treatment research were often based on biased samples. In addition to dropout and other well-known threats to validity, these authors discussed distortion introduced by varying definitions of alcoholism, by case selection from special populations, by the reputation of the treatment programme, and by some alcoholics' refusal to accept any help for their drinking problem. These and other factors endangering the representativeness of alcoholism treatment research will be dealt with in relation to specific studies later on.

Part I

Research in transition

Is alcoholism treatment more effective than no treatment at all? Are some types of treatment more effective than others? These are the questions discussed in Chapter 3. In this chapter outcome research in alcoholism treatment will be critically examined, and it will be compared with research on the outcome of psychosocial treatment for other health problems.

Part I also looks upon treatment in an historical perspective. Maybe psychosocial treatment has more to learn from the ancients and from the treatment of tuberculosis in the first half of the twentieth century than from modern medicine. A look back highlights the fact that alcoholism treatment is a culturally mediated phenomenon whose outcome is determined not only by the treatment approach, but also by the therapist and the patient. It will also help us to reconsider basic assumptions in psychosocial treatment research and to reorient its focus from the effects of specific techniques to natural healing processes, common therapeutic elements, and effects of client–treatment interaction. Parallel lines of development in psychotherapy research will be described as a recent background.

2 The Hippocratic tradition

2.1 Craftsmen and philosophers

Certain physicians and philosophers assert that nobody can know medicine who is ignorant what a man is; he who would treat patients properly must, they say, learn this. But the question they raise is one for philosophy; it is the province of those who, like Empedocles, have written on natural science, what man is from the beginning, how he came into being at the first, and from what elements he was originally constructed. But my view is . . . that one can attain this knowledge [i.e. of the nature of man] [only] when medicine itself has been properly comprehended, but till then it is quite impossible. (Hippocrates 1923, Vol. 1, p. 53)

This quotation is taken from one of the oldest scientific records we possess, the Hippocratic Collection. The cited treatise, *Ancient Medicine*, belongs to the end of the fifth century BC. It is the work of 'a wise eclectic and a careful empiric' (Jones 1946). Although his name is unknown, the dialect betrays that he was a Ionian Greek. The tract is, perhaps, the most important of the entire collection and has justly been described as one of the highest products of Greek culture (Farrington 1953).

The work and its background raises a question of great importance for treatment research, namely its relationship to clinical experience on the one hand and to various treatment philosophies on the other. In comparison with the biological medicine, research on psychosocial treatment is still in its beginning. Here, the relationship of science to empiricism and philosophical rationales is as crucial an issue today as it was in medicine 2400 years ago.

In the cited passage from *Ancient Medicine*, the author reverses the claim of the philosophers, that it is not possible to practice medicine if you do not know what a man is. He asserts instead that it is impossible to know what a man is without any knowledge of medicine in the broad sense. Man is said to be composed of a multitude of fluids and organs, each having its own special function. The human being is also under the constant influence of foods and drinks, his surroundings, the climate and the seasons. Therefore, if one is to learn about the nature of man, one must first study all that influences him.

This approach to treatment research, in which science builds upon observed facts and common sense-knowing, even though at best it goes beyond it, is referred to as the *empirical* or *Hippocratic* tradition. It stands in sharp opposition to the *rational* tradition in medicine, dating back to ancient physicians who deduced their treatment of cases from general principles.

The Greek author describes his art as ancient because he sees its origin in the oldest and humblest of all arts, namely the art of cooking. The practice of medicine had developed through man's observations of what influences promoted his nourishment, well-being, and health, rather than causing suffering, sickness and death (*Anc. Med.*, Ch. 3). Eventually, a body of knowledge and rules was built up concerning the symptoms and courses of diseases and the effects of drugs. During the fifth century BC, the teaching of medicine became concentrated to a number of medical schools, of which the ones on the island of Cos and in Cnidus, just opposite it on the mainland of Asia Minor, were the most famous. The members of these schools catalogued the practices and reworked the doctrines of traditional medicine. Like some other crafts, medicine was on its way to becoming a science.

Soon, however, rival medical schools in the West emerged, whose members did not have the same understanding of medicine as a practical art. These included the school of Empedocles at Agrigentum on Sicily, where it was assumed that man, like all physical bodies, consists of the four elements fire, air, earth, and water, whose characteristic qualities are those of being hot, cold, dry, or wet. Disease was said to be due to an excess or deficiency of one or other of these qualities, and the physician should, if he acted correctly, cure 'the cold' with 'the hot', 'the hot' with 'the cold', 'the wet' with 'the dry', and 'the dry' with 'the wet'. This was the foundation of humoral pathology, which was to dominate the practice of medicine all the way up until the last century.

Empedocles himself, referred to in the quotation above, was a remarkable and contradictory character. In many respects he was an ingenious thinker, but he was also most anxious to make an impression on the public with his wisdom. Robed in purple, girded in gold, crowned with a wreath of flowers and binders as an 'immortal god', he travelled from town to town as an itinerant philosopher, seer, and 'medicine-man'. He gathered thousands of adherents, and speculative natural philosophy gradually increased its influence. At the same time, his doctrines were diluted and coarsened. This paved the way for charlatans and adventurers, who covered the gaps in their dilettante knowledge with the veil of philosophy. A climate was created in which the ancient empirical schools of medicine, whose positive knowledge had been gained by means of sustained and meticulous observation, ran the risk of being stifled by newfangled philosophical doctrines.

It was to combat these doctrines, which made their *a priori* speculations about the elements a guiding principle for medical practice, that the treatise *Ancient Medicine* was written. From the very first sentence, the author leaps to the attack. He fiercely criticizes all who 'narrow down the causal principle of diseases and of death among men, and make it the same in all cases, postulating one thing or two' (Hippocrates 1923, Vol. 1, p. 13). This approach may work in natural philosophy, he concedes. But it is not advisable in medicine, which is 'an art, and one which all men use on the most important occasions, and give the greatest honours to the good craftsman and practitioners in it'. Here the pride of the craftsman is noticeable. Conscious of the richness of his factual knowledge, he is violently opposed to the intrusion of arbitrary assumptions or postulates into medicine:

I have deemed that [the art of medicine] has no need of an empty postulate, as do insoluble mysteries, about which any exponent must use a postulate, for example, things in the sky or below the earth. If a man were to learn and declare the state of these, neither to the speaker himself nor to his audience would it be clear whether his statements were true or not. For there is no test the application of which would give certainty. But medicine has long had all its means to hand, and has discovered both a principle and a method, through which the discoveries made during a long period are many and excellent, while full discovery will be made, if the inquirer be competent, conduct his researches with knowledge of the discoveries already made, and make them his starting-point. But anyone who, casting aside and rejecting all these means . . . asserts that he has found out anything, is and has been the victim of deception. (Hippocrates 1923, Vol. 1, pp. 13, 15)

In other words, back to the ancient art of medicine, undistorted by philosophical doctrines and based on reality, experience, and observation; but, mark well, the search must continue! The Hippocratic writers can be given the credit for having rescued medicine, albeit temporarily, from the clutches of metaphysical speculation and declared its independence. They also raised it from the status of a routine craft to a true art and a science based on sustained critical investigations.

The Hippocratic authors preserved a certain loyalty to the older, more modest folk medicine with its illiterate practitioner, who was aware of his inferior position. But by no means did they remain entrenched in the old drudgery, which merely piled facts upon facts and made use of rote-learned rules and techniques. These might very well be gained from experience and be practically useful, but they were not based on painstaking and systematic observation.

The Hippocratics did not content themselves with the knowledge that a treatment helps. They also enquired into the cause of its effects. Like the philosophers, whose role in the foundation and development of European science should not be underrated, they tried to find a theoretical explanation for the disease and not merely apply a routine cure to the individual case. The physician should concern himself with the individual case, but should at the same time strive methodically to find general rules governing its treatment. However, the explanations and guidelines should be tested by further appeals to sense-experience, they must not be taken for granted as an obvious truth. Thus did treatment research arise from the practical needs of the physician.

Another important issue, raised in ancient Greece, is the role of the therapist, the patient and the environment in bringing about healing. The Hippocratic view is eloquently expressed in the well-known aphorism:

Life is short, the Art long, opportunity fleeting, experience treacherous, judgment difficult. The physician must be ready, not only to do his duty himself, but also to secure the co-operation of the patient, of the attendants and of externals. (Hippocrates 1923, Vol. 2, p. 99)

Well aware of the limitations of ancient medicine, the Hippocratic writers advised against arbitrary interventions that might disrupt the natural healing process. The basic concept in their theory of medicine is that diseases are cured by nature itself and that the doctor should be a servant of nature, whose main task is to ascertain, and take into account, how climate, foods, modes of life, and other circumstances affect the human organism. The Hippocratic writings recognize that the physician cannot accomplish anything if he fails to secure the co-operation of the patient and his or her environment.

Adler (1988) made a useful distinction between operative and co-operative arts. In *operative* arts such as shoemaking and shipbuilding, painting and sculpture, the artist is the principal cause of the product produced. Nature may supply the materials and even models to imitate, but without the intervention of the artist, nature would not produce shoes, ships, paintings, or statues.

Healing, on the other hand, like farming and teaching, is a *co-operative* art. The co-operative artist merely helps nature to produce results that it is able to produce by its own powers. Fruits and grains grow naturally; learning would go on even if there were no teachers. The body has the power to maintain and regain health. The physician who adopts the Hippocratic conception of healing attempts to support and reinforce the natural processes of the body, just as the efficient teacher brings the natural process of learning to its fullest fruition.

By controlling the patient's regimen—his diet, his hours, his activities, his environment—the Hippocratic physician helped the body to heal itself by its natural processes. Administering drugs, i.e. introducing foreign substances into the body, was regarded as the least co-operative of medical treatments. Although sometimes justified, surgery was looked upon as a drastic measure to be resorted to only when all co-operative methods failed. According to Adler (op. cit.), it was regarded as an operative rather than a co-operative procedure. By analogy, psychotherapists who think of themselves as the principal, or even the sole, cause of remission in patients do not understand, as did the Hippocratics, healing as a co-operative art.

2.2   Therapy as a cultural phenomenon

Young sciences often split into rival schools of thought, each of which claims to have found the 'truth' while its opponents are in 'error'. Naroll (1983) asserts that shifts in the 'paradigms' or research strategies of less developed disciplines occur through changes in the interests of the scholars, often in response to changes in the climate of opinion.

Mature sciences change paradigms—i.e. the system of norms that regulates the researcher's choice of problems, concepts, and methods of investigation—only when rigorous observations show that the new paradigm fits the data better than the old one did. When a dispute arises in mature sciences, both parties usually agree that their viewpoints are tentative, pending further research. They also tend to agree on the nature of the studies needed to resolve the dispute, and to suspend final judgement until such studies are made.

Psychosocial treatment research is a developing discipline. The relationship of this research to empirical and rational traditions in treatment is brought to the fore by Peter Magaro, Robert Gripp, and David McDowell in *The Mental Health Industry: A Cultural Phenomenon* (1978). This book analyses the development of treatments in psychiatry, but its theses are applicable to alcoholism treatment as well. The authors try to demonstrate that psychotherapeutic methods at public mental hospitals and outpatient clinics have gained ground not so much due to their effectiveness in treatment, but because of their allegiance to dominant cultural ideas. They also argue that new concepts of pathology have arisen from changes in cultural beliefs more often than from scientific discoveries.

Clinical psychology is said to have rested heavily on postulates of what man is, i.e. the method the author of *Ancient Medicine* criticized for limiting our ability to perceive the diversity of human existence. When the culture's concept of human nature, and thereby its notions of deviant behaviour, changed, new professional groups with new rationales and treatments were able to gain prestige and influence.

A main thesis of the book is that 'the evidence confirming the success of a treatment decreases with the length of time the treatment is practiced' (Magaro *et al.* 1978, p. 15). Treatments seem to have a characteristic life cycle. Tourney (1970) reviewed the literature on a number of psychiatric therapies: medical, psychodynamic, and environmental. After having listed the success rate of each therapy over time, he drew the following conclusion:

Initial statistics often indicate results of 90 per cent recovery or marked improvement, whereas subsequent studies find these figures reduced to 50–60 per cent in psychoneuroses, and to 30–40 per cent in schizophrenia. Often such therapeutic developments become more like a religious movement, strongly identified with a particular leader—observed in psychoanalysis with Freud or insulin therapy with Sakel—than a scientific development. Rejected techniques are often reintroduced in new guises with new names and new theoretic foundations. This type of circular movement has been observed in the application of moral therapy, hospital treatment, psychotherapy, and drug and physical therapies. Too often psychiatric treatment reflects some of the social and political philosophies of the day, rather than a sound medical orientation applying the scientific laws of cause and effect. (Tourney 1970, pp. 6–7)

Magaro, Gripp, and McDowell thoroughly investigated the scientific support for psychosocial therapies, from the 'moral treatment' of the early nineteenth century to the milieu therapy and behaviour modification of recent decades in American psychiatric care. They found no convincing evidence for the universal effectiveness of therapies. They therefore interpret the advocacy of one treatment or the other as a *cultural phenomenon*. The credibility of a treatment method is undermined when the cultural world view changes, or when the method is spread to treatment settings with other values and assumptions than those of the innovators, and is applied to other treatment populations than it was originally intended for.

Along with a large number of critics since the mid-60s (Section 4.2), Magaro and colleagues call for a new way of formulating and solving treatment problems. Instead of trying to determine whether a given therapy is effective in a global sense, treatment should be conceptualized as an interactional process whose outcome is determined by a number of variables related to the therapy, the therapist, and the patient. This does not mean that a multidimensional matrix with hundreds of cells is required. It is possible, as the authors exemplifies, to begin on a much smaller scale.

The first step is to specify which patient characteristics and treatment variables are crucial and should be included in the model. Here, the model-builder must rely on available empirical evidence and his own theoretical orientation. The second step in the model-building process is to predict theoretically, with the support of empirical data, how the chosen variables will interact to achieve a desired result. The third step involves testing and modifying the model. Magaro, Gripp, and McDowell (1978) have not come that far with their own prescriptive treatment model, but they explain why it is important not to lose sight of the goal:

The prescriptive model offers a moderate solution [to the critique of the mental health industry and its therapies] by providing a data base concerning what treatments work for whom regardless of the cultural ideology of the day. It also requires the institution to give up its hope of consensus and enter into the conflict of ideas that could be resolved only through the effects on the residents. Hence the institution does become freer from the society and from internal domination by an administrative class no matter what their philosophy. (p. 213)

This approach is reminiscent of the one the Hippocratic writers advocated as a guiding principle for the art of medicine. Instead of first deciding what man is in general and then devising treatment methods accordingly, research should apply the empirical method. It should study everything that affects a man's health in order to arrive, via theoretical explanations, at a more accurate conception of the human nature.

To be sure, the Hippocratics had an imperfect understanding of how a theory is arrived at (Jones 1946). In a letter to Popper (1959), Einstein agreed that 'theory cannot be fabricated out of the results of observation, but . . . can only be invented' (p. 458). Thus, every research student must be a good guesser. But he should, *nota bene*, be aware of what he is doing. He must not—as the 'rational' physicians in antiquity—confuse his guesses with accurately observed facts, or with theories that have stood up to severe tests, nor think he has gained knowledge when he is only speculating.

Moreover, in some spheres of research deductive reasoning is the correct, and perhaps the only method. But as noted by the author of *Ancient Medicine*, the error lies in transferring this approach from spheres where it does apply to those where it does not. Narrowing down the explanation of psychiatric problems to one or a couple of mechanisms, whether they are related to neurophysiology, intrapsychic conflicts, or operant learning, may be acceptable in basic research, pending further advances. But it is not advisable in 'an art . . . which all men use on the most important occasions, and give the greatest honours to the good craftsman and practitioners in it' (Hippocrates 1923, Vol. 1, p. 13).

3 Outcome of alcoholism treatment

3.1 Review of outcome research

If Magaro and his co-workers (1978) are right, clinical psychology (Section 2.2) would profit from a re-evaluation in the Hippocratic spirit. The same may be said of alcoholism treatment. In 1976, Enoch Gordis, the present director of the US National Institute on Alcohol Abuse and Alcoholism (NIAAA), said that the treatment of alcoholism had not improved in any important way in 25 years. Seven years later this appraisal was reiterated by George Vaillant (1983b). Unfortunately, it is also confirmed by the following review of research on the outcome of alcoholism treatment.

In the first major survey of alcoholism treatment evaluation, Voegtlin and Lemere (1942) reviewed more than 200 studies published between 1909 and 1940. The authors were struck by the absence of statistical data by which the effectiveness of various programmes might be judged.

The reluctance to use experimental and quantitative designs was eventually overcome after the second world war. But it was not until the mid-1960s in the USA that outcome research came into its own. The purpose of evaluation was now defined as providing 'objective, systematic and comprehensive evidence on the degree to which the program achieves its intended objectives' (Hyman, Wright, and Hopkins 1962, p. 5).

Hill and Blane (1967) found 49 evaluations published between 1952 and 1963 that dealt with psychotherapy for alcoholics. They were unable to draw any conclusions about the value of these methods, since the research was far too deficient in a number of respects. The primary methodological weaknesses were poor planning, lack of control groups, biased selection procedures, inadequate criterion variables, unreliable measuring instruments, and deficient follow-up procedures. Similar shortcomings were found by Gillespie (1967) and Miller *et al.* (1970).

Conradsson and Holmgren (1974) carried out an extensive review of Swedish and international research on the outcome of treatment for alcoholics. They examined 231 reports published during the ten-year period 1965–74. Variation of outcomes tended to be large within treatments and small between treatments. It was not unusual for an average improvement rate of 45 per cent with a specific method to conceal a variation between different studies ranging from 10 per cent improved to 85 per cent improved. Like Emrick and Hansen in 1983, the authors found that the more stringent the design of an evaluative study, the less favourable were its conclusions.

Baekeland, Lundwall, and Kissin (1975) and Baekeland (1977) reviewed more than 400 reports on outcomes of alcoholism treatment published from 1953 to 1973. They were impressed with the dominant role played by the clients' pretreatment characteristics as opposed to the kind of treatment being used. Regardless of the treatment method, clients with higher socioeconomic status and social stability had improvement rates varying from 32 per cent to 68 per cent, whereas clients with lower status and stability (largely skid row alcoholics) had rates ranging from 0 per cent to 18 per cent.

Crawford and Chalupsky (1977) examined 40 reports published between the years 1968 and 1971 that evaluated some form of psychological treatment for alcoholism. They found that the quality of research had improved somewhat since Hill and Blane's (1967) review of evaluation in the 1950s and 1960s. In the early 1970s there was a greater use of control groups, a better description of the follow-up procedure, other outcome criteria besides abstinence, etc. Nevertheless, the authors concluded that most studies were both scientifically and practically unproductive.

Linda and Mark Sobell (1982) reviewed 37 evaluations of alcoholism treatment reported in the scientific literature between 1976 and 1980. Included were only studies of more than one client with a minimum of 12 months of treatment outcome data following either discharge from inpatient treatment or admission to outpatient treatment. As a result, two-thirds of all studies were excluded on methodological grounds from the start. However, the methodology of well-designed outcome studies had improved considerably over the few years since the review by Crawford and Chalupsky (1977).

Major advances included:

(1) using multiple information sources to gather outcome data;

(2) using multiple measures of life health functioning, in addition to drinking, to assess treatment effectiveness;

(3) using a minimum of a 12-month follow-up interval to assess outcome;

(4) using equal follow-up intervals for all subjects; and

(5) conducting multiple assessments throughout the follow-up interval.

In 1987 Mark Sobell and his co-workers published a new review including 48 outcome studies from 1980 to 1984. Significant improvements in outcome data had occurred with time. On the negative side, data on severity of dependence and other pretreatment characteristics were often lacking. This deficiency is considered to seriously impede attempts to compare studies or to reach definitive conclusions concerning treatment effectiveness.

Today's discussion is characterized by a growing awareness of the methodological problems associated with the evaluation of interventions for alcoholism (e.g. Jeffrey 1975; May and Kuller 1975; Schuckit and Cahalan 1976; Blane 1977; Nathan and Lansky 1978a; Sobell 1978; Mandell 1979; Caddy 1980; Tuchfeld and Marcus 1982; Moos, Cronkite, and Finney 1982; Emrick and Hansen 1983; Goldstein, Surber, and Wilner 1984; Nathan and Skinstad 1987; Lettieri 1988). This trend should enhance the quality of research and eventually lay a firmer foundation for alcoholism treatment.

The following review of the research concerning outcome of alcoholism treatment is restricted to *controlled studies*. It is based mainly on the results of experiments with randomly assigned treatment and control groups. The experiments have been randomized to compare the difference in outcome between two or more treatment groups or between a treatment group and a control group that has received minimal or no treatment. Two cited studies (Emrick 1975; Vaillant 1983b) have utilized a less rigorous type of control, namely comparison with studies of alcoholics that have received minimal or no treatment.

If the characteristics of alcoholics that relate to outcome had been well known and routinely reported, it would have been possible to draw conclusions about treatment effectiveness even from studies without control groups. However, the accumulation of knowledge on alcoholism treatment is still at an early stage, and the reporting of prognostic indicators is usually deficient. In a situation of this kind, the experiment is the most adequate method of eliminating alternative explanations for the outcome of treatment (Cook and Campbell 1979).

As is indicated by the discussion of control group effects below (p. 25), it is necessary in experimental studies as well to consider plausible alternatives to the hypothesis that the outcome was due to the particular treatment (see Cook and Campbell 1979). For this and other reasons, only preliminary conclusions can be drawn from reviews of outcome research in the field of alcoholism.

Furthermore, any assessment of the outcome of alcoholism treatment is dependent on what standard is used. The studies cited below have employed the most common criterion, namely *improved drinking behaviour after treatment*. Alcoholism treatment may also achieve important outcomes in the areas of health, subjective well-being, employment, family, etc., and cause changes that last only as long as the treatment is in progress. Data on such outcomes have been included, but are not the chief focus of attention in the following review.

The use of drinking behaviour as a major criterion of treatment efficacy is well-founded. Comparisons of group averages have demonstrated that drinking outcome tends to relate positively to outcome in medical, psychological, and social areas of functioning (Emrick 1974). Moreover, the correlation between continued heavy drinking and disabilities in other areas tends to increase with a longer follow-up period, especially with regard to physical and psychological health (Pettinati *et al.* 1982*a*; Fink *et al.* 1987; Babor *et al.* 1988).

Emrick (1975) summarized the results of 384 studies of psychologically oriented alcoholism treatment published between 1952 and 1973. He drew the conclusion that formal treatment increases an alcoholic's chances of reducing his drinking problem. Emrick calculated the average rate of improvement in 31 studies that met his requirements of at least three subjects, information on drinking behaviour, and a follow-up period of six months or more after termination of treatment. The result was *compared with* the change rate in five studies of alcoholics receiving *no or minimal treatment*. 'Minimal' treatment was defined as less than five outpatient sessions or two weeks of inpatient treatment. The improvement rate was in favour of the treatment groups, with 65 per cent as against 42 per cent in the groups with no or minimal treatment. Emrick's results can be interpreted as showing that formal treatment brings about, on average, 23 'successes' out of every 100 persons treated, beyond those 'successes' that would have occurred naturally.

However, this rather positive assessment of the chances for alcoholics who accept formal treatment is based on studies with, in most cases, only around six months' follow-up after treatment. The assessment turns out differently when treatment outcome is studied over a longer span. Mumford, Schlesinger, and Glass (1978; Schlesinger, Mumford, and Glass 1980; Glass *et al.* 1981) were able to find within alcoholism treatment 20 experiments comparing randomly assigned therapy groups and control groups. These experiments were reported in 15 studies: Clancy, Vanderhoof, and Campbell 1967; Ashem and Donner 1968; Gallant *et al.* 1968; Levinson and Sereny 1969; three studies by McCance and McCance 1969; Kissin, Platz, and Su 1970; Storm and Cutler 1970; Gallant 1971; Vogler, Lunde, and Martin 1971; Newton and Stein 1972; Cadogan 1973; Hunt and Azrin 1973; and Sobell and Sobell 1973.

The findings of these studies were summarized by means of a meta-analysis. The outcome at six months after therapy was similar to that observed by Emrick (1975). Mumford and her colleagues also, however, found a decay in the treatment effect over time (Fig. 3.1). Immediately after termination of treatment, there were 35 per cent more sober cases in therapy groups than in control groups receiving no or minimal treatment. At six months after discharge this difference had decreased to about 20 per cent. After one year there was virtually no difference at all between treated and and untreated alcoholics. Figure 3.1 shows a certain variation of the results at nought and six months, but after one year they have stabilized.

Emrick (1975) found 72 *comparative studies of two or more treatment programmes*. Among studies with a follow-up of more than six months, he was able to find only five showing that a given programme produces better results than another programme. These studies had been carried out by Ends and Page (1957), Pittman and Tate (1969), Tomsovic and Edwards (1970), Vogler *et al.* (1970), and Sobell and Sobell (1973).

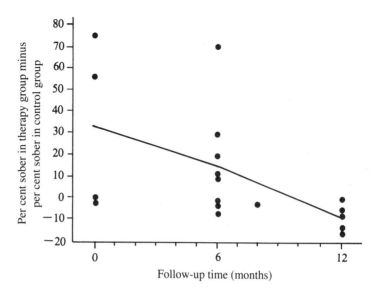

Fig. 3.1   Effect of psychosocial treatment of alcoholism related to follow-up time (solid line connects averages at 0, 6, and 12 months).

Edwards and his co-workers (1977*b*), however, maintain that only *one* of these studies deserves to be given further consideration. The others suffered from methodological shortcomings such as unsatisfactory methods of treatment assignment, a dropout rate of around 40 per cent, and inconsistent results. The exception was a much cited report by Sobell and Sobell (1973) on an attempt to teach severely alcohol-dependent persons (Gamma alcoholics) to drink in a controlled manner by means of an individualized behaviour therapy.

The Sobells' study has not passed unchallenged, however. Foy, Nunn, and Rychtarik (1984) replicated it, with more rigorous control of selection bias, etc. At six-month follow-up, the research team found that clients who had been trained in controlled drinking, in addition to standard treatment, relapsed to a significantly *greater* extent than clients who had received only standard treatment. At follow-ups 12 months and five to six years after termination of treatment, however, the difference in outcome was no longer statistically significant, indicating that even adverse effects of treatment are of short duration (Rychtarik *et al.* 1987).

Pendery, Maltzman, and West (1982) followed up Sobell and Sobell's (1973) 20 experimental subjects after ten years. They found no evidence that a single one of the experimental programme's Gamma (physically dependent) alcoholics had learnt to drink in a controlled manner. Only one subject, who apparently had never been alcohol-dependent or experienced physical withdrawal symptoms, continued to drink in a controlled manner. Nine subjects continued to drink excessively, four had died, and six had become abstinent.

A comparison with Vaillant (1983b, Ch. 3) shows that this outcome agrees with what could be expected merely through the passage of time. Thus, Sobell and Sobell (1984) are justified in asserting that it is probably not worse than in the control group. But it definitely does not support faith in the training of controlled drinking skills as a superior method for helping the more severely dependent majority of patients in alcoholism treatment.

Emrick (1975) points out that the Sobells' study, like the other four studies with positive outcomes, contains information indicating that subjects in the control groups may have felt neglected and deprived of their right to receive as appropriate treatment as possible. In the Sobells' study, for example, 60 per cent of the subjects in the control group felt rejected. The assignment to control groups can thus be harmful and delay remission.

In psychotherapy research this phenomenon is referred to as a control group effect or a reverse placebo effect. It has also been observed in 'no treatment control' groups consisting of alcoholics waiting for treatment (Kissin, Rosenblatt, and Machover 1968). Individuals put on a waiting list are probably not very inclined to turn to relatives and friends to get help with their problems (Eysenck 1983). Moreover, they may expect not to improve until therapeutic intervention is provided (Prioleau, Murdock, and Brody 1983). If a placebo can arouse hope in a desperate human being and bring about an improvement, a long waiting period may very well have the opposite effect.

A growing awareness of this risk has precluded the use of truly untreated control groups in the treatment of more severe problem drinkers. Instead, a few well-controlled randomized trials have *compared extended treatment with brief advice*. The first and most influential of these was carried out by Edwards, Orford, and their co-workers (1977b). They examined the outcome of the 'average package of help' for alcoholics that was offered at one of Britain's most renowned hospitals, Maudsley Hospital in London. The outcome one year after termination of treatment was found to be equivalent to the effect achieved in the control group by a single individualized counselling session that emphasized the alcoholic's own responsibility and the hospital staff's positive expectations.

This study was recently replicated by Chick, Ritson, and their co-workers (1988) in Edinburgh. Patients were randomly assigned to one session of advice or extended inpatient or outpatient treatment 'having much in common with elements of other programmes in the UK' (Chick and Ritson 1989, p. 817). Two years later, patients who had been offered extended treatment had accumulated less harm from their drinking, particularly as far as the family was concerned. Extended treatment did not, however, increase the likelihood of a patient achieving stable abstinence, or stable problem-free drinking, beyond that resulting from a brief counselling session.

Similar findings emerged from a New Zealand study by Howden Chapman and Huygens (1988). After inpatient detoxification, alcoholics were randomly assigned to either a six-week inpatient programme, a six-week outpatient programme, or a single confrontational interview. Outcome was assessed at six and 18 months after intake. On a variety of outcome measures, which included both levels of drinking and general functioning, no single intervention appeared to be consistently more effective than any other.

Nowadays the spouse and other family members are increasingly included in the treatment process. In an outpatient study at the Addiction Research Foundation in Toronto, Zweben, Pearlman, and Li (1988) evaluated the effectiveness of a short-term conjoint therapy that helped couples to adopt and maintain an interactional view of the drinking problem. As a control condition, the investigators used a single session of advice which also involved the spouse. At six, 12, and 18 month follow-ups there were no significant differences between the 'advice' and 'therapy' groups on any of the outcome measures, including both drinking behaviour and psychosocial functioning.

Advice, as described in these studies, should not be mistaken for no intervention at all. Edwards *et al.* (1977*b*), for example, report that patients gave a rather high subjective rating to the efficacy of the counselling session. The findings do suggest, however, that in the treatment of heterogeneous groups of alcoholics, extended treatment does not necessarily have an advantage over very brief intervention. This conclusion is confirmed, although in a less dramatic way, by several experiments *comparing programmes of varying length and intensity* (see reviews by Annis 1986, 1987; Miller and Hester 1986*a*, 1986*b*).

No significant difference in outcome has been found for alcoholics randomly assigned to inpatient programmes with a duration of five weeks versus three weeks (Page and Schaub 1979), of seven weeks versus two weeks (Walker *et al.* 1983), of three months versus nine weeks (Kish, Ellsworth, and Woody 1980) or three weeks (Willems, Letemendia, and Arroyave 1973), or even of either three to six weeks (Pittman and Tate 1969) or one month (Mosher *et al.* 1975; Eriksen 1986) versus seven to ten days of detoxification only.

McLachlan and Stein (1982), and Longabaugh and his colleagues (Longabaugh *et al.* 1983; McCrady *et al.* 1986; Fink *et al.* 1987), compared the outcome for patients randomly assigned to day-clinic treatment versus inpatient treatment. The operating cost of day clinics varied from one third to half of that of inpatient programmes. Evaluations after 12 months by McLachlan and Stein, and after six, 12, and 24 months by Longabaugh *et al.*, showed no significant difference between the two settings on measures of drinking or psychosocial adjustment. McLachlan and Stein found that alcoholics in the inpatient programme were readmitted to hospital significantly more often than day-clinic clients.

The efficacy of outpatient versus inpatient treatment has been compared in ten randomized trials, reviewed by Miller and Hester (1986b). For example, alcoholics who normally would have been admitted to inpatient programmes were randomly assigned to nine weeks of inpatient treatment versus an average of eight outpatient visits (Edwards and Guthrie 1966, 1967; Edwards 1970a) or four weeks of inpatient treatment versus an unspecified number of visits to community services (Stein, Newton, and Bowman 1975). In no study of a heterogeneous group of alcoholics seeking treatment was residential care found to yield superior improvement relative to treatment in a less expensive outpatient setting.

Thus, Annis' (1987) summary of the findings in unselected groups of alcoholics is justified:

The empirical evidence overwhelmingly supports the following conclusions: (1) inpatient treatment of a few weeks to a few months duration shows no better outcome than a period of brief inpatient stay; (2) day treatment or partial hospitalization is as effective as inpatient treatment; and (3) outpatient treatment produces comparable results to inpatient treatment. (p. 5)

Staff-intensive modalities have been compared with less heavily staffed alternatives in both inpatient and outpatient treatment. Stinson et al. (1979) randomly assigned clients to either intensive or peer-oriented incare combined with either organized network or informal outcare. There was 40 per cent less treatment staff in the peer-led programme. The only significant difference between settings over the course of 18 months, however, was that clients in the peer-led programme showed a greater improvement in drinking behaviour.

In another randomized trial, Galanter, Castaneda, and Salamon (1987) compared two ambulatory programmes recruiting largely homeless alcoholics: a control programme operated solely by professional staff, and an experimental one based on peer-led self-help. Although the self-help programme was staffed by only half as many therapists as the control programme, its clients achieved significantly better results with regard to social adjustment, and they improved as much as controls with regard to drinking over the course of the year of treatment.

Miller and Hester (1986a, 1986b) reviewed a dozen randomized trials in outpatient therapy. As with inpatient treatment, they found no advantage attached to more lengthy or intensive treatment. For example, Powell and her co-workers (1985) compared outcomes for 174 male alcoholics randomly assigned to one of three outpatient interventions: (a) a monthly medical examination; (b) the same as (a), plus Antabuse therapy and tranquillizer if necessary; (c) the same as (b), plus over 100 hours of individualized support in the form of individual counselling, marital or family counselling, vocational assistance, etc. One year after intake, no significant differences were found with respect to drinking behaviour or psychosocial functioning.

More recently, McLatchie and Lomp (1988*b*) evaluated 55 alcoholics who were randomly assigned to one of three alternatives following inpatient treatment: (a) four sessions of contracted aftercare, (b) aftercare at the clients' discretion, and (c) no aftercare. At three- and 12-month follow-ups, no outcome differences were observed. These findings lend further support to the conclusion that in unselected groups of alcoholics, improvements are unrelated to the intensity of treatment received.

Vaillant (1983*b*) has published a much-cited study on the long-term outcome of alcoholism treatment. He worked as a psychiatric consultant for what he considered to be 'the most exciting alcohol programme in the world' (p. 284). The programme was medically oriented with access to shelters, halfway houses, walk-in counselling round the clock, discussion groups, detoxification facilities, medical and psychiatric consultation, etc. Fuelled by his enthusiasm, Vaillant initiated a unique follow-up study that he hoped would prove the efficacy of the programme.

A group of 100 patients admitted for alcohol withdrawal were interviewed annually over a period of eight years (Vaillant 1983*b*; Vaillant *et al.* 1983). It is the first study in the field of alcoholism that both followed a treatment group for a period of more than four years and evaluated the outcome on more than one occasion. As the years passed, the patients were admitted for detoxification an average of 15 times and utilized the programme's other treatment and counselling options at least as many times.

The outcome was *compared with longitudinal studies of untreated alcoholics*. Comparisons at two and eight years revealed that the results of treatment were no better than the 'natural history' of the disorder. Vaillant (1983*b*) summarized: 'Perhaps the best that can be said for our exciting treatment effort at Cambridge Hospital is that we were certainly not interfering with the normal recovery process' (p. 285).

The conclusion that treatment of alcoholism did not alter the course of the disorder was corroborated by a comparison of three studies of 214 alcoholic patients who received no more than advice with four studies of 685 similar patients receiving inpatient treatment. At the end of a two-year period the proportions of significantly improved and unimproved alcoholics were roughly the same in the 'no treatment' and treatment studies. Likewise, at eight-year follow-up samples of persistently 'treated' alcoholics seemed to do no better than samples of essentially untreated alcoholics. Vaillant therefore generalized his findings, stating that: 'prolonged hospital treatment does little to alter the natural history of alcoholism. . . . Alcoholics recover not because we treat them but because they heal themselves' (p. 314).

This estimate of the long-term efficacy of treatment has been criticized for being too conservative (Nace 1989). The contrast between the optimism of the clinician and the dispassionate judgement of the researcher is nevertheless striking. It reminds me of a story told by the British philosopher and scientist Francis Bacon (1620, p. 56). It is about Diagoras, an ancient

Greek. On visiting a temple, he is shown a picture of those who have paid their vows and have subsequently escaped shipwreck. The visitor is asked whether he does not now acknowledge the power of the gods. 'Aye', he replies, 'but where are they painted who were drowned after their vows?'

Bacon comments that:

it is the peculiar and perpetual error of the human intellect to be more moved and excited by affirmatives than by negatives; whereas it ought properly to hold itself indifferently disposed towards both alike. Indeed in the establishment of any true axiom, the negative instance is the more forcible of the two. (ibid.)

As therapists, we may find comfort in anecdotal evidence of how people in a miserable condition have been helped by treatment. When conducting treatment research, however, we cannot content ourselves with such material. Like the sceptical visitor to the temple, we must also pay attention to those who were not improved by treatment and to those who improved without treatment.

Recently, Miller and Hester (1986a), Maisto and Carey (1987), and Riley, L. C. Sobell, and their colleagues (1987) have published scholarly reviews on the effectiveness of different approaches to treating alcoholism. Riley, Sobell, et al. (1987) identified 68 studies from 1978 to 1983 with a minimum of six months of treatment outcome data. A rigorous comparison was made with a review by Costello (1975b) of evaluative studies published between 1952 and 1972. The authors found that treatment outcome results had not changed appreciably, despite the radical shift in concepts and ideologies that has taken place over the last ten or 15 years. Their foremost conclusion was that 'treatments for alcohol problems with demonstrated enduring effectiveness do not exist, regardless of treatment orientations or treatment goals' (p. 107).

Maisto and Carey (1987) reviewed 26 controlled outcome studies, also published between 1978 and 1984. Only studies using prospective designs, and comparing matched or randomly assigned groups, were included. The survey was organized around length of follow-up interval. The authors found 'little evidence of short- or long-term differential treatment effects', but concluded that 'staying in treatment seems to be associated with benefits that may be maintained for some time' (p. 208).

Miller and Hester (1986a) started off with more than 900 treatment reports published up to the end of 1985. Their review was organized around specific treatment approaches. In contrast to an earlier survey by the same authors (Miller and Hester 1980), this one included only controlled research; that is, studies with either randomly assigned or matched control or comparison groups. Miller and Hester (1986a) diverged from most previous reviewers in concluding that certain treatment methods have demonstrated specific efficacy in the treatment of alcohol problems.

However, the techniques recommended by Miller and Hester (1986a) are not uncontroversial. The evidence in favour of behavioural self-control training comes from studies of persons who are not severely dependent on alcohol. The empirical support regarding the utility of aversion therapy (cf. McLellan and Childress 1985; AMA 1987), stress management (cf. Klajner, Hartman, and Sobell 1984), and marital or family therapy (cf. McCrady 1989), is equivocal, and indicates poor long-term effectiveness.

The outcome of social skills training has been more consistent, with positive effects demonstrated at one-year follow up (e.g. Eriksen, Björnstad, and Götestam 1986). However, few studies to date of this technique have been methodologically adequate. As regards the strength of scientific support, Miller and Hester (1986*a*; Miller 1988) are justified in putting the community reinforcement approach 'at the top of the list'. Here evidence of efficacy is provided by a series of well-controlled studies (Hunt and Azrin 1973; Miller 1975; Azrin 1976; Azrin *et al.* 1982; Mallams *et al.* 1982; Sisson and Azrin 1986). Yet, Hester, Miller, *et al.* (1990) failed to replicate the favourable outcome reported by previous research.

Among other candidates for superior efficacy, no one has truly met the criterion of replicated findings. This is also true of the much-publicized Minnesota Model. It is true that outcome figures in uncontrolled research appear to be 'equivalent to or even better than those of other treatment programmes' (Cook 1988, p. 741). But in a well-controlled randomized trial (Keso 1988), the positive trend in measures of improved drinking did not reach statistical significance one year after treatment. Unfortunately 'the power of the study was not very good' (Keso and Salaspuro 1990, p. 588).

In summary, controlled studies of unselected groups of alcoholics with improved drinking behaviour as the outcome criterion have *generally demonstrated only weak and short-term effects of alcoholism treatment*. An average of around twenty treatment-related 'successes' per hundred persons six months after treatment, and virtually no effects remaining after one or two years, is a reasonable estimate. The question of whether treatment is more effective than no treatment at all must consequently be answered in the negative, if by 'effective' is meant permanent improvement in drinking behaviour.

Does this imply that treatment of alcoholism is of no value? Certainly not! Weak and short-term improvements are definitely preferable to no improvements other than those produced by natural healing processes alone. Even if psychosocial treatment does not 'cure' alcoholism, it may contribute to making life more tolerable for many alcoholics and their families. In this humanitarian sense, treatment is more valuable than no treatment at all.

The question of whether some types of treatment are consistently found to be more effective than others can be answered in the negative, too, as it was done, incidentally, by a recent committee of the US Institute of Medicine (IOM 1989). Programmes of varying theoretical orientation, length, and intensity have been compared in more than a hundred studies, but no single treatment has been found superior for all alcoholics. Findings definitely show that more treatment or more expensive treatment is not necessarily better treatment.

To be sure, some approaches to treating alcoholism have more logical and empirical appeal than others. Azrin's community reinforcement approach (Section 10.4 below) is one of these. What is impressive here is not only the empirical support, but the pervasive focus on modification of the client's social environment. What Azrin and his colleagues actually did was not so much to treat individual alcoholics as to identify and harness healing processes in their natural environmental situation. The fruitfulness of this perspective will be elaborated in Chapter 25.

Finally, this chapter is a review of alcoholism treatment and its outcome. Preventive measures for problem drinkers having little or no documented physical dependence have not been discussed here. If interventions of the latter type had been included, then the conclusions should have been far more sanguine. In fact, there is ample evidence demonstrating that brief interventions may be modestly but reliably effective in helping the less serious type of problem drinker (see review by Babor, Ritson, and Hodgson 1986).

3.2   Are the conclusions plausible?

The plausibility of my conclusions can be judged from several viewpoints. One way is to compare the effectiveness of alcoholism treatment with the efficacy of psychosocial treatment of other clinical populations. Bergin and Lambert's (1978) comprehensive review of research on outcome in psychotherapy compared improvement rates in treated and untreated groups of neurotics. Their results were in favour of the treatment groups, with 65 per cent 'successes' as compared to 43 per cent in control groups who had not received any formal treatment. This assessment and the estimate by Emrick (1975) above (p. 23) suggest a remarkable similarity between the efficacy of psychotherapy as applied to neurosis and the effectiveness of alcoholism treatment.

However, the maintenance of treatment gains may be a more common outcome in psychotherapy than in alcoholism treatment. Meta-analyses by Landman and Dawes (1982) and Nicholson and Berman (1983) compared results obtained at post-treatment with results at follow-up, within the same studies of mainly neurotic disorders. They found that improvement following treatment was generally stable over many months.

In conclusion, trials in treatment populations other than alcoholics have typically demonstrated small, albeit clinically meaningful, improvements as a result of psychosocial treatment. These gains may be maintained over longer periods of time than those achieved by alcoholism treatment. Even though individuals representing different value orientations tend to evaluate research studies differently (see review by Garfield 1983), most experts would probably agree with Philip Gallo's (1978) appraisal that 'psychotherapy has a real, measurable, and quite weak effect upon the adjustment scores that constitute the dependent measure' (p. 516).

Several research reviews have summarized the results of studies that compared specific treatment methods. Meltzoff and Kornreich (1970) examined 38 studies of this kind and found no evidence that one method is more successful than another.

Luborsky, Singer, and Luborsky (1975) conducted a detailed analysis of more than 100 comparative studies of psychotherapy in a paper whose subtitle alluded to the 'dodo bird verdict' in *Alice in Wonderland*: 'Is it true that "Everyone has won and all must have prizes"?' They added up the number of methodologically adequate studies that supported individual therapy versus group therapy, time-limited therapy versus time-unlimited therapy, pharmaco-therapy versus psychotherapy (combined in different ways), client-centred therapy versus other psychotherapy, and behaviour therapy versus other psychotherapy. The main conclusion arrived at was that it is not possible to identify any one-prize winner when different psychotherapeutic methods are compared.

Similar results have since been obtained in a traditional research review by Bergin and Lambert (1978), and in meta-analyses by Smith and Glass (1977), Smith, Glass, and Miller (1980), and Shapiro and Shapiro (1982). Research reviews by Kazdin and Wilson (1978) and Rachman and Wilson (1980), and a meta-analysis by Andrews and Harvey (1981) have, on the other hand, concluded that behaviour therapy often is more effective. But in a comprehensive review of reviews, Stiles, Shapiro, and Elliott (1986) believed that this relative superior showing 'may well be due to a systematic bias resulting from experimenter allegiance' (p. 167–8). On the whole then, Kendall and Norton-Ford's (1982) characterization of the research situation seems justified:

To date, however, authors of cumulative analyses have drawn similar conclusions: essentially, it appears that . . . no therapeutic intervention has emerged as consistently and dramatically superior to all its competitors. (p. 454)

Studies of alcoholism treatment indicate that the length of therapy does not affect the outcome. Similar results have been reported for other patient populations in research reviews by Bergin (1971; Bergin and Lambert 1978), Luborsky *et al.* (1975), Butcher and Koss (1978), and Johnson and Gelso (1980), and in meta-analyses by Smith and Glass (1977), Smith *et al.* (1980), and the Shapiros (1982). The latter three studies, together with a traditional review by Durlak (1979) and a meta-analysis by Hattie, Sharpley, and Rogers (1984), have also demonstrated that paraprofessionals and trainees achieve clinical outcomes that are equal to or better than those obtained by trained, experienced therapists. Although these studies do suggest that a hope-engendering, morale-enhancing relationship may be useful in many settings beyond formal therapy, definitive studies on this matter are yet to be done (Lambert, Shapiro, and Bergin 1986).

In a review of the development and current state of psychotherapy, Garfield (1981*b*) concluded that no real breakthroughs have occurred. Despite claims to the contrary, those innovations and modifications that have been introduced have not produced any truly remarkable results. Garfield summed up by saying that the fact that there are so many variants of psychotherapy suggests rather that the development of psychotherapeutic procedures is still at an early stage. Viewed in this light, the conclusions arrived at on the basis of outcome research in the field of alcoholism treatment (Section 3.1) are neither implausible nor surprising.

4 New directions in research

4.1 Issues in treatment research

Numerous solutions have been proposed to resolve the paradox that different psychosocial treatments have tended to yield equivalent outcomes (see Stiles, Shapiro, and Elliott 1986). Kazdin and Wilson (1978), among others, remarked that outcome research had relied far too much on 'comparisons of ill-defined treatment approaches applied to heterogeneous disorders using unsatisfactory global measures' (p. 174). Studies of this nebulous character are very difficult to interpret and have few counterparts in more mature disciplines.

There is, however, a growing recognition that the methodological flaws were largely a consequence of the way in which psychosocial treatment had been conceptualized. Thus, from Cronbach (1957) until the present time, researchers have challenged the conceptual framework in which problems of treatment were formulated.

Kiesler (1966, 1971) drew early attention to the theoretical shortcomings of psychotherapy research. Three theoretical formulations dominated research during the 1960s. They were Freud's psychoanalysis and theory of psycho-pathology, Carl Rogers' client-centred therapy and hypotheses about therapeutic change, and behaviour therapy based on behaviouristic learning theory. Kiesler did not believe that these formulations provided adequate guidelines for research.

According to Kiesler (1966), the traditional formulations were not sufficiently comprehensive. They did not provide an exhaustive description of known facts and variables in the domain of research. The existing theories were either too specific (behaviour therapy) or too general (psychoanalytical and Rogerian therapy).

Nor did any of the formulations adequately allow for individual differences between clients or therapists. Earlier therapy research was based on the implicit assumption that there is one ideal form of therapy for all patients. The function of research was to tell us which of the proposed models best approximate this ideal.

Kiesler denied the possibility of finding a psychosocial panacea. With reference to Stein (1961), he noted that different theoretical formulations and techniques were originally derived from work with different types of patients. This has probably contributed to the often-related difficulties of replicating and generalizing results of treatment studies. Stein wrote:

One source of difference between schools of psychotherapy that is often overlooked and which needs to be made explicit is the difference in types of patients on which the founders of the different schools based their initial observations. Maskin summarizes this point rather well when he says: 'Freud used hysteria as the model for his therapeutic method, depression as the basis for his later theoretical conjectures. Adler's clinical demonstrations are rivalrous, immature character types. Jung's examples were constructed to a weary, worldly, successful, middle-aged group. Rank focussed upon the conflicted, frustrated, rebellious artist aspirant. Fromm's model is the man in a white collar searching for his individuality. And Sullivan's example of choice is the young catatonic schizophrenic.' To this one might add that Rogers' original formulations were based on college students. (pp. 6–7)

According to Kiesler (1966), previous research strategies were based on the *uniformity assumption myth*, that is, the belief that all patients are essentially alike. He and others (Paul 1967; Strupp and Bergin 1969) criticized the majority of studies for treating therapists and patients as homogeneous groups. In actuality, the reverse was probably true. Different therapists (even within the same therapeutic orientation) effect different changes in different kinds of patients (even within the same diagnostic group). Studies of average outcome in a heterogeneous treatment population were not considered to permit any definite conclusion as to how the treatment works. This outcome may mask a variability which suggests that some clients are influenced differently by the treatment than others (Bergin 1971).

The critics of psychotherapy research advocated a *multivariant* approach, whereby treatment is perceived as a process during which a number of influences interact. Research was faced with the dual task of identifying which influences are of crucial importance and defining how these interact to bring about a specific outcome. Individual case studies in a natural setting, as well as experimental analogue studies under more or less artificial conditions, were recommended as ways of achieving greater insight into the mechanisms of therapeutic change.

The arguments for a multivariant approach to research and treatment were summarized in an influential work by Bergin and Strupp in 1972. In a review published a few years later, Strupp (1978) found that the quality of research had improved and that there was now cause for some optimism about the future. Above all, there was a willingness to reject the traditional question 'Is psychotherapy effective?' and to ask instead, in response to Paul's (1967) admonition, what kinds of treatment produce what kinds of changes in which kinds of individuals under what conditions. The trend towards greater specificity was becoming the hallmark of well-designed research.

However, Strupp's optimism was based on the profession of the need for specificity rather than on a major breakthrough in research. In fact, despite more than two decades of advocacy of a multivariant approach, and occasional research on the interaction between patient, treatment, and outcome (e.g. Gunderson 1978; McLean 1981; Magaro and DeSisto 1981; Öst et al.

1981, 1982; Frank and Gunderson 1984; see also Chapter 21), psychotherapy research has still not succeeded in answering complex questions such as the one posed by Paul (1967). As noted by Stiles *et al.* (1986), there has been no easy progress toward fitting treatments to clients.

It is impossible on the basis of present-day knowledge to formulate any more than preliminary hypotheses to guide the choice between psychosocial treatment methods and settings (see e.g. Magaro *et al.* 1978; Beutler 1979, 1983, 1989; Frances and Clarkin 1981; Almond 1983; Norton, Dinardo, and Barlow 1983). Thus, it is not yet possible to predict with any certainty which treatment best matches the specific characteristics, problems, and needs of the individual client (see reviews by Berzins 1977; Gomes-Schwartz, Hadley, and Strupp 1978).

In his retrospect on the 1970s, Strupp (1978) further observed that debates within and across theoretical systems were becoming more issue-oriented and less polemical. There were signs that the ideological struggles between adherents of behavioural and psychodynamic orientations, in particular, were giving way to a more open-minded and scientifically argued communication. In the 1980s, rapprochement and integration have become issues of growing concern, as manifested by an ever-increasing number of articles, books, and conferences. Important contributions to the discussion have been compiled and reviewed by Goldfried (1982) and Norcross (1986). Noted researchers and therapists have joined the Society for the Exploration of Psychotherapy Integration (SEPI), a steadily growing international network devoted to bringing about a dialogue across different orientations.

A readiness to engage in such a dialogue was expressed by Lazarus (1977), a pioneer of behaviour therapy, in the following Hippocratic fashion:

I am opposed to the advancement of psychoanalysis, to the advancement of Gestalt therapy, to the advancement of existential therapy, to the advancement of behavior therapy, or the advancement of any delimited school of thought. I would like to see an advancement in psychological knowledge, an advancement in the understanding of human interaction, in the alleviation of suffering, and in the know-how of therapeutic intervention. (p. 553)

To date, Goldfried, Greenberg, and Marmar (1990) remarked, the theme of integration has given rise to more dialogue than research. However, behaviourally and dynamically oriented therapists have initiated an examination of empirical data for the purpose of identifying points of similarity and dissimilarity. Dynamically oriented therapists have begun to acknowledge the utility of certain behavioural techniques, while behaviour therapists are in the process of recognizing the importance of the therapeutic relationship. Furthermore, the cognitive influence that began in the 1970s, and the growing literature by behaviour therapists on self-control and mastery, have led to a shift away from behaviourism in its original form and towards a greater emphasis on what occurs within the person. Cognitive-behavioural therapy, with its already more than twenty variations (Dobson 1988), has become part of the mainstream.

4.2   Changing notions of treatment

Since the 1960s, Mansell Pattison has consistently advocated the use of a multivariant approach to alcoholism and treatment. He did not believe that any psychotherapy was absolutely superior, nor did he accept the conclusion that all therapies are equivalent. According to Pattison (1974), the latter impression may be artefactual and arising from the fact that so little work has been done to pin down specific psychotherapy methods that will be applicable to the various subpopulations of alcoholics.

In his comprehensive review of alcoholism treatment research, Emrick (1975) drew the following widely quoted conclusion:

Whether or not long-term beneficial effects will ever be demonstrated, the weight of present evidence is overwhelmingly against technique variables being powerful determinants of long-term outcome, whatever the valence. It would seem that continued efforts to develop techniques having uniquely positive posttreatment outcome will bear little fruit. A wiser expenditure of resources might be in the area of developing strategies to involve alcoholics in therapy, any kind of therapy, since all approaches seem generally helpful to the majority of patients. (pp. 94–5)

The assumption that the benefits of treatment are more or less independent of the specific characteristics of the method being used, is called the *non-specific hypothesis*. This interpretation of the outcome of psychosocial treatment was put forward by Rosenzweig (1936) more than 50 years ago. It has since been elaborated in particular by the psychiatrist Jerome Frank, to whom I shall return below. However, the quoted paragraph contains yet another assumption, which I have previously called the matching hypothesis. Emrick (1975) went on to suggest that:

rather than seek an outstanding treatment, therapists might give attention to matching each alcoholic with the setting and approach which meshes best with his views on the causes, nature and treatment of alcoholism (Pattison *et al.* 1969). Such endeavors should advance the field of alcoholism treatment more than further proliferation of techniques used to help alcoholics once they are involved in therapy. (p. 95)

On the basis of their much-publicized finding that conventional alcoholism treatment did not result in better outcomes than an individualized counselling session, Edwards and Orford (1977) concluded that many more people should be offered much less intensive help than had previously been thought adequate. They also called for a closer study of those forces in the alcoholic's environment that promote 'spontaneous' remission, i.e. the process by which some alcoholics achieve remission whether they receive treatment or not (Orford and Edwards 1977).

Vaillant (1983*b*) devoted a chapter of his seminal study of the causes and treatment of alcoholism to what he called the doctor's dilemma: How do we retain an open mind to the sobering findings of treatment research without losing confidence to deal with those patients who expect our help? Like Orford and Edwards (1977), he stressed the importance of investigating 'natural' healing processes, since what proper treatment can do is primarily to facilitate these processes.

Vaillant compared the situation to that which existed within medicine before a specific cure had been found for tuberculosis. Treatment was then concentrated entirely on identifying and capturing those factors that contributed to the resistance of the patient. Instead of getting out of the business of treating tuberculosis, the doctors carefully observed what psychological and social factors could alleviate and improve the condition of their patients. According to Vaillant, alcoholism treatment has a great deal to learn from the way in which medicine dealt with tuberculosis before 1950.

Like Magaro, Gripp, and McDowell (1978; Section 2.2 above) in psychiatry, Vaillant discloses an affinity with the Hippocratic tradition in medicine. The Hippocratics understood healing as a co-operative art. Vaillant (1983*b*) brings an analogous insight to alcoholism treatment, whose scientific underpinnings recall those of ancient medicine insofar as no specific cures are forthcoming.

Vaillant's analysis is based on Jerome Frank's classic monograph, *Persuasion and Healing* (1961), which outlines a transcultural model for psychosocial treatment that is non-specific for illness or patient. Frank's conclusions are based both on reflections upon his and other's clinical experience and on an array of data from anthropology, comparative religion, experimental psychology, and psychotherapy research. According to Parloff (1986) and others, his formulation is the most systematic and thoughtful elaboration of the non-specific hypothesis.

Frank (1973, 1974*a*) believes that whatever their symptoms, most, if not all, patients who enter psychotherapy suffer a comparable state of mind identified as *demoralization*, that is, a feeling of subjective incompetence, coupled with distress which he or she cannot adequately explain or alleviate. Although most patients present themselves with specific symptoms, much of the improvement resulting from psychotherapy springs from its ability to restore the patient's morale.

According to Frank (1971, 1973, 1982), all therapies are beneficial because they have in common healing components which are also shared by age-old procedures of psychological healing (cf. Singer (1984) on commonalities of spiritual healing and family therapy in alcoholism treatment). These components are construed as means of combating demoralization. The first and foremost of them is an emotionally charged, confiding *relationship* and a *setting* which itself arouses the patient's expectation of help. The importance of a good therapeutic relationship and favourable expectations was recognized in the Hippocratic writings and is a recurring theme in the treatment literature (Chapter 25 below).

The second of Frank's prerequisites for successful therapy is a *rationale* that provides a plausible explanation for the patient's symptoms and prescribes a procedure for relieving them. To be effective, the rationale must be compatible with the cultural world view shared by patient and therapist. In the Middle Ages, Frank (1974*a*) goes on, what we call psychotherapy was based on demonology. This doctrine offered a conceptual scheme which was, in fact, almost as elaborate as modern therapeutic philosophies (Clark 1984). In many primitive societies the underlying rationale of psychosocial treatment is shamanism. In Western society today, psychotherapy has mainly invoked the symbols of science.

Linked to the rationale is a *ritual* that requires the active participation of both patient and therapist and that is believed by both to be the means for restoring the patient's health. Frank suggests that persons who have previously encountered and conquered the same problem are particularly effective in restoring hope and combating isolation, especially if they suffer from a stigmatized condition such as alcoholism.

Vaillant's (1983*b*, Chs. 4–5) study of recovery from alcoholism confirms Frank's theses:

Time and time again, both evangelists and behavior therapists have demonstrated that if you can but win their hearts and minds, their habits will follow. In other words, if we can but combine the best placebo effects of acupuncture, Lourdes, or Christian Science with the best attitude change inherent in the evangelical conversion experience, we may be on our way to an effective alcoholism program. (pp. 287–8)

In an early review of research on the outcome of alcoholism treatment, Voegtlin and Lemere (1942) warned against an over-enthusiastic reception of new, apparently exceedingly effective methods that have not been subjected to the test of time (cf. Section 2.2 above). They mentioned as an example the injection of atropine and strychnine, which in the 1920s was said to cure 60 per cent of alcoholics (Hare 1924). Two decades later, however, these drugs had lost their extraordinarily therapeutic ability.

Vaillant (1983*b*) pointed to other examples of treatments which initially showed improved drinking behaviour among 50 to 85 per cent of the alcoholics two years after termination of treatment. What, he asked himself, could emetine aversion conditioning in the 1940s at the Shadel Clinic (Shadel 1944) have in common with Antabuse and group therapy at the world-famous Menninger Clinic in the 1950s (Wallerstein 1956), attendance at Alcoholics Anonymous coupled with indigenous Calypso singing on Trinidad in the 1960s (Beaubrun 1967), and behaviour therapy aimed at controlled drinking at Patton State Hospital in the 1970s (Sobell and Sobell 1976)?

Vaillant's answer was that each programme maximized the power of those healing components which, according to Frank (1961), characterize successful therapy. It applied the newest method of its decade. As trained and sanctioned healers, the staff brought hope, provided a rational explanation for mysterious suffering, and then created a framework for sharing that suffering with others. Each programme prescribed a daily ritual. Shadel's patients were given a sign—'There is one thing I cannot do'—which they should hang by the mirror while they shaved. The Menninger patients had their daily Antabuse ceremony. The patients on Trinidad had to attend AA meetings several times a week. The Sobells' patients were given a wallet-sized card of 'Dos' and 'Don'ts' to keep with them at all times.

To the question of why history has been so unkind to these treatment programmes and why no apparently superior outcome has been widely replicated, Vaillant (1983*b*) replied with an anecdote about Sir William Osler, the legendary physician of the nineteenth century. A friend had told him about his successful treatment of tuberculosis. Osler wrote back: 'That is a fine record . . . I'm afraid there is one element you've not laid proper stress upon—your own personality. Confidence and faith count so much in these cases' (Cushing 1925). Obviously Vaillant meant that alcoholism treatment today is what the treatment of tuberculosis was prior to 1950, a culturally mediated phenomenon whose outcome is determined not only by the treatment method, but also by the therapist and the patient.

4.3   Basic assumptions reconsidered

Assumptions in alcoholism treatment research can be classified into four major categories depending on how they respond to the following crucial questions: (a) Is treatment effective? (b) Do therapies vary in efficacy? (c) Is there a superior therapy? (Table 4.1).

The technique hypothesis implies an affirmative answer to all of the three questions:

(a) treatment is certainly considered to be more effective than no treatment at all;

Table 4.1   Assumptions regarding the treatment of alcohol problems

	Is treatment effective?	Do therapies vary in efficacy?	Is there a superior therapy?
The technique hypothesis	Yes	Yes	Yes
The matching hypothesis	Yes	Yes	No
The non-specific hypothesis	Yes	No	—
The natural healing hypothesis	No	—	—

(b) therapies are believed to vary in efficacy, i.e., some therapies are likely to be more effective than others; and

(c) one of them is assumed to be superior in the sense of being uniquely effective in helping everybody with a particular problem.

In short, one expects to find a specific therapeutic technique or setting that is effective and better than other treatment for all patients with a given diagnosis. This assumption is the traditional basis of research on the effectiveness of psychotherapy.

The matching hypothesis presupposes the existence of interaction effects, i.e. effects of a reciprocal influence of patient and treatment variables on each other. This hypothesis gives an affirmative answer to two of the questions posed above: treatment is considered to be effective, and therapies are believed to vary in efficacy. It is assumed that treatment outcome will improve if a consistent pairing of patient characteristics and treatment approaches is carried through. Instead of searching for a programme that is uniquely effective for all, research should try to find out which patients are likely to respond to to what treatments.

The non-specific hypothesis is based on a belief that treatment is effective; but since therapies apparently do not vary in efficacy, it makes no difference which one you employ. All therapies produce beneficial and equivalent results. The benefits of treatment are assumed to be an effect of active ingredients that are common to a variety of treatment approaches. Consequently, it is argued, research should identify and clarify these therapeutic components so that their power can be enhanced in the context of specific therapies.

The natural healing hypothesis, taken in isolation, implies that all benefits of treatment are illusory. Those improvements that are observed after termination of any treatment episode are assumed to be no greater than the expected rate of spontaneous remission, i.e. remission due to natural healing and other influences that are beyond the direct control of the therapist. However, it is often recognized that research on remission that is due to influences other than formal treatment may provide valuable clues as to how treatment could accelerate and facilitate 'spontaneous' or 'natural' healing processes.

It is true, of course, that one seldom comes across these basic assumptions in isolation. Almost all researchers take the occurrence of spontaneous remission into account. Most recognize the therapeutic power of features common to various forms of treatment, and many undoubtedly agree that a given treatment method tends to be more appropriate for some types of patients than for others. However, a research strategy based on the technique hypothesis assumes that a specific therapy will be found that produces results which override the effects of natural healing, non-specific components, and patient–treatment interaction.

Studies based on this assumption—which has prevailed in psychotherapy research—often control for effects that can be attributed to interaction, common elements, or spontanous remission. But these effects are chiefly regarded as noise to be filtered out of 'real' effects. Only after hundreds of trials and errors guided by the technique-centred assumption have researchers begun to take an active interest in the other three assumptions presented above.

In the mid-1960s, the psychologist Gordon Paul formulated the matching hypothesis in an eloquent way. Since the mid-1970s the efficacy of non-specific therapeutic components has evolved into a clearly delineated area of interest. Today, it is becoming increasingly popular to study those forces beyond formal treatment which are effective in accelerating natural healing processes.

The matching and non-specific hypotheses are both reasonable research strategies in a situation where only weak effects of treatment have been demonstrated. Personality psychologists such as Mischel (1973; 1981, Ch. 20) have pointed out that when subjects are exposed to weak treatments, individual differences should exert significant effects. Conversely, when treatments are powerful, the role of individual differences will be minimized. The relevance of the matching hypothesis is thus inversely proportional to the potency of the treatment methods. A similar line of reasoning can be followed regarding the non-specific hypothesis. The weaker the effect of treatment is compared with no or minimal treatment, the greater is the likelihood that a number of treatment methods can achieve the same outcome, and that the outcome is actually brought about by elements that are common to different kinds of treatment.

Jerome Frank, who emphasizes the therapeutic role of non-specific elements, also advocates, in keeping with the above logic, research on interaction effects and a careful matching of client characteristics to treatment approaches (Frank 1978, p. 17 f.; Frank 1974b, 1979). Telch (1981), however, criticized these suggestions in a debate with Frank (1979). Telch recommended that rather than attempting to identify under what conditions weak treatments will produce favourable results, reseachers should strive to develop more potent psychological procedures. He hoped that the future would bring a new and more optimistic *Zeitgeist*.

In his reply to Telch, Frank (1981) agreed that the more potent the therapy, the less important the personal qualities of patient and therapist become. However, he based his more pessimistic assessment of psychological methods on other premises than the spirit of the time, writing:

Medicine abounds with examples, such as tuberculosis. Interest in the personality variables affecting susceptibility to and convalescence from this disease virtually vanished when potent curative drugs were discovered. The chances, however, that any psychotherapy will prove to be as powerful as streptomycin are remote. (p. 477)

Perhaps psychosocial treatment research has started at the wrong end. Instead of moving from the top downward in Table 4.1, it might be more profitable to proceed from the bottom up. If Frank is right, the benefits of psychosocial treatment are an effect of its power to facilitate natural healing processes and support the patient and his environment in their 'spontaneous' efforts to cope with the drinking problem. Hence the attempt to define what influences, within or outside of formal treatment, have been effective in the actual recovery of alcoholics would be a better way than the technique-centred one to clarify which ingredients are active in treatment and prevention. As these ingredients become better known, it will be easier both to match the 'right' client with the 'right' intervention and to specify and evaluate various approaches to treatment and prevention.

In the meantime it is recommended that alcoholism treatment research should adopt a diversified strategy, with its main focus reoriented from the effects of specific techniques to natural healing processes, common therapeutic elements, and effects of client-treatment interaction. The significance and implications of these strategic options will be elaborated in Part III of this book.

In Part IV, I will concentrate on effects of client–treatment interaction observed by research on alcoholism treatment. Part V formulates a set of hypotheses about which are the common elements in successful alcoholism treatment. These hypotheses are suggested as an explanation of the empirical findings about which kinds of clients benefit from what kinds of treatment. They are ultimately based on a Hippocratic conception according to which treatment supplements natural healing processes, rather than the other way around.

In Part II, however, I will examine how alcoholism has been conceived. The choice of theoretical perspective is not a merely academic issue. The notion that one superior method exists for all alcoholics is usually based on the assumption that alcoholism is a unitary phenomenon. If no convincing support exists for this assumption, a differential approach to treatment seems warranted.

Part II

Conceptions of alcoholism

The public, professionals, and politicians employ a number of models to understand and explain alcoholism (see Siegler, Osmond, and Newell 1968). Conventional notions concerning the nature of alcoholism are seldom clear and unambiguous. Caddy, Goldman, and Huebner (1976*a*, 1976*b*), however, claimed that they can be conceptually clustered into the three general categories of physical disease, underlying psychological illness, and learned pattern of behaviour. To these concepts, Brower, Blow, and Beresford (1989) and Meyer and Babor (1989) added the understanding of alcoholism as a social career, as well as a number of integrative models. Brower *et al.* also brought the moral model up-to-date.

The debate on conceptual issues has been intense during the last few years. However, I have not yet seen any dispassionate analysis reviewing in depth the spectrum of data and concerns pertinent to different conceptions and their treatment implications. Such an analysis should address topics like: (a) why people begin drinking; (b) how and why their drinking escalates to abuse; (c) why people maintain harmful drinking; (d) why and how people stop drinking; and (e) why people relapse after a period of abstinence.

Part II reviews current psychosocial research on alcoholism. Special attention is paid to the question whether there is any scientifically valid support for the assumption that alcoholics are essentially alike and have more or less the same treatment needs. Five conceptions of alcoholism are examined: the moral model, the disease model, the symptomatic model, the learning model, and the social model. In conclusion a biopsychosocial synthesis of knowledge is proposed. A separate chapter clarifies the concept of alcohol dependence, which is of central importance in emergent models of alcohol problems and their treatment.

5 The moral model

In the initial stage of treatment interventions, alcoholism was regarded as a sin or a vice. Temperance was propagated primarily from a spiritual or moral point of view. Characteristic of the moral model is its view of the alcoholic as an individual with a weak or bad character. According to a variant called the *legal model* (Dunham and Mauss 1982), a person has freedom of choice and is able to control his own action, if he only makes an adequate effort. The focus is upon control of behaviour through presumably deterrent punishments, including, where necessary, incarceration. However, since the scope of this study is limited to treatment in voluntary forms, the use of legal coercion as a protective and preventive measure will not be discussed.

An advantage of the moral model, pointed out by Brower *et al.* (1989), is that it holds people accountable for the consequences of their substance abuse. Although blaming someone for being dependent on alcohol is generally counter-therapeutic, holding people accountable for consequences may be useful in overcoming denial and increasing commitment to change (see Hallek 1982; Fingarette 1988). Protecting alcoholics from the consequences of their drinking often 'enables' them to continue drinking. On the other hand, while being continuously reminded of the importance of change is probably necessary, it is not sufficient to alter the course of an individual's life. Vaillant (1983*b*, 1988) found that at least one of three other conditions must also be fulfilled: (a) a substitute for alcohol; (b) powerful new sources of self-esteem and hope; or (c) the acquisition of a new stable relationship.

Alcoholics Anonymous (AA) and other twelve-step programmes combine elements of both the moral and the disease model. Although these programmes prefer to describe themselves as spiritual programmes, Brower *et al.* (1989) rightly consider the *spiritual model* to be a variant of the moral model. It attributes chemical dependency to the substance abuser's misalliance with God and the universe. According to AA, the alcoholic is alienated from God, stubbornly self-willed, and trying to dominate and control the outside world. Therefore, treatment aims at helping him to adopt a more 'complementary' view of his relationship to others and to the universe or God.

In the terms of psychoanalysis, systems theory and existential philosophy, the alcoholic's admission that he is 'powerless over alcohol' (the first step of AA) has been described as a reduction of narcissistic ego components (Tiebout 1961) and as a change to a more correct epistemology (Bateson 1971) or to a more accurate understanding of the limitations of the human condition (Flores 1988). However, many alcoholics are either unwilling to concede the premise of being powerless over alcohol or they accept it only briefly during the remorse following a binge. Given the variant nature of excessive drinkers, Emrick (1987) concluded that AA is the most appropriate option only 'at certain times' and 'for certain individuals'. According to Ogborne (1989), AA is of use primarily for 'drinkers who have experienced loss of control, who believe in the need to abstain, and who believe that AA can help them' (p. 62).

In his influential psychiatric textbook, Kraepelin (1883) described the dominant symptom of alcoholism as a 'general withering away of those continuous incentives for action that are summed up as "moral standards" or "character"' (p. 32; translated from German). In simplistic moralizing on alcoholism, 'low moral standards' or 'bad character' is actually regarded as a major *cause* of the disorder. However, prospective studies of samples from a general population followed from pre-adolescence to adulthood (Kammeier, Hoffmann, and Loper 1973; Vaillant 1980*a*; Vaillant and Milofsky 1982*b*) show that antisocial behaviour is normally a consequence rather than a cause of alcoholism. In other words, it seems to be the drinking behaviour itself that sometimes leads to a spiritual state which can, using a biblical metaphor, be compared to 'the troubled sea, when it cannot rest, whose waters cast up mire and dirt' (Isaiah 57:20). 'At bottom', most alcoholics are not more alienated from the mainstream values than others.

The notion that alcoholism is a symptom of personality disorder is further analysed in Chapter 8. The next chapter discusses a theoretical model that has arisen as a reaction to such spiritual, moral, or psychological views that do not give adequate consideration to the specific pharmacologic actions of alcohol.

6 The disease model

Among the earliest advocates of alcoholism as a disease were three physicians: the American Benjamin Rush (1785), the Briton Thomas Trotter (1804), and the Swede Magnus Huss. Huss (1849–51) introduced the term *alcoholism*, by which he meant

the complex of disease manifestations from the nervous system, including its psychic, as well as its motory and sensitive spheres . . . that is prevalent among persons who have, for an extended period of time, persistently and excessively indulged in alcoholic beverages. (1849, p. 33; translated from Swedish)

The disease concept was expanded on by medical writers such as Emil Kraepelin (1883) and by the temperance movement. However, it was not until after the second world war that the public and legislators began to conceive of habitual drinking as a disease. Impetus was provided by Alcoholics Anonymous (AA) and other sources in the USA, where numerous disease conceptualizations have appeared (e.g. Alcoholics Anonymous 1939, 1957; Jellinek 1952, 1960; AMA 1961; Keller 1962, 1976; APA 1968, 1980; Mann 1968; Gitlow 1973).

6.1 The classical model

The most complete and rigorous formulation of the disease concept was provided by Morton Jellinek (1960) in *The Disease Concept of Alcoholism*. Jellinek presented his theory as a working hypothesis. In view of the scientific evidence available, Jellinek cautiously wrote: 'For the time being this may suffice, but not indefinitely' (op. cit., p. 159). Many people, however, accepted Jellinek's preliminary theses as established truth. These came to have a great impact on public opinion, often in highly simplified versions (e.g. Glatt's (1972) Addiction Chart).

The *classical model* of alcoholism as a disease was formulated in Jellinek's most influential work, the article 'Phases of alcohol addiction' from 1952. In the book published eight years later, this model corresponds to *Gamma* alcoholism (loss of control), which Jellinek says is the predominating species of alcoholism in Anglo-Saxon countries. At the same time, he identifies four other species of alcoholism characterized by different drinking patterns. However, only one or two of these (*Delta*: inability to abstain; *Epsilon*: episodic use) are designated as diseases. Moreover, Jellinek points out that one would need the entire Greek alphabet, and perhaps several other alphabets, for labelling all species of harmful drinking.

Jellinek's refinement of the original disease concept passed relatively unnoticed. The ensuing discussion mainly focused on the Gamma species of alcoholism, with incidental remarks that alcoholism is not a unitary disease as mere lip service. This is unfortunate, since Jellinek's (1960) attempt to characterize *different* kinds of drinking patterns is of great theoretical interest whether one accepts his disease concept or not.

According to Pattison, Sobell, and Sobell (1977), the classical disease model can be summarized in the following propositions:

1. There is a unitary phenomenon which can be identified as alcoholism.
2. Alcoholics and prealcoholics are essentially different from nonalcoholics.
3. Alcoholics may sometimes experience an irresistible physical craving for alcohol, or a strong psychological compulsion to drink.
4. Alcoholics gradually develop a process called 'loss of control' over drinking, and possibly an inability to stop drinking.
5. Alcoholism is a permanent and irreversible condition.
6. Alcoholism is a progressive disease which follows an inexorable development through a distinct series of phases. (pp. 2–3)

Advocates of the disease concept often recommend a non-medical rehabilitation approach, especially participation in AA. This organization is guided by four basic concepts (Malikin 1973). The first is to show alcoholics that they can be accepted and loved. The second concept is that of inspiring hope in its members. The third concept involves the alcoholic's recognition of the fact that he has a physiological disease and that 'even one drink is too many'. The fourth concept is that the alcoholic must learn to live one day at a time without taking a drink. By attending AA meetings and verbalizing problems, he strengthens his resistance to drink and gradually reconstructs his lifestyle to rid himself of dependency on alcohol.

It may seem paradoxical to claim on the one hand that alcoholism is a physical disease beyond the individual's control and on the other hand advocate a psychosocial approach to rehabilitation. However, the disease concept was not the result of any scientific discovery. It was originated for a political and humanitarian purpose (Room 1972). Jellinek hoped to change the general attitude towards alcoholics from one of blame and punishment to one of concern and treatment. Other deviant behaviours have undergone a similar medicalization, probably leading to greater compassion and more humane treatment (Ausubel 1961).

The disease concept was, furthermore, heavily lobbied by the alcohol industry (Cahalan 1988). By supporting the position that the alcohol problem lies in the individual, not in the bottle, it made it easier for this burgeoning industry to fend off restrictions on aggressive marketing, the threat of higher taxes on alcoholic beverages, and other constraints.

The medical definition made it possible to shift the burden of dealing with the alcohol problem away from regulatory over to care-providing agencies.

A dramatic expansion of treatment services for problem drinkers has taken place since the late 1960s in the industrial world; detoxification facilities for inebriates have proliferated; welfare agencies have been charged with increasing responsibility in dealing with alcohol problems; public drunkenness has been decriminalized; industry-based programmes designed to identify and manage problem drinkers have expanded, etc.

6.2   Scientific critique

In recent years, social and behavioural scientists in particular have begun to question the justification of applying the disease concept to behavioural disorders of a more or less deviant nature (e.g. Szasz 1964, 1970; Ullman and Krasner 1969). In this connection, growing criticism has been levelled at the conception of alcoholism as a disease (e.g. Bratt 1953; Verden and Shatterly 1971; Robinson 1972; Room 1972, 1983; Szasz 1972; Davies 1974; Hershon 1974; Pomerleau, Pertschuk, and Stinnet 1976; Pattison *et al.* 1977; Heather and Robertson 1981; Peele 1985; Hill 1985; Miller 1986; Fingarette 1988).

Jellinek's disease concept was saddled with many *methodological problems.* The concept of a unitary natural history with different phases (Jellinek 1946, 1952) was, for example, based on a postal questionnaire with open-ended questions directed at members of Alcoholics Anonymous. It is probable that the responses were coloured by the special philosophy and membership composition of this, at that time, rather small movement (Seiden 1960). Moreover, only 98 (6 per cent) of the returned questionnaires were completed in such a manner that it was possible to analyse them at all.

Numerous more refined studies have failed to confirm Jellinek's theses. Jellinek's (1952) original assumption that a distinct physical mechanism is involved in *loss of control* was clear and unambiguous:

Loss of control means that any drinking of alcohol starts a chain reaction which is felt by the drinker as a physical demand for alcohol. This state, possibly a conversion phenomenon, may take hours or weeks for its full development: it lasts until the drinker is too intoxicated or too sick to ingest more alcohol. (p. 679)

The hypothesis of 'loss of control'—the main criterion of alcoholism according to the classical disease model—was tested experimentally during the 1960s and early 1970s and was rejected. Research on the ability to drink in a controlled manner (see review by Heather and Robertson 1981) has shown that this is determined to a large degree by *cognitive* factors (e.g. what the person believes he has drunk) and by *environmental* factors. The ability also varies among chronic alcoholics. Loss of control is not a necessary corollary of alcoholism.

Mello and Mendelson (1971), for example, have demonstrated that an alcoholic who is given an opportunity to work for alcohol often remains abstinent all day in order to store up a sufficiently large supply for his next bout. During these 'white days', his blood alcohol level approaches zero. Withdrawal symptoms can be observed, and still the alcoholic refrains from drinking. Such abstinent days can be described as periods of self-control.

Hospitalized alcoholics have been found to control their drinking if excessive drinking is associated with a loss of privileges (Cohen, Liebson, and Faillace 1971), and some alcoholics are able to return to controlled drinking in periods after discharge (e.g. Davies 1962; Orford, Oppenheim, and Edwards 1976; Armor, Polich, and Stambul 1978). The drinking alcoholic is still a sensible human being who is capable of making decisions and—at least to some extent—being influenced by his own resolve and the pressures of those around him. To be sure, the ability of an alcohol-dependent person to control his drinking is impaired, as is his responsiveness to normal processes of social control. But the differences between drinkers are a question of degree, not of 'self control' versus 'loss of control' in the absolute sense that Jellinek (1952) attached to the concepts.

Jellinek described alcoholism as a disease characterized by a number of 'phases' with different patterns of symptoms. The idea of describing alcohol abuse from a developmental perspective has proven to be very fruitful. But Edwards (1980, 1984) emphasizes that we need to separate out the ideas of *natural history* and *career*. Natural history is the development of the individual's reactivity to alcohol, while career pertains to the evolution of the individual's role.

Natural history is an idea borrowed from medicine, and underlies Jellinek's 'phases of alcoholism'. It implies a biological condition with a tendency, once established, towards a march of symptoms and progression. Individual characteristics and environmental factors only determine the pace of progression. However, advocates of the medical model admit the possibility of fluctuation and 'spontaneous regression'.

The career concept draws attention both to the individual and to the culture and society which surrounds, constrains, and encourages certain behaviours. Social scientists have shown how drinking careers are influenced by the individuality of the drinker, by the perceptions and reactions of those around him, by society's definition of the drinker's condition, and by individual and social processes of the most diverse kinds.

The biologically rooted concept of natural history and the psychosocial concept of career represent, according to Edwards (1980, 1984), *supplementary* perspectives. Edwards believes that alcohol dependency is a result of an interaction between biological processes and aberrant learning. Once the individual has developed a tolerance for alcohol and has begun to experience key symptoms of withdrawal (tremors, nausea, sweating, mood disorders), biological processes may have been set in motion that gradually alter the individual's tissue and body-system reactivity to alcohol. And once drinking has been cued to withdrawal relief and avoidance, learning processes may have been initiated that are reinforced and elaborated in a predictable manner if the person continues to drink.

From a psychological viewpoint, the development of withdrawal symptoms (i.e. 'physical dependence') and repeated drinking to relieve or avoid these symptoms can reinforce the disposition to drink, through operant and classic conditioning. Minimal symptoms of withdrawal (e.g. trembling) or merely the expectance of withdrawal symptoms become stimuli which trigger a craving for alcohol (Rankin and Hodgson 1977; Hodgson, Rankin, and Stockwell 1979). On the basis of behavioural theory, we can expect the drinking behaviour to be gradually reinforced. For the severely dependent person, the attempt to cut short a brief drinking binge may lead to actual or expected, biologically or psychologically determined withdrawal symptoms, which could evoke a feeling of 'loss of control'. Edwards and Gross (1976) assume:

Reinstatement of tolerance and of withdrawal symptoms suggests that a biologically determined change in response to alcohol may be brought about by certain patterns of exposure. But repeated relief of withdrawal (and of subacute withdrawal), or repeated fear of withdrawal, results in an abnormal drive towards repeated experience of high alcohol intake. The learning process is very incompletely understood, but dependence *should perhaps be seen as being in the same group of disorders as phobic and obsessional states*, with *a potent, complicating biological factor*. (p. 1061; italics added)

One characteristic of a behaviour that has been learned well and repeated many times is a *tendency towards stereotyping*. This has been demonstrated in animals (Solomon and Wynne 1953), in humans with obsessions (Rachman and Hodgson 1980), and in compulsive gamblers (Dickerson 1977). Edwards and Gross (1976), who have contributed a preliminary description of the alcohol-dependence syndrome (Chapter 7), regard stereotyping of the drinking pattern (narrowing of the drinking repertoire) to be a symptom of dependence.

The ordinary drinker's consumption and beverage will vary from day to day and from week to week. He may have a beer at lunch on one day, nothing to drink on another, share a bottle of wine at dinner one night, and then go to a party on a Saturday and have a lot to drink. A person who is in the process of getting caught up in heavy drinking may at first widen his drinking repertoire as well as the range of cues that signal drinking. As dependence advances, the cues are increasingly related to relief or avoidance of alcohol withdrawal, and the person's drinking repertoire becomes increasingly narrowed. The dependent person begins to drink the same whether it is workday, weekend, or holiday. The nature of the company or his own mood makes less and less difference.

It is possible, according to Edwards and Gross (1976), to assess the degree of dependence by questioning about how far this process has advanced. With advanced dependence, the individual has a daily schedule planned to maintain a high concentration of alcohol in the blood. He is able to recount where and when each drink of his daily ration was bought and consumed. However, even when dependence is well established, some capacity for variation remains. Change in personal circumstances such as a new job or a new living partner may for a time constrain the drinking. Price policy and sales restrictions may also influence the consumption of alcohol-dependent persons (Bruun *et al.* 1975; Kendell, de Roumanie, and Ritson 1983).

On the basis of principles of conditioning, it is reasonable to assume that craving or the urge for alcohol will vary in intensity with the degree of dependence. It is therefore not surprising that Edwards and Gross (1976) list the *salience of drink-seeking behaviour* over other subjective motives as a symptom of dependence. At the same time as the drinking becomes increasingly stereotyped, the urge to drink becomes more important than other pleasures or interests.

Indeed, the failure of unpleasant consequences to deter the individual from drinking may be a clinical indicator of the degree of dependence. The wife's distressed scolding—once effective—is later regarded by the drinker as evidence of her lack of understanding. Income that had previously provided for many needs is eventually sacrificed on the altar of drink. Gratification of the urge for alcohol may become more important for the patient with liver damage than even considerations of survival, the motto being: 'A short life and a merry one'.

Edwards (1980; Edwards and Gross 1976) finds, in summary, that essential dependence symptoms, such as narrowing of the drinking repertoire and salience of drink-seeking behaviour, can be explained on the basis of general behavioural principles of learning and conditioning. Consequently, he rejects the classical disease model's notion of a natural history. The idea of natural history, if taken in isolation, he says, will lead to a 'mechanistic' and 'hopelessly insensitive' analysis of the unfolding story of the individual's life. Variations between different alcoholics are so great that drinking patterns, life situations, and potentials for change must be studied individually. At the same time, Edwards emphasizes that psychological and social studies of drinking careers will fall short if they neglect to take into account developments over time in biological responses to alcohol. The aberrant learning processes take place in individuals who are far from being 'blank pages' as regards their biochemical reactivity to alcohol.

Alcohol abuse has been found by other scientists as well to be too complex a social, psychological, and biological phenomenon to be pinned down by the one-dimensional categories of the classical disease model. When it was introduced, Jellinek's working hypothesis had a salutary effect on alcohol research. Today, many researchers regard it as a potential obstacle to the advancement of knowledge and the emergence of interdisciplinary approaches to alcoholism.

6.3   Social consequences

The biological disease model has been effective in furthering the establishment of treatment facilities for alcoholic persons, making alcoholism a morally acceptable condition, and raising funds for research. Alcoholics Anonymous, who in North America are the primary agents of alcoholism treatment, consider the disease concept to be helpful in dealing with denial and minimization.

However, the concept of alcoholism as a disease has had distinct disadvantages from the political and clinical viewpoints as well. One is that it has not only absolved alcoholics of blame and punishment; in contrast to the interpretation of disease given by AA, the concept has also tended to declare the individual alcoholic incapable and exempt from responsibility. In fact, common conceptions concerning the nature of being ill (see Robinson 1971) still agree with Talcott Parsons' (1952) classic definition of the *sick role*:

1. The sick person is temporarily exempted from normal social responsibilities in order to promote recovery.

2. The sick person cannot be expected to recover by his own effort. He is in a condition that must be 'taken care of'.

3. The sick person construes his condition as undesirable and wants to recover as expeditiously as possible.

4. The sick person is willing to seek professional help and ready to cooperate in the treatment process to the best of his ability.

No one any longer questions—as they did in Jellinek's time—the alcoholic's right to adequate treatment of complications related to his drinking. What is unfortunate, however, is that alcoholics, physicians, and the general public have, to a great extent, come to confuse detoxification and other medical care for alcoholics with alcoholism treatment. Programmes that treat alcohol-related disabilities, but ignore the social matrix of drinking can, in fact, contribute towards locking the alcoholic in a passivating sick role. They can thereby help to maintain the alcoholic's drinking pattern.

Naturally, the opportunity to sober up in detoxification centres has been appreciated by public inebriates. However, decriminalization of public drunkenness also has another side. Police officers traditionally maintained the sobriety of the most deteriorated of alcoholic populations by seeking to 'install themselves . . . and let the consciousness of their presence play the part of conscience' (Bittner 1967, p. 708). The disengagement of the police from dealing with public drunkenness has relaxed social controls on the drinking of chronic inebriates. As a consequence, more drinking and a deterioration in health has been reported, with the drunks becoming more, rather than less, entrenched in their deviant lifestyle (Fagan and Mauss 1978; Giffen and Lambert 1978; Giesbrecht *et al.* 1981).

Ironically, Jellinek himself warned forty years ago that a broadening of the disease concept to include all excessive drinking—'whether or not there is any physical or psychological pathology involved in the drinking behaviour'—could legitimize drunkenness. Jellinek (1952) said:

Such an unwarranted extension of the disease conception can only be harmful, because sooner or later the misapplication will reflect on the legitimate use too and, more importantly, will tend to weaken the ethical basis of social sanctions against drunkenness. (p. 674)

The concept of alcoholism as a disease has probably made it easier for problem drinkers to speak openly with fellow employees about their plight. Such conversations have great potential, Trice and Sonnenstuhl (1988) point out, since the workplace can bring effective pressures to bear on deviant drinking behaviour. But a 'rush to treatment', prolonged sick leaves, and disability pension, instead of being offered adequate help while staying on the job and being held responsible for one's behaviour, may very well legitimize, exacerbate, or even perpetuate the abnormal use of alcohol (Roman and Trice 1968; Trice and Beyer 1981, 1982, 1984).

Furthermore, the redefinition of excessive drinking from a societal problem to an individual problem has promoted the substitution of alcoholism treatment for preventive policies aimed at the control of alcohol. A group of WHO investigators have even described the rapid growth of alcoholism treatment in the western world from the end of the 1960s as 'a kind of cultural excuse' for the relaxation of controls on the drinking behaviour of the 'normal' majority (Mäkelä *et al.* 1981, p. 65). According to Seldon Bacon (1973), founder of the US National Council of Alcoholism and an early advocate of the disease concept, the notion that alcoholism is 'only' or 'predominantly' a disease has had consequences that are 'both humanitarian and *massively* nonhumanitarian':

Twenty-five years ago this belief acted to tear down the walls of avoidance, denial, ignorance, cruelty, and hopelessness. Today, however, I see signs of its being used as a copout. For example: 'Let's turn the whole problem over to the doctors: it's a disease, isn't it?' This can be seen in efforts of law enforcement agencies to relieve themselves of responsibility. This can be seen in terms of friends, associates, and relatives, who can explain away their possible responsibilities by this new magic just as they could escape by such old magics as ideas of lack of will power, of sin, or of biological inheritance. (p. 24)

Bacon points out that research, manpower training, and facilities for alcoholics have been given a medical slant, and he concludes: 'In the past we turned over these problems to the churches, to the schools, to legislative sales controls, to policemen and jails. Now it will be medicine's turn, as it looks like a nice new copout' (ibid.).

The Scottish psychiatrist and WHO investigator R. E. Kendell (1979) broadened the critical perspective on the classification of alcohol abuse as a disease:

The disease concept of alcoholism may be out of tune with the facts and a serious obstacle to rational solutions, but it has the great attraction of embodying assumptions that are convenient to almost everyone concerned. It allows us to drink happily, secure in the belief that normal people like ourselves do not become alcoholics; it allows the alcohol industries to do their best to persuade us to drink more without any suggestion that this is dangerous; and it allows politicians to avoid electorally unpopular decisions. Even alcoholics stand to gain: they are offered treatment for their 'illness' and by implication reassured that it is not their fault that they have become ill and that it is someone else's job to get them better. (p. 370)

Public attitudes research (Crawford and Heather 1987; Crawford et al. 1989) has challenged the assumption that the disease concept of alcoholism is still a powerful vehicle for the promotion of humanitarian attitudes. The assumption that it is useful for the handling of all kinds of drinking problems can be questioned as well. Deteriorated alcoholics, in particular, are rarely able to satisfy the expectations associated with the sick role (Kurtz and Regier 1975). As a rule they will not actively seek help or co-operate in promoting their recovery. On the other hand, heavy drinkers who do not fit the pattern of symptoms that define the disease may be provided with a rationalization for denying that they have a problem.

6.4   Alcoholism—a disease?

The strength of the classical disease model in comparison with the moral model is that it calls attention to the addictive effect of alcohol or the evolution of the individual's reactivity to alcohol. Its fundamental weakness is a tendency to absolve the individual drinker from responsibility for his behaviour and to minimize the importance of psychological, cultural, and environmental factors in the aetiology and maintainance of drinking patterns.

As suggested above, the disease concept has been applied to treatment in more than one way. Alcoholics Anonymous place a great emphasis on individual responsibility and a supportive social environment as prerequisites for successful rehabilitation. The individual is assumed to take an active part in his or her own recovery. With this attitude they introduced a non-Parsonian sick role, which, although it has counterparts in somatic medicine (see Mäkelä 1980), has not yet permeated the public mind.

The disease concept has been given different interpretations in the scientific discussion as well. As shown above, evidence does not support the biological disease model introduced by Jellinek (1952). Whether alcoholism as a multidimensional phenomenon is to be classified as a disease, a behavioural disorder, or merely a deviant behaviour is, however, ultimately a public policy decision rather than a scientifically meaningful question (Seeley 1962; Edwards 1970*b*; Conrad and Schneider 1980).

There are two current trends with regard to this issue. One denies the usefulness of disease models in describing and explaining alcoholism. This critique focuses on the common beliefs alluded to by Parsons (1952), that is, the *technological* conception of health and illness (WHO 1986) emphasizing biological processes and professional help. The other trend attempts to place disease (including 'alcoholism as a disease') in the context of social living conditions and individual patterns of behaviour, as determined by sociocultural factors and personal characteristics. This *ecological* conception of health and illness, promoted by WHO (1986), emphasizes not only preventive measures but also the individual's responsibility for his own health. Its recent coming of age illustrates a tendency which Zola (1972) observed: 'At the same time as the label "illness" is being used to attribute "diminished responsibility" to a whole host of phenomena, the issue of "personal responsibility" seems to be re-emerging within medicine itself' (p. 491).

From logical and empirical viewpoints, it makes no difference whether alcoholism is regarded as a behavioural disorder with biological components or as a disease with behavioural components. The choice between these two conceptions is primarily a political and ethical decision, which should be based on a thorough evaluation of its consequences for the individual and for society.

The criticism voiced above applies to the classical disease model, not to an ecological disease concept that views alcoholism from a biopsychosocial perspective (cf. Chapter 11). In the next chapter, alcoholism is defined as a dependence syndrome, which is described in both behavioural and medical terms. This concept permits a less biased assessment of the need of alcoholics for both support (including medical attention) and social controls than the 'sin' and 'vice' concepts or the biological disease concept.

7 Alcohol dependence

'Alcoholism' is currently in the process of being abandoned as a diagnostic term. The World Health Organization, WHO, instead recommends the term *alcohol dependence*, defined as a condition in itself. The concept of dependence was introduced by WHO in 1965 to emphasize the fact that 'addiction' or 'habituation' to a wide variety of chemical substances belongs to the same family of disturbances (Eddy *et al.* 1965). The specific influences on the central nervous system range from stimulation to depression; but all drugs were considered to have one effect in common: in certain individuals, they are capable of creating a particular state of mind called 'psychic dependence'.

The term 'alcohol dependence' has given rise to and been the focus of considerable research in recent years. During the period 1972 to 1975, a group of investigators within WHO worked on definitions of alcohol-related disabilities, resulting in a document (Edwards *et al.* 1976, 1977*b*) that is still regarded as normative. The group's report served as a basis for the ninth revision of the International Classification of Diseases (WHO 1977), where the term 'alcohol-dependence syndrome' has been substituted for 'alcoholism'. Alcohol-dependence syndrome is defined as follows:

A state, psychic and usually also physical, resulting from taking alcohol, characterized by behavioural and other responses that always include a compulsion to take alcohol on a continuous or periodic basis in order to experience its psychic effects, and sometimes to avoid the discomfort of its absence; tolerance may or may not be present. (WHO 1977, p. 198)

In a draft to the tenth revision of the International Classification of Diseases (WHO 1989*a*), the concept of 'dependence syndrome' is further elaborated along the guidelines provided by Edwards and his colleagues in the 1970s:

A cluster of physiological, behavioural and cognitive phenomena in which the use of a drug or a class of drugs takes on a much higher priority for a given individual than other behaviours that once had higher value. A central descriptive characteristic of the dependence syndrome is the desire (often strong, sometimes overpowering) to take drugs . . . , alcohol or tobacco. There may be evidence that return to substance use after a period of abstinence leads to a more rapid reappearance of other features of the syndrome than occurs with non-dependent individuals. (p. 54)

Recently, a dependence syndrome construct has been adopted also by the American Psychiatric Association (DSM-III-R; APA 1987). 'Alcohol dependence' in accordance with WHO's definition should not be confused with alcoholism in any of its usual definitions: *harmful drinking, heavy drinking*, or *physical dependence*.

7.1   Alcohol-related disabilities

The most common definition of alcoholism centres on the harmful effects of habitual drinking. The 1989 edition of *The New Encyclopaedia Britannica* thus states that the term alcoholism is used to denote 'a repetitive intake of alcoholic beverages to an extent that causes repeated or continued harm to the drinker' (Vol. 13, p. 224). The disabilities referred to may be of a physical, psychological, or social nature.

In socio-political investigations, the terms 'alcohol abuser' or 'problem drinker' are often used as synonyms for 'alcoholic'. Terms such as 'alcohol abuse' and 'problem drinking' as well as alcoholism as 'harmful drinking' are, however, all ambiguous, since they may refer to either the state of dependence itself or the harmful effects of the alcohol consumption, or both. WHO's group of investigators (Edwards *et al.* 1977*b*) instead define two

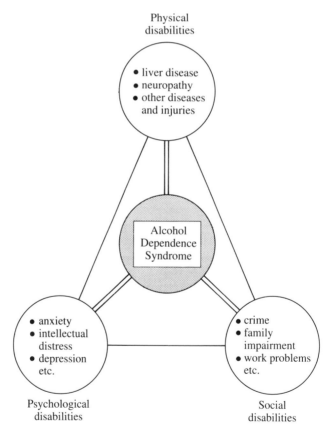

Fig. 7.1   The WHO's differentiation of the alcohol dependence syndrome from alcohol-related disabilities.

conditions, an *alcohol-dependence syndrome* and *alcohol-related disabilities* in a broader sense (Fig. 7.1).

With this distinction, the group wishes to stress the fact that an individual may have contracted pancreatitis, committed drunkenness offences, or have other alcohol-related problems without being alcohol-dependent. The scope and nature of the alcohol-related disabilities are determined not only by the severity of the dependence, but also by the individual's general physical, psychological, and social resources as well as by societal values, norms, and sanctions.

Edwards (1977) says:

It is possible for a person to be in some degree dependent on alcohol while having sustained no interference with physical and mental health, or social or economic function. Similarly, it is eminently possible for a drinker to be in no way abnormally dependent on alcohol, but to have sustained major disabilities in several dimensions of his life. (p. 140)

In general, however, there is a close correlation between the degree of dependence and the extent of the alcohol-related disabilities (Polich *et al.* 1981; Skinner and Allen 1982; double lines in Fig. 7.1). The WHO group of investigators therefore emphasizes the importance of identifying and treating the alcohol-dependence syndrome itself in cases where disabilities appear to be related to alcohol. It is not enough—as is usual today (Holt *et al.* 1980; Hingson *et al.* 1982; Moore *et al.* 1989; Yersin and Paccaud 1989)—to focus on the physical, psychological, or social disorders that cluster around the syndrome.

7.2 Quantity of consumption

An increased awareness of the scope of 'hidden' alcoholism has led some researchers and clinicians to classify drinkers according to quantity of consumption only. A few authors even think it would be a good idea to omit such terms as 'alcoholic' and 'alcohol abuser' from our language, since they are generally based on the incorrect assumption that a clear limit exists between harmful and harmless consumption. In fact, virtually all alcohol consumption is harmful, and there is a well-substantiated correlation between the total amount of alcohol consumed in a society and the number of heavy drinkers.

In socio-political analyses a classification according to level of consumption is often convenient. Here the problem is how disabilities caused by alcohol can be reduced in the general population. In clinical contexts, however, the severity of alcohol dependence has proven to be a more reliable indicator of future alcohol problems (Polich *et al.* 1981, Ch. 3; Polich 1980).

Heavy drinking and severe alcohol dependence do usually go hand in hand. But the importance of quantity of consumption for blood alcohol level and development of dependence is affected by a number of individual parameters, such as body volume, eating habits, and distribution (or concentration) of drinking in time (Edwards *et al.* 1977*b*). Furthermore, there are people—such as bartenders, travelling salesmen, and brewery workers—who regularly consume a large quantity of alcohol on the job or in the company of friends without being psychologically dependent. Drinking for these individuals has not taken on a much higher priority than other sources of gratification. Nor is their drinking characterized by the three qualities which, according to both Rachman and Hodgson (1980) and the WHO (1989*b*, p. 49), are key indicators of compulsive behaviour:

(1) experienced pressure to act in a particular manner;

(2) an unwillingness to comply with this pressure;

(3) an internal source of the pressure.

These persons run just as great a risk as alcohol-dependent heavy drinkers of sustaining physical, psychological, or social disabilities, but they have a relatively favourable prognosis for treatment.

WHO's distinction between an alcohol-dependence syndrome and alcohol-related disabilities helps to prevent confusion between questions relating to individual rehabilitation and questions relating to the effects of preventive measures (sales restrictions, tax increases, etc.). This makes it easier to take both of these views of the alcohol problem into consideration. With a concept of alcoholism that is based on a narrow definition of 'harmful drinking', there is a risk that the social alcohol problem will be reduced to a question of treatment and other forms of intervention for individual alcoholics. On the other hand, a classification based on the quantity of consumption alone runs the risk of ignoring the specific problems and needs of the alcohol-dependent consumers.

7.3   Physical dependence

Physical dependence is defined as an adaptive state that manifests itself in the form of intense physical disturbances when the administration of the dependence-inducing drug is suspended (Eddy *et al.* 1965, p. 723). Physical dependence is a very common and conspicuous accompaniment of alcoholism. It also contributes towards reinforcing psychological dependence. In some medical writings on alcoholism withdrawal distress and morning drinking are considered sufficient to define the condition.

It should therefore be emphasized that 'alcohol-dependence syndrome' is not merely a synonym for 'physical dependence'. WHO's dependence concept describes a system of determinants that includes both biological and psychological components. But what above all unites alcohol-dependent persons, according to the definitions given above (p. 59), is a *psychological dependence* defined as a 'compulsion' (WHO 1977) or a 'desire (often strong, sometimes overpowering)' (WHO 1989*a*) to take alcohol.

By stimulating the brain directly and centrally, substances of abuse may, in susceptible individuals, offer more powerful euphoric effects than can be attained by food, sexual partners, or the beauty of nature, art, and music (Wise and Bozarth 1987; Wise 1988). Such positive affective states constitute, according to Seevers (1969) and Bejerot (1972*a*, 1972*b*, 1975*a*, 1977, 1980), the primary biological basis for 'psychological' dependence on alcohol. Like Keller (1969), these writers reduce physical dependence to an alcohol-related disability, an incidental 'complication' or 'side effect' of drinking.

Their argument is intriguing and echoes Trotter's (1804) classic view that 'the habit of intoxication belongs to the mind' (p. 175–6). Admittedly, physical dependence may contribute towards maintaining alcohol abuse, but so do other complications of drinking such as depression, divorce, etc. Furthermore, the relief of withdrawal distress has not been effective in treating alcohol dependence. Edwards and his colleagues (1977*b*) do, however, regard withdrawal symptoms as one component of the dependence syndrome.

7.4   Dependence as a syndrome

The WHO group of investigators (Edwards *et al.* 1976, 1977*b*) do not take any position on the question of whether the alcohol-dependence syndrome should be considered a disease or not. The term 'syndrome', the investigators point out, merely means that a number of phenomena tend to cluster sufficiently often to constitute a recognizable pattern. The diagnosis 'alcohol dependent' should, according to their guidelines, be based on the following kind of criteria:

1. *Altered behavioural state*: including an increase in drinking that breaks with social norms and previous behaviour. There is a diminished variability in the pattern of consumption. It eventually becomes limited to two types: either complete abstinence or very heavy continuous drinking. Eventually, the individual ceases to care about what people around him think of his drinking. In the final stages, he continues his drinking despite very painful consequences such as physical illness, break-up of the family, economic embarrassment, or penal sanctions.

2. *Altered subjective state*: impaired control over alcohol consumption and the presence of 'craving', i.e. a greatly heightened desire for alcohol or an inner compulsion to ingest alcohol. These impulses, which occur with varying intensity, are brought on by alcohol ingestion or other cues that vary from

person to person. A mental obsession with alcohol known as 'drink centredness' often sets in. But it is important to remember that an altered subjective state and behavioural alterations may be difficult to recognize in sociocultural situations where more or less continuous drinking is allowed, the WHO group points out.

3. *Altered psychobiological state*: appearance of withdrawal symptoms, from relatively trivial discomforts such as trembling, sweating, and retching in the morning through unpleasant affective disturbances such as anxiety, depression, and irritability to, in rarer cases, fully developed and life-threatening delirium tremens. The order of occurrence, combination, strength, and frequency of these withdrawal symptoms can vary considerably. An important confirmation that the individual really has experienced withdrawal symptoms is his report that such symptoms have been relieved by further drinking, such as 'morning drinking'. A high alcohol tolerance is a prerequisite in order for the individual to attain sufficient blood alcohol concentrations to induce withdrawal states. Tolerance usually increases as the alcohol dependence advances, but may decrease in the later stages of the dependence, so that the individual will become drunk on a small quantity of alcohol.

It is not necessary for all of the criteria enumerated above to be present simultaneously in order for an individual to be diagnosed as alcohol dependent. The dependence may be of different degrees, from a mild dependence that has only an insignificant effect on the individual's behaviour to a severe dependence that controls the individual's entire life or large portions of it. Thus, each sign and symptom can be more or less pronounced along a continuous scale. According to WHO's group of experts, the existence of different 'types' of alcoholism (Jellinek 1960) can best be interpreted as culturally, environmentally, or personally patterned manifestations of the same fundamental alcohol-dependence syndrome.

The fact that a person has stopped drinking or has reduced his consumption does not necessarily mean that his previously developed alcohol dependence no longer exists. In such situations, the WHO group prefers to speak of 'remission' rather than 'recovery' from the dependence condition. Comparison is made with asthma, where recovery from an attack should be distinguished from recovery from the actual condition of asthma, i.e. the tendency to suffer asthma attacks.

The term 'syndrome' raises the question of whether the pattern described above occurs regularly in reality. Shaw (1980, 1985) and Heather and Robertson (1981) have criticized the concept of dependence, which they regard as being ultimately based on a medical point of view and as merely a new and more sophisticated attempt to rescue the disease concept and its advocates from an increasingly massive, empirically founded criticism. Hodgson (1980*a*) admits that the term 'syndrome', with its medical connotations, can cause misunderstanding. But he emphasizes that empirical support exists for the hypothesis of a uniform dependence state, characterized by a drinking pattern that differs qualitatively from the norm.

Edwards and Gross (1976), two members of the WHO's group of investigators, have, in a thorough examination of the concept of alcohol dependence, identified the following components that are said to occur together with some regularity:

(1) narrowing of the drinking repertoire;

(2) salience of drink-seeking behaviour;

(3) increased tolerance to alcohol;

(4) repeated withdrawal symptoms;

(5) relief or avoidance of withdrawal symptoms by further drinking;

(6) subjective awareness of compulsion to drink; and

(7) reinstatement of the syndrome if the client begins to drink again after a period of abstinence.

In contrast to Jellinek (1952), Edwards and his colleagues (1977a) do not believe that psychological dependence necessarily implies a total loss of control:

There is evidence that even dependent drinking is influenced by environmental cues; it is a mistake to accept the over-simple view of dependence as necessarily implying a total lack of responsiveness. What has been referred to as loss of control over drinking would be more aptly termed *impaired control*. (p. 10)

The description of the biological and psychological components of the alcohol-dependence syndrome provides a theoretical basis for measuring the degree of dependence. WHO has given high priority to attempts to develop and test standardized instruments, which are being pursued at research centres in London, Edinburgh, and Toronto, among other places. Interview and questionnaire surveys, as well as behavioural techniques, have shown that the main elements of the syndrome can be reliably assessed. A number of these elements form a cluster and correlate both with clinical severity ratings and symptoms of dependence severity not embraced by the given instruments (see reviews by Hodgson and Stockwell 1985; Edwards 1986).

The degree of alcohol dependence is important to know for a number of reasons. The WHO investigators point out that the diagnosis 'alcohol dependent' can say something not only about an individual's current status but also about his prognosis. Moreover, it has been found that a reliable assessment of the degree of alcohol dependence can influence or alter the interpretation of empirical findings (see Chapter 22). The varying severity of dependence appears to be a reality that will have to be taken into account in research and treatment. It will not suffice to determine whether a person is an 'alcoholic' or not (Edwards 1974, 1977, 1986; Hodgson *et al.* 1978; Hodgson 1980*a*; Hodgson and Stockwell 1985).

The question of whether WHO's dependence concept is prognostically more useful than other recent attempts to divide alcoholics into subgroups—for example, primary and secondary (Goodwin and Guze 1981; Schuckit 1985) or 'milieu-limited' and 'male-limited' (Cloninger 1987)—can, however, not be answered until further systematic, comparative studies have been conducted. From such studies more powerful 'hybrid models', integrating the alcohol dependence dimension with neurobiological or psychosocial categories, may very well emerge (see Morey, Skinner and Blashfield 1984; Morey and Skinner 1986).

In conclusion: the concept of dependence neither underestimates the excessive drinker's changing reactivity to alcohol nor absolves the individual of responsibility for his behaviour. By distinguishing between alcohol dependence and alcohol-related disabilities, it decreases the risk of confounding causes and consequences of drinking with essential elements of the syndrome itself.

This specification facilitates a biopsychosocial explanation of the condition, which, in addition to chemical and physiological factors, also takes into account environmental influence, cognitive and behavioural factors, etc. By taking into account the varying degree of dependence, it is also possible to analyse how the interaction between biological factors on the one hand and psychological and social factors on the other changes during different phases of addiction. However, since the concept of psychological dependence is defined in terms of the 'compulsion' or 'desire' to take alcohol, it cannot *in itself* explain habitual drinking.

8 The symptomatic model

Early in this century, the psychiatric literature generally considered alcoholism to be symptomatic of another primary mental disorder (Bowman and Jellinek 1941). Notably, Knight (1937), a well-known psychoanalytic writer, stated that 'alcoholism is a symptom rather than a disease . . . There is always an underlying personality disorder evidenced by obvious maladjustment, neurotic character traits, emotional immaturity or infantilism' (p. 234). Knight also suggested the possiblity of a true cure in some alcoholics. Once the basic problem has been uncovered and resolved, the alcoholic may again be able to drink socially.

In Hayman's 1956 study of American psychiatrists' alcoholism treatment practices, insight-oriented psychotherapy was employed by 85 per cent of those reporting and supportive psychotherapy by 82 per cent. With the advent of the disease concept, however, penetration into the alcoholic's unconscious was increasingly questioned. At an American Psychiatric Association (APA) meeting in 1949, for instance, Tiebout (1951) accused his colleagues of side-stepping the drinking as 'merely' a symptom. Alcoholism, he contended, is a symptom which has become a disease in itself.

Galanter (1986), in a recent APA editorial on 'Why therapists fail', expressed a similar concern:

Relatively few therapists are experienced in offering proper care to addicted persons. Instead of setting abstinence as the goal, many engage the patients in exploratory therapy, hoping that a resolution of his internal conflict or social stress will end his substance abuse. (p. 769)

Much has changed since the 1950s, however. In Miller and Frances' 1986 study of American psychiatrists' practices concerning substance abuse, 60 per cent used supportive psychotherapy frequently and only 33 per cent reported that they were using insight-oriented therapy frequently. The latter figure would have been even smaller in Europe, except perhaps for Germany and surrounding nations, where symptomatic conceptualizations of alcoholism are still common (Miller 1986). Supportive therapy of alcoholics focuses on guidance and persuasion, generally through seeking alternatives to drinking and setting up realistic goals which are continually reviewed (e.g. Öjehagen and Berglund 1986; Okpaku 1986).

Another indication of change is the increasing number of therapists from the psychodynamic camp itself who are challenging symptomatic notions of alcoholism. For example, Brickman (1988) commented that psychoanalytic theory has failed to integrate more recent findings from other biobehavioural disciplines. 'The basic misconception', he noted, 'is that substance abuse is a secondary phenomenon to underlying psychopathology *and thus amenable to being influenced by psychoanalytic insight*' (p. 360; italics in original). As a consequence, he contended, substance abuse encountered in psychoanalytic practice is frequently mismanaged. In this chapter, the symptomatic model will be evaluated in the light of research data and their clinical implications.

8.1 Prospective studies

Many researchers, particularly during the 1940s and 1950s, have devoted considerable time, effort, and imagination to trying to find specific personality traits that precede alcoholism (see reviews by Barry 1974; Hoffmann 1976; Barnes 1979, 1983; Freed 1979; Neuringer 1982; Cox 1987; Nathan 1988; Sutker and Allain 1988). These studies have produced contradictory results, and critical reviewers (Sutherland, Schroeder, and Tordella 1950; Syme 1957; Armstrong 1958) early agreed that alcoholics do not comprise a unique type of personality. Keller (1972) summarized the research in a widely quoted maxim: 'Alcoholics are different in so many ways that it makes no difference' (p. 1147).

But even if no one has demonstrated the existence of any single *prealcoholic personality* with a unique constellation of personality traits, many researchers maintain that a number of characteristics are sufficiently common to be deserving of attention. Several studies have drawn the conclusion that characteristics such as emotional insecurity, anxiety, and unsatisfied dependence needs (e.g. Simmel 1948; Blane 1968), chronic depression (e.g. Winokur, Clayton, and Reich 1969), or sociopathy (e.g. Robins 1966) in particular predispose certain individuals to use alcohol as a means of dealing with their life circumstances.

Such conclusions, however, generally suffer from either of two major methodological flaws (Vaillant 1984). First, they are often based on *retrospective* findings, i.e. data collected after the fact from the alcoholic himself, from his family and friends, or from sources that may not have been intended for research purposes, for example official records. However, data obtained from the authorities may cause systematic errors, as exemplified by a comparison between official and self-reported criminal records (Short and Nye 1962). Data based on the alcoholic's own reconstruction of the past contain an even greater margin of uncertainty. Vaillant (1984) writes: 'As water refracts the passage of light and so produces visual illusions, so do lives passing through time bend memory and understanding and thus produce cognitive illusions' (p. 265).

A growing number of studies have demonstrated the impact of mood states on the recall of past events. Lewinsohn and Rosenbaum (1987), for instance, studied distorted memory in clinically depressed persons randomly selected from the general population. They found that whereas the currently depressed subjects recalled their parents as having been more rejecting and unloving, the remitted depressed, regardless of how many past episodes of depression they had, did not differ from the never-depressed controls in their recall of parental behaviour. Thus, whether early childhood is recalled as happy or unhappy may reflect current mood states more than reality.

Alcoholism takes a heavy toll on psychological well-being and jeopardizes social stability. Like an episode of depression, it is therefore likely to distort a person's memory of past events. This makes the follow-back study of alcoholics potentially misleading or confusing when used to elucidate cause and effect relationships.

Another important bias in studies of aetiological factors in alcoholism derives from the assumption that individuals who attend clinics or come to the attention of social agencies are representative of alcoholics in general. Alcoholics who die, spontaneously recover, or have other social supports do not present for treatment or become registered by agencies. Moreover, recidivists will be overrepresented in a random sample selected from a clinic or an official record. In clinical samples, alcoholics tend to be more dependent, more physically ill, and more psychologically vulnerable; in official records, they tend to have a wider range of antisocial behaviours.

The proper way to investigate antecedents of alcohol dependence is the *prospective*, longitudinal study. Studies of this kind ideally start with a random sample representing the general population. The sample should be selected at an early age, before drinking patterns have been established, and be followed forward to a point when some individuals in the subject group probably have developed drinking problems. The problem drinkers are then compared with the other subjects in the random sample with regard to alleged antecedents. Information on childhood and family should have been collected in advance for the purpose of research. With this methodology, which takes advantage of 'nature's own experiment', it is possible to control for biases that tend to occur as a result of distorted memory or skewed samples of non-representative subjects.

More than a dozen prospective studies have been carried out to date (see reviews by Vaillant 1984; Zucker and Gomberg 1986; Fillmore 1988). These studies have more or less serious methodological problems of their own. The problems include samples that are not represenative of the general population, small subject groups, incomplete inventory of possible causal factors, a late start in life, a short follow-up interval, a high dropout rate, restriction to alcohol abusers known to the authorities, and lumping together of alcohol abuse and other manifestations of psychosocial maladjustment.

Among prospective studies, the sophistication of George Vaillant's (1983*b*; Vaillant and Milofsky 1982*b*) follow-up of 456 men from Boston's Core City (previously studied by Sheldon and Eleanor Glueck 1950, 1968) is outstanding. Vaillant studied the development of an exceptionally large number of nonantisocial subjects. They were followed up from early adolescence (age 14 ± 2) well into adulthood (age 47), which is a longer period than that covered by previous studies. The attrition rate, 13 per cent of the surviving subjects, is remarkably low. The severity of drinking problems, including both 'hidden' problems and those known to clinics and agencies, was rated from a two-hour semistructured interview as well as recent psychiatric, medical, and arrest records. Childhood and familial data are extremely comprehensive and provide information on, for example, ethnic background, alcoholism in first and second degree relatives, relationship with parents, adolescent adjustment, emotional problems, and family relations. Moreover, in contrast to many colleagues, Vaillant separates antecedents of alcoholism from those of other unfavourable adult outcomes. The major limitation of Vaillant's study is the absence of data on the life course of women alcoholics.

At some point in their adult life 71 men (18 per cent) met the DSM-III criteria for alcohol dependence (APA 1980), and 32 met the criteria used for the diagnosis of sociopathy. As soon as one disorder was present the second was likely to follow, with alcoholism more often being the 'horse' than the 'cart' (Vaillant 1983a). But alcoholism and sociopathy as primary disorders appeared to have different aetiologies (cf. Cadoret et al. 1985). A problematic, unhappy childhood was associated with sociopathy in adult life. But it did not in itself increase the risk of future alcohol dependence.

The most important predictors of alcoholism were: (a) *drinking practices* related to ethnicity, and (b) *alcoholism in relatives* (Beardslee, Son, and Vaillant 1986; Vaillant 1986; Drake and Vaillant 1988). Men of Anglo-Irish or northern European descent were at higher risk of developing alcohol dependence than men whose parents had grown up in the Mediterranean cultures. Men of Irish extraction were seven times more likely to manifest alcohol dependence than men of Italian, Syrian, Jewish, Greek, or Portuguese descent. Italians, for example, learned from an early age that drunkenness is not tolerated. In contrast to the Irish, who preferred drinking in pubs, they drank with the family and at meals.

Yet, cross-cultural research has shown that alcohol-related mortality is higher in the Mediterranean than in northern Europe. This may be attributed to the greater availability and lower cost of alcoholic beverages in wine-growing nations. Bruun and his colleagues (1975) have demonstrated a high correlation between alcohol-related disabilities and the *availability of alcohol*. The conclusion of Vaillant's study must therefore be conditional: in a given geographical region during a given period of time, drinking practices and acceptance of drunkenness are major determinants of the risk of developing alcohol dependence.

Among men of Irish descent, familial alcoholism played an insignificant role for the development of alcoholism. Many Irish subjects with alcoholic relatives became lifelong teetotallers. Among other ethnic groups, including southern Europeans, alcohol dependence occurred five times as often in men with several alcoholic relatives as it did in men with no alcoholism in the family. This result agrees with estimates based on adoption studies of how genetic factors influence the risk of alcoholism (see Goodwin 1985).

However, recent findings indicate that learning about alcohol and its appropriate contexts of use takes place early in the child's life (see review by Zucker and Noll 1987). In Vaillant's study, alcoholism in the environment of the developing child and a family history of alcoholism independently contributed to adult alcohol dependence. When environment was controlled for, men with alcoholic relatives were only twice as likely to manifest alcohol dependence as other men. Adoption studies, too, are likely to underestimate the importance of the environment, because of the elimination of extreme environments by a careful selection of adoptive families (Cadoret 1986) and a sparse or inadequate inclusion of environmental variables (Searles 1988). Therefore, saying that an inherited susceptibility doubles the risk of developing alcohol dependence may be the most realistic estimate of the importance of alcohol-specific endogenous factors (cf. Peele 1986).

Ethnicity and alcoholism in relatives did not influence the risk of sociopathy as a primary disorder. The only variable that predicted both alcoholism and sociopathy in a significant way was *antisocial behaviour*. Youths with school behaviour problems and truancy ran four times as great a risk as their peers of developing alcoholism. This result agrees well with prospective studies indicating a relationship between youthful antisocial behaviour and later drinking problems, at least in the most disadvantaged segments of society (e.g. Magnusson 1988; see review by Fillmore 1988).

Alcoholism predicted by antisocial behaviour tended to have an early onset. In a prospective study of a large Swedish sample followed from the age of 11 to the age of 27, Cloninger, Sigvardsson, and Bohman (1988a) recently confirmed that individuals with antisocial personality traits, including low harm avoidance, high novelty seeking, and low reward dependence, were at increased risk of developing early-onset alcoholism. In fact, the variables of novelty-seeking and harm-avoidance distinguished groups of individuals who showed a 19-fold variation in risk. On the basis of this and other findings, Cloninger (1987; Cloninger *et al.* 1988b) has proposed two types of alcoholics, one of which is much less prevalent (perhaps 25 per cent of those diagnosed for alcoholism in early adulthood and 10 per cent of those diagnosed in middle life) and characterized by both antisocial personality traits and alcoholism onset before the age of 25 (see Section 19.4). A similar distinction between 'affiliative' and 'schizoid' alcoholics, or 'developmentally cumulative' and 'antisocial' alcoholics, has been suggested by Morey, Skinner, and Blashfield (1984) and Zucker (1987), respectively.

Disturbed childhood environment has been cited as a risk factor for alcoholism in both retrospective and prospective studies. Vaillant, however, found that familial cohesion and relationships with parents explained less than 0.1 per cent of the variance in subsequent alcohol dependence, when the contribution of ethnicity and parental alcoholism was controlled. That is, of men who had a stable childhood but who did have an alcoholic parent, one fourth became alcohol-dependent as adults; of the men with an unstable childhood but no alcoholic parent, only one of 20 became alcohol-dependent. Interestingly, McCord (1988) recently found that sons of alcoholic men were even more likely to become alcoholics if their mothers showed high esteem for their fathers. McCord believes that those alcoholics actually may have been taught that their fathers' behaviour was acceptable or, at least, forgivable.

Applying Ockham's razor, i.e. the principle that a simple explanation is preferable to a more complicated one, Vaillant dissects an earlier conclusion by the McCords (1960) that a dominant father, immigrant Catholicism, and low social status protect against future alcohol abuse. The McCords failed to note, he points out, that in the population studied most such individuals were first- and second-generation Italians. It may have been the drinking attitudes and practices among this group of immigrants, rather than other and more imaginative factors, that protected the children from alcoholism later in life.

The McCords' blindness to the social and cultural context of drinking is typical. Before Vaillant's landmark study, investigators were often so convinced that alcoholism *must* be a symptom of underlying personality disorder that it simply did not occur to them that it might be an affliction with a life of its own and with other antecedents than poor mental health.

Vaillant's data show that the differences frequently observed between alcoholics and non-alcoholics as regards social status, unemployment, educational level, and mental illness in fact appeared *after* the development of alcoholism. Although as adults the alcohol-dependent men suffered from personality disorders and were socially inadequate, as children they had neither more severe emotional problems, lower intelligence, poorer parental relations, or a more underprivileged status in society than their peers who were subsequently to drink socially.

Evidence from Vaillant's study also demonstrated that the 21 alcoholics who had abstained for at least three years and remained abstinent at follow-up were functioning about as well psychologically as those for whom alcohol had never been a problem. Nor did they differ from unremitted alcoholics with regard to those factors that predicted who would develop alcoholism. Similar improvements, with securely abstinent alcoholics being no more depressed than community controls, have been reported in long-term follow-ups by Moos, Finney, and Chan (1981) and Pettinati, Sugerman, and Maurer (1982b).

From their own study and a critical review of the literature, Vaillant and Milofsky (1982b) drew the following conclusion:

Available prospective studies suggest that if one controls for antisocial childhood, cultural attitudes towards alcohol use and abuse, for alcohol heredity, and most especially for the *effects* of alcohol abuse then many of the childhood and adult personality variables to which adult alcoholism has traditionally been attributed will appear as carts and not horses. (p. 502)

The absence of a correlation between an unhappy childhood and adult alcoholism has been confirmed by Vaillant (1980a; Beardslee and Vaillant 1984) in a prospective investigation of 184 men who were initially studied during their college years. The men's childhood environment was assessed by eight psychiatric interviews and a careful social history taken on a visit to their parents. The subject group was reinterviewed at the age of 47. Attrition was negligible.

Vaillant found in this more privileged group as well that a bleak childhood significantly predicted poor adult mental health but not alcoholism. Alcohol dependence, on the other hand, tended to evoke pessimism, passivity, self-doubt, dependence, and other 'oral' traits that were formerly considered to characterize the prealcoholic personality.

In a research review, Vaillant (1984) raises the question of whether *adult* depression, and dependency perhaps nevertheless favour the development of alcoholism. To find an answer, he followed Vaillant's (1980a) prospective study of college men until the age of 60. Estimates of psychopathology, chronic depression, and dependence were available from follow-ups at the ages of 20 and 47. Since more than half of the alcohol abusers became so after the age of 45, Vaillant was able to study the extent to which the abuse was a symptom of underlying psychiatric problems in adulthood. He found, however, that those men who eventually abused alcohol before the age of 60 did not exhibit more dependence or personality disorder between the ages of 20 and 47 than those who continued to drink socially. But once college men began to abuse alcohol, oral dependence traits became very common.

The conception of alcoholism as a symptom of a problematic or unhappy childhood and of underlying personality disorder is based, according to Vaillant, on a *retrospective illusion*. Prospective studies do not support the once popular slogan that 'alcoholism does not lie in the bottle, but in the man'.

George Vaillant (1980a) maintains that alcohol abuse may be more analogous to any intractable habit (e.g. smoking or fingernail biting) than to mental illness and may develop independently of pre-existing psychiatric problems. Prealcoholics are assumed to be no more different from the rest of the population than heavy smokers. Vaillant's and others studies of male alcoholism, in particular, indicate that a family history of alcoholism as well as cultural attitudes and drinking practices mean a great deal more for the development of alcoholism than early childhood environment and personality disorder as conceptualized in the psychoanalytic literature. However, certain behaviours associated with antisocial personality, notably low harm avoidance and high novelty seeking, seem to play a significant aetiological role for a less prevalent form of alcoholism characterized by early onset.

The outcome of prospective studies does not, however, mean that psychological susceptibility is generally unimportant in the genesis or treatment of alcoholism. It is more appropriate to conclude that the relationship between alcohol dependence and personality is much more complex than the symptomatic model would have us believe, and that personality disorder is much more often an effect than a cause of alcohol abuse.

Heavy drinking fairly consistently decreases self-esteem, interferes with normal sleep patterns, leads to depression and suicidal thoughts, and often produces increased anxiety and social isolation (McNamee, Mendelson, and Mello 1968; Tamerin, Weiner, and Mendelson 1970; Nathan *et al.* 1970; Allman, Taylor, and Nathan 1972; Logue *et al.* 1978). Psychiatric problems of this kind can probably accelerate the evolution of alcohol abuse and make remission more difficult. The alcoholic who finds that alcohol provides immediate relief from tremulousness, fearfulness, and dysphoria produced by brief abstinence can start to use alcohol as a panacea for a wide variety of unpleasant internal states and distressing external circumstances (Ludwig, Wikler, and Stark 1974; Goodwin 1979). In conditioning theory, this process is called *stimulus generalization*. However, the widespread belief that such a drinking pattern is merely a symptom of personal problems confuses cause and effect.

8.2   Dynamic psychotherapy

The definition of alcohol abuse as predominantly a form of *self-medication* or a way to alleviate underlying distress has obvious implications for treatment. Above all, it has inhibited the emergence of treatment techniques which, at least in an initial phase, are directly and primarily aimed at analysing and modifying the drinking behaviour itself. Instead treatment has been geared toward helping the patient to gain psychological insight and to improve his self-image. The hypothesis has been: treat the basic disorder and the dependency on alcohol will fade and disappear. Since alcohol is not the problem but an attempt at self-help, it will no longer be needed once the patient has improved his mental functioning.

As might be expected from the aetiological literature, this approach has yielded disappointing results. Although controlled research on the efficacy of insight-oriented psychotherapy is largely lacking, the evidence available suggests that such therapy has 'a high drop-out rate and lower or at best equivalent effectiveness in comparison to alternative treatment methods' (Miller and Hester 1980, p. 46). For example, in a long-term study of outpatient clinics, some of which applied dynamic psychotherapy, Gerard and Saenger (1966) concluded: 'The less the clinic became involved in the intricacies of the determinants of the patient's symptoms, relationships, or defences, the more likely was the clinic to succeed in supporting change in drinking behaviour' (p. 192).

Levinson and Sereny (1969) compared a six-week programme focusing on underlying psychological problems with an equally long programme which simply provided the alcoholics with a period of rest and diversion. At follow-up after one year, the recreational programme was 'unexpectedly' found to be at least as effective as the programme geared towards establishing psychological insights.

In a randomized controlled trial, Olson *et al.* (1981) compared the effectiveness of insight-oriented therapy (transactional analysis) and behavioural therapy with inpatient alcoholics. Drinking outcome was assessed over five follow-up periods from discharge to four years after treatment. Strong and consistent trends emerged favouring the behavioural approach on both abstinence and improved drinking measures across all periods. In fact, the insight-oriented treatment group did worse than the control group, which had not received any additional therapy.

Freud avoided treating addictions, which he felt were not accessible to customary analytic therapy (Harding 1975). In a standard textbook on dynamic psychotherapy, Lewis Wolberg (1967) takes the same position. He thinks that insight-oriented treatment is usually futile in alcoholism, since the alcoholic's

capacity to integrate and to utilize his insight in a constructive manner is impaired. The alcoholic patient will dig out fascinating dynamic structures during psychotherapy, but this effort will have little influence on his drinking. (p. 971)

An impaired capacity for complex cognitive tasks such as abstraction, problem-solving, and learning has been reported even in heavy drinkers with early symptoms of dependence (e.g. Bergman 1985, 1987). The ability to reason by analogy, which is pivotal for the gaining of psychological insights, is often impaired too (Yohman and Parsons 1987). In alcoholics with mild reductions of intellectual capacity, a prolonged abstinence over a period of several months enables the brain to recover most of its normal capacity (see reviews by Goldman 1983; Porjesz and Begleiter 1983; and a long-term, prospective study by Muuronen *et al.* 1989). As a consequence, alcoholics in stable remission, without severe brain damage, may well benefit from therapeutic activities demanding satisfactory cognitive functioning. Before that, however, it will often be more sensible to 'keep it simple'.

The French psychoanalyst Saliba (1982) maintains, in a study of patterns of recovery, that abstinence (even when externally imposed) is a prerequisite. Without abstinence lasting behavioural change, much less any change of intrapsychic structure, cannot take place. Abstinence is not the ultimate goal, Saliba points out, but it creates scope for change. Among English-speaking psychiatrists there is also an emerging consensus that the alcohol disorder should be treated first (Cohen 1985).

Vaillant (1981) contends that even if certain alcoholics—like certain non-alcoholics—have actually had problems with their parents, the period during which they give up alcohol is not the right time to work on these problems. Once an alcoholic has achieved stable sobriety, he has the same capacity to benefit from explorative psychotherapy as any other member of the population. But until then, the situation seems to be quite different. He underscores his point with facts from the lives of 268 men, prospectively followed from their first year in college until the age of fifty (Vaillant 1980a):

Twenty-six of these men at some point lost control over their use of alcohol. One-half sought psychotherapy and on the average received about two-hundred hours of psychotherapy. With time, one-half of these men have achieved stable remission from their alcoholism—usually through abstinence. In only *one* case did psychotherapy seem to be related to the remission; in many cases it seemed to deflect attention away from the problem. (Vaillant 1981, p. 54)

Vaillant illustrates the danger of psychotherapy with a case study of a male alcoholic who had received over one thousand hours of psychotherapy. Over the course of two decades his diagnosis deteriorated from inadequate personality to schizophrenia. However, therapy helped neither the man himself nor any therapist to realize that his core problem was actually the alcohol, not the secondary personality disorders or his allegedly disturbed relationship with his mother. Eventually the man actually gave up alcohol and his ego functioning matured considerably—as a result of his coming into contact with AA.

Brickman (1988), a Californian psychoanalyst, confirms that substance abuse is a serious impediment to successful psychotherapy. His conclusion is based on a systematic review of 20 years of practice. In most cases the extent of the patient's use of substances came to light incidentally during the unfolding treatment process. If the therapist and the patient cannot agree that the substance abuse is a serious issue that must be faced independently of the psychotherapy, Brickman considers therapy a waste of time. By nurturing the myth that therapy will help, the therapist may, in fact, interfere with patients' natural recovery through the experiencing of the adverse consequences of drinking. *Psychotherapeutic enabling* is Brickman's apt term for such an unwitting support of continued drinking.

Drawing from ideas in the literature and from experience, Levy (1987) outlines how traditional psychotherapeutic theory and technique must be modified when applied to the treatment of an alcoholic population. 'The first modification of critical importance when initially treating an alcoholic', he contends, 'is the need to focus on the patient's drinking as a problem without attempting to explore with the patient the reasons for the drinking' (p. 787). If the drinking is out of control, insights will not improve or change anything. In fact, things may very well be getting worse. A number of reasons, discussed in depth by Levy, indicate that reconstruction of the patient's past—the

the cornerstone of psychoanalytic therapy—is contra-indicated until sobriety is more firmly in place.

Ewing (1977), a psychoanalyst with 25 years of experience working with alcoholics, similarly states that 'psychoanalysis is contraindicated in the treatment of the average alcoholic' (p. 26). Too many patients after years of analysis and 'full of insight' hopefully resume drinking, only to find that disruptive, malignant drinking patterns soon reappear.

In a paper on 'Psychopathology produced by alcoholism', Bean-Bayog (1986) reckons that an alcoholic ordinarily needs three years to cope with the effects of stopping drinking. Brown (1985), drawing on an in-depth study of people who stopped drinking, Bean-Bayog (1985) and Brickman (1988) see an initial role for AA as the primary treatment agent, with psychotherapy serving as an adjunct. Rosen (1981) proposed a variant of the sequential approach. After initial treatment in AA, patients are provided with a substitutive attachment to the therapist, with whom they can work through a process of separation.

Levy (1987) proposes bringing AA to patients via the one-to-one therapeutic relationship. During the early stages of treatment, advice and suggestions, generally eschewed by clinicians trained within a psychodynamic model, are recommended. Dodes (1988) believes that with proper attunement to the patient's drinking and to the need to be abstinent, postponement of psychotherapy until after a lengthy sobriety may not be necessary. He considers the psychology of combining dynamic psychotherapy and AA, and, like the other clinicians above, he emphasizes the alcoholic's need for external support and structure.

These reports all signal a change in orientation, which may give dynamic psychotherapy a new role in the treatment of alcoholics. The revival, however, is likely to be contingent on a successful integration of recent prospective research findings, leading in turn to an abandonment of traditional, symptomatic conceptions of alcoholism and treatment.

8.3   Alcoholism—a symptom?

It is justified to assume, as Vaillant (1983b) and Schuckit (1986) do, that in the vast majority of cases, patients who say they drink because they are unhappy and anxious are in fact unhappy and anxious because they drink. Without being aware of it themselves, they are diverting attention from the real problem: their uncontrolled drinking.

Patients and therapists are as prone as researchers interviewing alcoholics after the fact to fall victim to the retrospective illusion, that is, the view that most alcoholics have been severely disturbed or distressed from the very beginning. The resultant interpretation of heavy drinking as a form of self-medication facilitates collusion with the patients' denial that drinking is a serious problem in its own right. The danger of interfering with natural recovery in this way is evident from outcome studies and clinical experience. Therefore, active alcoholism should be regarded as a *contra-indication* for insight therapy, i.e. treatment focusing on underlying dynamic structures.

The symptomatic model should, however, be commended for stressing the importance of diagnosing and treating coexisting psychiatric problems when present. Current trends in psychiatry indicate that the symptomatic model is yielding to a *dual diagnosis* model, that is, the idea that treatment may be required both for alcoholism and those psychiatric problems that persist after four weeks or more of abstinence (Attia 1988; Brower *et al.* 1989; Ridgely 1989; Evans and Sullivan 1990).

Most symptoms of anxiety (Brown, Irwin, and Schuckit 1991) and depression (Brown and Schuckit 1988) that are present prior to this phase of recovery, however, appear to be a function of a *protracted abstinence syndrome* rather than a psychiatric comorbidity. Some withdrawal (abstinence) symptomatology, such as disrupted sleep (Wagman and Allen 1975), may persist even for several years. Thus, the old notion that withdrawal is an acute episode lasting only about a week has proven to be incorrect.

Alcoholism and affective disorder are now conceived as two separate and distinct disorders, with little evidence of overlapping aetiology (Vaillant 1983*b*; Schuckit 1986). Male alcoholics do not seem to have a higher prevalence of primary affective disorder than the general population. However, among women attending an alcoholism treatment programme, the rate of primary affective disorder with secondary alcoholism may be as high as 10 to 15 per cent (Schuckit and Winokur 1972). Rounsaville *et al.* (1987) found that these 'negative affect alcoholics' (Zucker 1987) had better posttreatment outcome than other female alcoholics. This finding is consistent with the observation that depression is usually associated with a better prognosis than alcoholism. It also suggests that psychiatric diagnoses should be included in future prognostic studies, especially those focusing on patient–program matching.

9 The learning model

The learning model differs from the disease model and the symptomatic model in a number of respects. It is primarily concerned with how human behaviour is acquired, maintained, and changed. Deviant behaviour is not classed differently from normal behaviour. This model is not based on any assumption concerning disease processes or underlying disorder; instead, it assumes that both deviant and normal behaviour are learned and that the events influencing this process can be identified, measured, and altered.

Treatment interventions often teach alternatives to self-destructive or socially unacceptable habits. *Behaviour therapy* provides learning experiences that promote constructive and adjusted behaviour. The behavioural approach no longer ignores the mind and cognitive strategies, but its advocates emphasize that personal change is sometimes easier to accomplish by first altering behaviour and restructuring environments.

A drinking problem is regarded as a learned behavioural disorder of the same kind as overeating, heavy smoking, and sexual deviations. The learning model cites antecedent cues, reinforcing consequences, modelling, expectancies, and so on to explain how these behaviours are learned. All alcohol consumption is assumed to exist along a continuum with regard to frequency and duration, the amount of alcohol consumed, the degree of inebriation, and the resultant damage. Thus, no sharp borderline is drawn between social drinking and alcoholism.

Behavioural psychology has had a growing influence on alcoholism treatment research in recent years. In the process, its perspective has progressed from simple 'black box' models to increasingly sophisticated mediational explanations for excessive drinking.

9.1 Conditioning approaches

The learning model of alcohol abuse has evolved through a number of stages from classical conditioning to tension-reduction theory, operant conditioning and cognitive-behavioural theory (see George and Marlatt 1983). Ivan Pavlov (1927) suggested the importance of conditioned reflexes in addictive disorders. A *classical conditioning* approach has later been used by Ludwig and Wikler (1974; Ludwig, Wikler, and Stark 1974) to explain craving, relapse, and loss of control drinking. Their theory postulates that exposure to cues previously associated with either heavy drinking or withdrawal experiences (conditioned stimuli) elicits an anticipatory 'miniwithdrawal' (conditioned response), which is often interpreted as craving by the alcoholic.

Recently, Ludwig (1985) reported that alcoholics on the verge of relapse could almost taste or smell a cold beer or experience the warm glow or light-headed effect of a cocktail as they *imagined* themselves consuming these beverages. This mental imagery induced a powerful urge to drink. In contrast, recovering alcoholics experienced either negative associations to drinking, such as disgust, embarassment, physical discomfort, and nausea, or initial positive associations which became progressively more unpleasant as their train of thought continued.

These observations, as well as Ludwig and Wikler's caveat that the 'miniwithdrawal' is not invariably interpreted by the alcoholic as craving, suggest the role of cognitive modifiers. A conditioned withdrawal response presupposes, furthermore, that the drinker has experienced many prior withdrawals. As suggested by Ludwig, Wikler, and Stark (1974), their 'hard-core, multiadmission, hospitalized' subjects may not be representative of other excessive drinkers. Thus, even if conditioned effects of alcohol and of alcohol withdrawal probably play some role in eliciting the desire to drink in abstinent alcoholics, cognitive mediators and other factors must also be taken into account (see Marlatt 1978). Cognitive processes may also be responsible for some of the success reported with aversive conditioning procedures (Miller and Hester 1980).

The *tension-reduction theory* originated from animal experiments (Conger 1951, 1956). This once very popular theory claims that alcohol consumption mainly serves as a means of reducing tension or stress in its various aversive manifestations, such as fear, anxiety, conflict, and frustration. However, later findings from experiments with both animals and human beings were not able to provide a clear-cut answer to the questions of whether alcohol really does reduce tension and of whether people drink more when they are feeling tense or stressed.

Cappell and Herman (1972), Mello (1972), Cappell (1975), Marlatt (1976), Nathan and Lisman (1976), and Lindman (1980) examined the literature and drew the conclusion that the tension reduction hypothesis is insufficient to explain why alcoholics drink. Cappell and Herman (1972) summarize: 'while the tension reduction hypothesis may be plausible intuitively, it has not been convincingly supported empirically' (p. 59).

Reviewing the literature subsequent to the mid-1970s, Cappell and Greeley (1987) conclude that even if alcohol is a tension-reducing agent, it is a relatively ineffective one, primarily because it has other actions which negate its ability to reduce tension, especially in higher doses. Expectancies might explain why alcohol can reduce tension for one person but not for another (Young, Oei, and Knight 1990).

Stockwell and his co-workers (1984) suggested that therapies directed at alternative ways of managing stress would be indicated only after an analysis of the functional relationship between drinking and anxiety in each patient. To be sure, they found that patients diagnosed as both alcoholic and phobic attributed tension-reducing properties to alcohol and believed that drinking was an effective coping mechanism. But a significant majority also reported that a heavy drinking bout worsened their fears. Similar issues arise in a consideration of the relationship between depression and alcoholism (Schuckit 1986), or between dissatisfaction with life and heavy drinking (Newcomb, Bentler, and Collins 1986), thus supporting the hypothesis that tension and stress is more often an effect than a cause of alcohol abuse (see Section 8.1).

The tension reduction theory and other early attempts to explain alcohol dependence, e.g. the traditional disease model, the symptomatic model, and classical conditioning, generally missed the point that alcohol problems are multivariant by nature. They also tended to overemphasize a single factor in the complex interaction of learning and biological processes. In contrast, the *operant conditioning* approach addresses both antecedent and consequent influences on drinking and provides a framework for their integration.

Peter Miller and Eisler (1975) suggested an operant analysis for both the acquisition and maintenance of alcohol abuse. Within a social-learning framework, alcohol and drug abuse are viewed as socially acquired, learned behaviour patterns maintained by numerous antecedent cues and consequent reinforcers that may be of a psychological, sociological, or physiological nature. Such factors as reduction in anxiety, increased social recognition and peer approval, enhanced ability to exhibit more varied, spontaneous social behaviour, or the avoidance of physiological withdrawal symptoms may maintain substance abuse, they contend.

Broad agreement exists today that almost no behaviour is so simple that it is acquired in accordance with a single learning mechanism. Caddy (1978) gives the following examples of contingencies that reinforce alcohol abuse and dependence:

1. Positive reinforcement associated with the psychopharmacological properties of alcohol (e.g. euphoria and relaxation).

2. Positive reinforcement associated with the social aspects of alcohol use (e.g. acceptance into a drinking group).

3. Negative reinforcement associated with aversive environmental aspects (e.g. relief of boredom or temporary escape from unpleasant living conditions).

4. Negative reinforcement related to aversive physical states induced by alcohol use (e.g. relief from the physical discomfort of the withdrawal state) or by other causes (e.g. relief of chronic or acute pain due to injury or illness).

5. Negative reinforcement related to attempts to alter the drinker's psychological state (e.g. removing anxiety or inducing a temporary change in self-concept).

The incentives to drink are assumed to occur, with varying intensity, in virtually as many combinations and variants as there are individuals. Therefore, no single treatment method is recommended for all excessive drinkers. It is believed that therapy must be preceded by a *behavioural analysis* of which functions drinking serves for which individuals in which contexts (Albrecht 1973; Davis *et al.* 1974; Miller 1976; Sobell, Sobell, and Sheahan 1976; Lovibond 1977; Pattison *et al.* 1977; Sobell and Sobell 1977, 1978; Rönnberg 1979). The operant approach to alcohol abuse has given rise to systematic descriptions and analyses of drinking patterns and what influences them as well as the adoption of individualized and refined evaluation methods.

Eclectic treatment programmes intended to fit each individual have been designed. Excessive drinkers have been found to attribute relapse primarily to frustration and an inability to express anger, an inability to resist social pressure or interpersonal temptation to drink, and intrapersonal negative emotional states (Marlatt 1978). As a consequence, social skills training and assertiveness training have dominated the past decade of behavioural alcoholism treatment research (Ingram and Salzberg 1988).

The teaching of more effective and appropriate interpersonal coping behaviours has been used both as the primary treatment strategy and as one of a number of components in broad-spectrum therapies. Interestingly, social skills training has also been used to help alcoholics perform the recovery steps of AA (Anderson and Gilbert 1989).

9.2   Alcohol expectancies

The importance of cognitive factors for alcohol dependence was long a neglected field of research. However, recent studies indicate that cognitive processes are more important predictors of drinking behaviour than had previously been imagined (see reviews by Goldman, Brown, and Christiansen 1987; Critchlow Leigh 1989). This line of research was originally influenced by anthropological evidence (MacAndrew and Edgerton 1969) showing that alcohol-induced transformations in behaviour vary widely from culture to culture and in the same culture across time periods. Such observations suggested that the effects of alcohol on behaviour are culturally learned rather than the direct result of pharmacological action.

Experimental studies have separated actual alcohol ingestion from the belief that alcohol has been consumed. In one of the earliest of these studies, Marlatt, Demming, and Reid (1973) established a laboratory analogue of Jellinek's (1952) loss-of-control hypothesis. They assigned alcoholics and

Table 9.1 Total amount of beverage (in fluid ounces) consumed by alcoholics and social drinkers, as a function of expected and actual alcohol content

	Alcoholics ($N = 32$)		Social drinkers ($N = 32$)	
	Told tonic	Told alcohol	Told tonic	Told alcohol
Given tonic	10.94	23.87	9.31	14.62
Given alcohol	10.25	22.13	5.94	14.44

social drinkers to a task that involved rating the taste qualities of a number of beverages. The subjects were randomly divided into two groups. One group was led to believe that their drinks would contain vodka and tonic, while the other group was told that their drinks would contain only tonic. In actuality, half of the drinks in each group contained vodka, while the other half contained no alcohol at all. According to Jellinek's hypothesis, alcoholics who received alcohol would show the greatest beverage consumption regardless of what they were told about beverage content.

Table 9.1, however, shows that both alcoholics and social drinkers drank more when they believed that their drinks contained alcohol. Also, alcoholics drank significantly more than social drinkers. But the actual presence or absence of alcohol did not influence the consumption. These and other research findings (see reviews by Maisto and Schefft 1977; Marlatt 1978) indicate that loss of control is partly determined by the drinker's expectations, which serve as a self-fulfilling prophecy.

Other studies have used the same *balanced-placebo design* to evaluate the role of alcohol expectancies in emotional experiences. These studies, largely based on samples of male college students, have demonstrated that regardless of the actual content of the drink (vodka and tonic or only tonic), persons who believe that they have consumed alcohol tend to become less inhibited, more easily sexually aroused, more aggressive, etc. (see reviews by Hull and Bond 1986; Crowe and George 1989).

9.3 A cognitive-behavioural model

The *cognitive-behavioural* or cognitive-social learning approach emphasizes the interaction between personal dispositions and situations as well as the necessity of assessing the contribution of cognitions and emotions to drinking behaviour (Marlatt and Gordon 1985; Abrams and Niaura 1987; Wilson 1988). Marlatt's (1979; Marlatt and Donovan 1981, 1982) model of relapse has been described as the most well articulated statement of this approach. It predicts that the probability of excessive drinking will vary in a particular situation as a function of the following factors:

1. The degree to which the drinker feels controlled by or helpless relative to the influence of another person, a group, or environmental events, e.g. social pressure to conform, peer-modelling, personal evaluation or criticism by others, or being frustrated or angered by others. Situations which threaten the drinker's perception of control are defined as high-risk situations.

2. The availability of an adequate coping response as an alternative to drinking in these high-risk situations. If the person fails to perform an appropriate coping response to resolve the situation, perceived self-efficacy is lowered, which further reduces the perception of control.

3. The availability of alcohol and the constraints upon its use within the particular situation.

4. The person's expectations about the potential effects of alcohol in the stressful situation he has to cope with. These expectations can centre around alcohol's presumed role in directly bringing about reinforcing consequences (e.g. relaxation or sexual arousal) or in enabling behaviours that will be reinforced (e.g. assertiveness).

A test of the cognitive-behavioural approach to excessive drinking has been conducted by Cooper, Russell, and George (1988). Problem and non-problem drinkers were drawn from a general population sample. Path analysis was used to investigate how some variables may influence alcohol use indirectly, through other variables. In this study, drinking as a strategy to cope with emotion emerged as a powerful predictor of abuse, with alcohol expectancies being relatively less important.

A comprehensive cognitive-behavioural relapse prevention model has been developed by Marlatt and his colleagues (Marlatt and Gordon 1980, 1985; Marlatt and George 1984; Brownell, Marlatt, *et al.* 1986). However, most forms of therapy based on learning theory, cognitive psychology, and related disciplines (see review by Ingram and Salzberg 1988) focus on two or more of the stages in the sequence described above.

Such treatment generally begins with a behavioural assessment (Bellak and Hersen 1988), i.e. an identification of high-risk situations, behaviour deficits, and psychological conflict areas (*stage 1*). It then continues with attempts to initiate and maintain behaviour patterns that are alternatives to and incompatible with alcohol abuse (*stage 2*). This may involve everything from a global life-style intervention to the training of specific behaviours that can serve as alternatives to abusive drinking in high-risk situations (see reviews by O'Leary, O'Leary, and Donovan 1976; Van Hasselt, Hersen, and Milliones 1978).

A supplementary treatment strategy (*stage 3*) aims at making alcohol less accessible and applying behavioural contracting. For example, the drinker's social environment can be taught to reward sobriety and to allow alcohol use to be systematically followed by withheld rewards (e.g. Hunt and Azrin 1973; Miller 1975; Azrin 1976). Finally (*stage 4*), methods have been developed that can be used to alter expectations, enhance self-efficacy, and influence other cognitive factors associated with drinking (e.g. Marlatt 1985; Sjöberg and Samsonowitz 1985; Annis and Davis 1988).

9.4   Alcoholism—a learned behaviour?

Alcoholism can cogently be conceptualized as a learned behaviour. The learning models presented to date have not, however, answered the more complex questions raised by the alcohol literature. Alcohol dependence represents a typical interdisciplinary subject of study. Yet the majority of theories are still either medical or behavioural and social. There is a great need for a biopsychosocial theory that can describe and explain the interaction between biological and psychosocial processes during the various phases of the addictive cycle.

Without a holistic perspective, there is a risk that certain research results will be overinterpreted. For example, some authors have, from Marlatt's and his co-workers' (1973) laboratory analogue of the loss-of-control hypothesis (Section 9.2) and similar experiments, drawn the conclusion that excessive drinking is merely a result of culturally-induced beliefs about the effects of alcohol.

Such a conclusion is untenable. The expected consequences of drinking and the pharmacological effects of alcohol are not independent of one another. The fact that an alcoholic drinks a large quantity and feels euphoric when he believes that the drinks of tonic he has been given contain vodka must be interpreted in a longer perspective than that of the individual trial. This will most likely reveal that the individual's expectancies are influenced by previous experiences associated with the pharmacological effects of alcohol.

The evidence from experiments by Stockwell and his co-workers (1982) and Laberg (1986) confirm that both cognitive and pharmacological factors are significant. Severely dependent subjects were reacting more strongly to the pharmacological effects of alcohol than less dependent alcoholics. These findings support a classical conditioning interpretation of loss of control and the perception of intoxication (see also Marlatt and Rohsenow 1980, pp. 191 f.).

What Marlatt and others have shown is that expectancies are of importance for drinking behaviour, not that they are decisive. In her recent review of alcohol expectancy research, Critchlow Leigh (1989) believes that:

expected consequences may play a greater part in influencing a teenager's first drink than in influencing an alcoholic's millionth drink. Whereas the new drinker, with no direct drinking experience, might be swayed by the symbolic power of alcohol, the experienced drinker may drink more from habit or addiction. (pp. 370–1)

The role of expectations on any given occasion is determined by complex and relatively poorly understood interactions of biological, psychological, and social influences. Marlatt and Rohsenow (1980) point out that research concerning the expectancy effect raises more questions than it answers. In order to explore these and other issues raised by the learning model, prospective studies are needed. With only cross-sectional data, no valid inferences can be drawn about the causal relationships hypothesized by the model.

The behavioural analysis of the functions of alcohol use undoubtedly represents an improvement over Jellinek's schematic phase model, according to which alcoholism is a progressive disease with a predictable course. Jellinek's phase model has proved to be oversimplified. The behavioural theories, on the other hand, run the risk of getting lost in specifics and becoming too static, if they fail to take into account the biological processes triggered and accelerated by alcohol consumption. According to Edwards and his colleagues (e.g. Hodgson 1980a), an assessment of the degree of dependence is essential as a complement to the information provided by a behavioural analysis.

It is reasonable to assume that Marlatt's cognitive-behavioural model (Section 9.3) will be capable of predicting the probability of excessive drinking in an individual case only if the severity of dependence is known. At an early stage, social pressure to drink, notions of alcohol as a 'disinhibitor', and testing personal control seem to exert a crucial influence on the amount and frequency of alcohol consumption. Later, excessive drinking may become increasingly associated with relief or avoidance of both physical complications (withdrawal symptoms) and emotional, interpersonal, and social complications of drinking. It then enters a new phase, where psychobiological processes are becoming more dominant and drinking gradually emerges as a generalized coping strategy. As time goes on, the availability of alcohol and the constraints upon its use will probably take on a more important role relative to the other factors enumerated by Marlatt, such as stressful events, skills deficits, and expectancies.

A reliable assessment of the severity of the alcohol dependence—in contrast to the conventional categorization into 'alcoholics' and 'non-alcoholics'— has already proved to be of value for prediction of the outcome of behavioural self-control training (see Chapter 22).

Similarly, Annis and Davis (1988; 1989b) taught alcoholic clients appropriate coping responses in high-risk situations and provided mastery experiences so that their self-efficacy would be enhanced. Clients were randomly assigned to receive this relapse prevention training or more traditional counselling. In analysing the outcome at six month follow-up, Annis and Davis (1989*a*) categorized clients as having either a *generalized profile* of drinking risk situations, i.e. similar drinking across all types of situations, or a *differentiated profile*, i.e. greater drinking risk in some types of situations than in others. Results for clients with generalized profiles showed no differences across the two treatment conditions in typical daily quantity of alcohol consumed; however, clients with differentiated profiles showed a substantially lower typical daily quantity after relapse prevention training than after traditional counselling.

This client–treatment interaction effect accounted for over 30 per cent of the outcome variance on the drinking outcome measure, which is an exceptionally high figure. Thus, Annis and Davis' study supports both the predictive validity of the 'narrowing of the drinking repertoire' criterion of alcohol dependence (see Section 6.2; Edwards and Gross 1976) and the relevance of the latter concept in treatment considerations. Their study suggests that relapse prevention training should be a key component in the treatment of the less dependent drinker.

While it has definite advantages, the learning model also displays a weakness in that the drinker's changing reactivity to alcohol and the personality-disabling consequences of excessive drinking are often not sufficiently recognized. There is also a tendency to ignore the irrationality of human beings. This may cause the therapist to overrate the abilities of his client and encourage unrealistic expectations with regard to treatment results. To his positive appraisal of Marlatt and Gordon's (1985) seminal work on relapse prevention, Edwards (1987) wisely added the following caveat:

Those of us who labour in the clinical field . . . know that Mr Jones just may not turn up at the clinic tomorrow, may not bother with the 'homework' which has been set, may be too drunk to discuss our cunning behavioural analysis. Happily, the next outpatient session is not always so gloomy, but the light of pure reason and rationality, of benign effect following sharply identified cause, is not always there either. (p. 319)

The cognitive and social learning model will have to be supplemented with a psychobiological perspective that includes genetic, pharmacological, and longitudinal considerations. Without such an interdisciplinary approach, no satisfactory explanation is likely to be provided for why a given type of behavioural modification prevents relapse in one individual but not another. As suggested in Chapter 8, the therapist must also take into account the patient's psychiatric problems. The importance of these for the prognosis will be elaborated on in Section 16.3.

10   The social model

Traditionally, models of alcoholism sought explanations 'inside' the individual, in his or her personality or biological constitution. In contrast, proponents of the social model emphasize relations 'between' individuals, in the social context where problem drinking develops and is maintained. According to this view, successful rehabilitation must address the environmental, cultural, social, peer, or family matrix of drinking (Beigel and Ghertner 1977).

This model is often inspired by sociology and theories of prevention. The sociologist Ole-Jørgen Skog (1989), for example, recently suggested that concepts such as 'social integration', 'informal social control', and 'the social network', which have proved so useful in understanding problem drinking at the societal level, may prove quite useful at the individual level as well. Furthermore, they may help us to 'link together the micro-level and macro-level', that is, to combine biopsychological and socio-cultural theories of drinking and drinking problems.

Another sociologist, Robin Room (1989), reported that about one third of a US adult sample had pressured others to cut down their drinking in the previous year. Such informal efforts to control drinking are far more widespread than formal treatment. Indeed, Room contended, it seems that few people enter alcoholism treatment without having been pressured by family or friends about their drinking. Informal pressures may even be a precondition for formal treatment. These observations highlight the importance of considering the interaction of community and treatment responses to alcohol problems.

In this chapter, I will review current trends of research that demonstrate the utility of a comprehensive focus on the problem drinker's environment. First, however, some earlier conceptions of alcoholism as 'merely' a symptom of social disruption should be discussed.

10.1   Symptomatic conceptions

A study of Swedish cause-of-death statistics (SPRI 1983) illustrates the point made in Chapter 8, i.e. that the relationship between alcoholism and its concomitants is generally much more complex than the symptomatic model would have us believe. This study showed large differences in the risks of death between married and single men (unmarried, divorced, widowers). Married men generally had very low death-risk figures, while singles ran much greater risks. This applied to most causes of death, although the difference was especially great for alcohol-related disorders. A divorced man aged 45–49 years, for instance, ran a ten times greater risk of dying of cirrhosis of the liver than a married man of the same age.

At first glance, these findings might seem to support the familiar notion that loneliness and a lack of family obligations increases the risk of alcohol-related disorders and death. A closer look, however, reveals that divorce was probably much more often an effect than a cause of alcohol abuse. At the same time, it is reasonable to assume that even if alcohol abuse preceded the divorce, drinking problems would tend to increase after the break-up of the family. The assumption of such a reciprocal relationship is confirmed

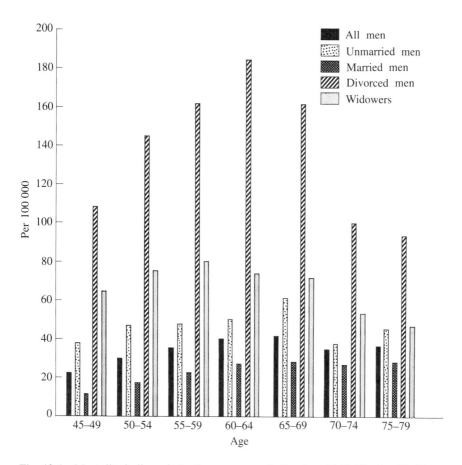

Fig. 10.1 Mortality in liver cirrhosis among men in Sweden, 1969–78, classified by marital status and age.

by the data on mortality in liver cirrhosis for men in various age groups categorized according to their marital status during the period 1969–1978. Figure 10.1 shows that widowers had a higher mortality than unmarried men, irrespective of age. On the other hand, they had a much lower mortality than divorced men across all age groups.

To complicate the matter even further, Lindberg and Ågren (1988) reported that divorced female alcoholics had a lower mortality than other females, i.e. the converse of the relationship described for men. This finding is attributed to the fact that alcoholic females are often married to excessive drinkers, so divorce may also entail breaking off a destructive pattern of drinking.

Like divorce, unemployment is a common concomitant of drinking problems. In a review of the Scandinavian literature, however, Jyrkämä (1980) concluded that unemployment seldom leads to heavy drinking. On the contrary, statistics from Sweden in the thirties and Finland in the seventies showed declining sales of alcoholic beverages at times of high unemployment. A common explanation is that reduced incomes make alcoholic beverages more difficult to afford. In fact, the greatest increase in alcohol consumption and abuse in Sweden took place in the prosperous sixties, which were characterized by full employment, real wage increases, and social reforms.

On the other hand, studies quoted by Jyrkämä (1980) indicated that persons who were already serious problem drinkers changed for the worse after losing their jobs. A similar 'polarisation of drinking patterns' has been reported by others (see review by Crawford, Plant et al. 1987). However, few studies have employed the prospective, longitudinal design that would permit causal statements about the effects of job loss upon drinking behaviour.

In a seminal study, Kendell, de Roumanie, and Ritson (1983) prospectively analysed alcohol consumption in Scotland during a period of unemployment which coincided with an increase in excise duty on alcoholic beverages. They found that physically dependent drinkers reduced their alcohol consumption at least as much as light and moderate drinkers.

A prospective study by Iversen and Klausen (1986) investigated alcohol consumption among laid-off workers before and after closure of a Danish shipyard. The main finding was that, irrespective of age, the unemployed workers reduced their alcohol consumption more than the re-employed workers. Iversen and Klausen believed that two mechanisms may have been operative: loss of income and the dissolution of an occupational subculture involving drinking. Thus, the consequences of unemployment for the heavy drinker are complex. They depend on, for example, his or her disposable income (including social security benefits), the price of alcoholic beverages, and occupational drinking practices.

The role of distinctive drinking practices was emphasized by Cosper (1979) in an incisive critique of the literature on occupational differences in drinking. Cosper noted that the assumption that job stresses lead to alcoholism has become part of popular culture. Stress theories view drinking as symptomatic of tensions and frustrations of various kinds. However, these theories ignore the fact that in certain occupational subcultures, such as those of businessmen and miners, heavy drinking may be a valued activity that indicates conformity rather than deviance or pathology.

According to one popular notion, alcoholism predominantly afflicts people who lead boring and monotonous lives or have dull and unpleasant jobs. The primary difficulty with this and other explanations focusing on negative life-events (see critical review by O'Doherty and Davies 1987) is that they are generally invoked after the fact. When a high rate of drinking problems is observed in a particular social group, it is tempting to point to stresses to which the group is subject. However, problem drinkers in the general population seldom attribute increased drinking to greater tensions and other problems of living. In a follow-up study by Cahalan (1970), these drinkers instead emphasized financial ability, peer pressures, and having more opportunities or time for drinking.

It may also be argued that drinking problems are most common among people with independent and interesting jobs such as writers, journalists, actors, musicians, artists, doctors, diplomats, restaurant personnel, and seamen (see reviews by Murray 1975; Plant 1977, 1979a; Whitehead and Simpkins 1983). What all of these high-risk professions have in common is that their practitioners are able to drink on the job without being noticed by a supervisor, or that their working hours are free and irregular.

Perhaps the highest rate of alcoholism reported for any defined group is that among Americans who have won the Nobel Prize for literature. Of the seven American prize-winners, five (Sinclair Lewis, Eugene O'Neill, William Faulkner, Ernest Hemingway, and John Steinbeck) were alcoholics according to standard diagnostic criteria (Goodwin 1988). Rather than attributing this fact to 'psychological aloneness', 'tortured sensitivity', and the like, Room (1984) suggested some plausible social explanations. He noted that more than half of the alcoholic American writers in the first half of this century spent time in Paris in the 1920s. This literary generation, he contended, may have been pushed into heavy drinking by several concurrent factors, such as inexpensive alcoholic beverages, a cosmopolitan style of drinking ('cocktails before meals like Americans, wines and brandies like Frenchmen, beer like Germans, and whiskey-and-soda like the English'), a French cultural avant-garde for whom drunkenness symbolized defiance of bourgeois morality, and a community of expatriate writers congregating in the cafés of Montparnasse ('the school of the Rotonde').

In a comprehensive review of the literature, Whitehead and Simpkins (1983) drew the following conclusion concerning occupational factors in alcoholism:

the structural characteristics of the occupations that are most associated with high rates of heavy drinking and alcoholism are characteristics that have to do directly with drinking, for example, social pressure to drink heavily, the opportunity to obtain alcoholic beverages inexpensively, and peer sanction of drinking on the job. This finding is in somewhat marked contrast to a good deal of the literature on alcoholism in industry, where the typical suggestion is that drinking is simply a symptom of the complex set of personal and environmental circumstances in which the individual finds himself or herself and that the features of the person's occupation that contribute to this drinking are fairly esoteric (e.g. nebulous production goals) or vague (e.g. stress). (pp. 485–6)

The question then arises: Do certain occupations encourage heavy drinking, or do they simply attract a high proportion of people who were already heavy drinkers? Plant (1979b) suggested that in the alcohol industry at least, both tendencies are important. Furthermore, alcohol producers who left the drink trade for a job in a 'drier' occupational setting reduced their alcohol consumption. Apparently, a selection effect was involved here as well. Some persons stated that they left because they did not like to drink heavily. Social pressures in the new occupational setting may also have been operative in motivating the leavers to moderate their drinking.

By and large, it is very difficult to find any social disadvantages that increase the risk of alcoholism. In a review of a large number of surveys, Park (1983) found no consistent relationship between the indexes of problem drinking and social class. In fact, the observed prevalence of alcoholism in different social strata varied depending on how the problem was defined. If alcoholism was defined in terms of alcohol-related social disorders (e.g. trouble with spouse, friends, job, and police), the problem seemed to be greatest in lower social strata. But if alcoholism was defined as psychological dependence (e.g. inability to abstain), the problem appeared to be greatest in the upper classes.

However, none of the surveys reviewed by Park (1983) had a sufficient sample size to make possible a detailed breakdown in terms of specific drinking patterns and specific social subgroups. In this respect, Knupfer (1989) recently made a unique contribution by analyzing ten US surveys combined. Her study demonstrated that it is necessary to take several factors into account simultaneously to get a correct picture of the prevalence of various drinking patterns. Figures on social class alone without age and sex, for example, will give invalid results.

If age and sex were not taken into account, the proportion of persons who were drunk at least once a week seemed to change very little across different socio-economic status groups. This does not, however, mean that their proportion is apt to be the same no matter what the cultural influences. Among males aged 18–34 the proportion of frequent drunks went steadily up as socio-economic status went down, from 13 to 37 per cent. Among young females, the change was from 5 to 13 per cent. Among older age groups these differences disappeared.

By contrast, the proportion of moderate-to-heavy drinkers went down from 60 per cent for males in the highest socio-economic group to 28 per cent in the bottom group. For females the change was from 50 per cent to 15 per cent. Knupfer (1989) interpreted these differences in terms of distinctive social contexts and cultural definitions of drinking. In the upper classes such customs as serving wine with dinner, giving cocktail parties, etc. are more common, she said. In the lower classes, especially in the younger age groups, the idea that if one drinks at all, the goal must be to get drunk is probably more prevalent. The large and consistent differences between the sexes are attributed to traditional gender roles.

At the general societal level the risk of alcoholism is affected mainly by social norms regarding drinking and by legal and economic constraints on access to alcohol (Bruun *et al.* 1975; Mäkelä *et al.* 1981; Colón, Cutter, and Jones 1982; Moskowitz 1989). Rural regions in Sweden with a strong temperance tradition have a lower mortality in alcohol-related diseases than other regions (SPRI 1983). Similarly, the agricultural American Southeast, where fundamentalist and proscriptive attitudes are prevalent (e.g. Alabama, Georgia, Mississippi), has a lower alcohol-related mortality than other parts of the country (Colón *et al.* 1982).

In summary, there is little evidence to support the common assumption of a causal and direct association between divorce, unemployment, occupational stresses, or other social problems and heavy drinking. Alcohol abuse and alcoholism seem instead to constitute a relatively independent social problem, which is heavily influenced by (a) alcohol *availability*, and (b) the *cultural values*, *attitudes* and *mores* that regulate the use of alcohol.

According to the social model, the socio-cultural setting of drinking can be modified by direct interventions both at the individual and the societal level. The assumption that nothing can be done until 'underlying' stresses and strains have been removed is misleading. However, even though the symptomatic conception must be rejected, the combination of heavy drinking and severe social problems can exacerbate the drinker's situation and make recovery more difficult. In such cases, of course, both sets of problems have to be focused on.

10.2 Patterns of recovery

Several convergent lines of research illustrate the potential importance of environmental factors for alcoholism treatment (see reviews by Ogborne, Sobell, and Sobell 1985; Vuchinich and Tucker 1988). Laboratory studies, for example, have demonstrated the significance of role modelling and environmental contingencies associated with drinking. Epidemiological studies have emphasized the role of economic and legal constraints on access to alcohol as well as alcohol-related values, attitudes, and mores.

Other evidence that suggests the importance of the natural environment derives from a growing body of studies showing that many alcohol abusers and alcoholics recover without the aid of any formal treatment. A general population study by Saunders and Kershaw (1979) suggested that remission from problem drinking and alcoholism is often precipitated by changes in life circumstances, such as marriage or a new job, which may exert effective controls on the use of alcohol. Tuchfeld (1981) found that few, if any, alcoholics recovered 'spontaneously', that is, without external influences such as informal social controls and non-alcohol-related leisure activities.

In a retrospective study of skid row inebriates, Giesbrecht (1983) reported that affiliation with abstainers and moderate drinkers via AA groups or religious organizations was the best predictor of stable abstinence. Similarly, Stall (1983) found that the support of family and non-drinking friends or a religious group was essential for remission and maintenance of sobriety. Finally, in a long-term clinical follow-up, Nordström and Berglund (1986) noted that 70 per cent of the recovered alcoholics attributed their improvement mainly to the negative social consequences of abuse, changes in social circumstances, and social pressure to stop drinking.

Ludwig (1985), however, avoided listing specific life events or external circumstances. He concluded that external life changes were less important as motivators for abstinence than the alcoholics' reactions to them. A given event can mean different things to different individuals or different things to the same individual at different times. Since most respondents had experienced profound personal humiliation, shame, despair, or meaningful loss prior to the radical change, Ludwig considered 'hitting bottom' as essential in the process of recovery.

Vaillant (1980b, 1983b) and Edwards et al. (1987) have taken our understanding of attributions of change a step further still. Instead of merely listing discrete factors contributing to remission, and attributing these to either external or internal conditions, they analysed separate *patterns of recovery* which overcome the external/internal dichotomy.

Edwards et al. (1987) used a 70-item Attributions Inventory in the follow-up of 66 married male alcoholics one decade after their admission to a clinical trial. A factor analysis revealed two factors which were labelled, respectively, *active* and *responsive* attribution of good drinking outcomes. Active attribution implied some sort of positive personal action, commitment, or working for a change, such as avoidance of wet environments, AA participation, experience of personal responsibility, and taking an interest in other people. This style of attribution was associated with *high* alcohol dependence. Responsive attribution reflected a reaction to actual or threatened consequences of drinking. This style of attribution of good outcomes was associated with *low* alcohol dependence.

Vaillant (1980b, 1983b) interviewed those 110 out of 456 Boston men who at some time during the course of 35 years had developed drinking problems. Of these 110 men, 49 had achieved at least a year of abstinence and 22 men had been able to return to social drinking. Eighty-two per cent of those who became abstinent were Gamma (loss-of-control) alcoholics as against only 12 per cent of those who returned to social drinking. Interviewers were instructed to systematically look for contingencies which might be important in altering drinking habits.

For those problem drinkers who returned to social drinking, effective confrontation and will-power often seemed to be treatment enough. For those Gamma alcoholics who became abstinent, the experience of having something to lose if they continued drinking was of little use in itself. Much more important was either AA or religious involvement or some other substitute for alcohol offering new sources of self-esteem and new people to care about. These findings are consistent with those of Edwards and his co-workers (1987). They corroborate the latter's hypothesis that 'different programmes and different coping, cognitive and reality strategies will on the whole be required for less as opposed to more dependent subjects' (p. 544).

The patterns of recovery described by Vaillant (1983b) and Edwards et al. (1987) provide some clues as to what is called for in helping drinkers at various stages of alcohol dependence. Since the highly dependent drinker differs from the less dependent one mainly in terms of a more impaired control over his drinking, a digression on the concept of control is warranted. Interestingly, this concept is especially apt to reconcile external and internal attributions of recovery from alcoholism.

Beauchamp (1981), a sociologist, has challenged the idea that control over alcohol is solely or principally a personal achievement. According to Beauchamp, this idea ignores the contexts that make the term 'control' meaningful. Before we can claim that most drinkers have some personal ability to control their drinking, we would need evidence that if they were exposed to a wet environment they would still be able to avoid drinking problems. The empirical relationship between per capita consumption and heavy drinking (Bruun et al. 1975; Mäkelä et al. 1981) and the conclusions arrived at in Section 10.1 do not support such an assumption.

The absence of problems in the population at large may therefore simply be due to widespread and enduring social controls over the use of alcohol. The ability of less dependent drinkers to capitalize on 'actual or threatened consequences of drinking' (Edwards et al.) or 'effective confrontation' and 'will-power' (Vaillant) may reflect the involvement of these drinkers' social environment in efforts to constrain and channel their choices about alcohol. Like control, 'will-power' is largely a social phenomenon.

In an incisive analysis of the therapeutic power of AA, Khantzian and Mack (1989; Mack 1981) have approached the concept of control from the standpoint of psychodynamic theory. 'Alcoholics Anonymous is effective', they claim, 'because it appreciates that the underpinnings of self are connected with social structures and institutions' (p. 76). With excessive and prolonged drinking the alcoholic develops an injured sense of self resulting in alternating attitudes of self-serving grandiosity and wallowing self-pity. AA confronts the alcoholic's conviction that he can solve life problems alone or, worse still, that they are not solvable at all. It helps him to see that the self never functions as a solitary entity:

By placing the alcoholics' inability to control their alcohol as the central focus, AA creates a basis to address a fundamentally important reality, namely, that as human beings we do not and cannot survive and grow on our own and that governance of our lives as well as our behaviors is intimately linked and involved with other people. Once alcoholics 'surrender' to the human reality of interdependence through AA and accept their 'powerlessness' to control their alcohol alone, other beneficial aspects of AA begin to provide a basis to address, repair, and/or strengthen other vulnerabilities involving deficits and dysfunctions around one's feeling life and behaviors. (Khantzian and Mack 1989, p. 86)

Thus, the highly dependent drinkers' attribution of recovery to 'fresh self-esteem', 'taking an interest in other people', and the like may indicate a subjective reappraisal of the interdependence of self and others. This psychological shift, which has been described by other writers as well (e.g. Tiebout 1961; Bateson 1971; Brown 1985; Flores 1988), is probably facilitated by the availability of a 'social cocoon' (Emrick 1989) such as AA, a religious group, or a cohesive, non-drinking primary group.

10.3   Environmental resources

Notwithstanding the heuristic value of retrospective attributions, the difficulty of distinguishing between these and causality should be kept in mind. Still another line of evidence linking environmental factors to treatment outcomes focuses on patients' posttreatment environmental resources. The best known research in this area has been conducted by Moos and his colleagues (see reviews by Billings and Moos 1983; Moos, Finney, and Cronkite 1990).

Moos *et al.* (1990) emphasize the 'need for a fundamental shift' in thinking about alcoholism treatment programmes and their effects. They advocate a more long-term phase of treatment following the alcoholic's return to the community. Today, treatment does not substantially influence the social context and coping responses that are closely linked to the process of remission and relapse. This conclusion is based on extensive six-month, two-year, and ten-year follow-ups of a large clinical sample.

Moos and his colleagues systematically evaluated the relationships between environmental resources and treatment outcomes for a variety of populations and treatments. Their studies showed that patients with stable family or work environments prior to treatment or follow-up had a significantly better drinking and psychosocial outcome than those patients who lacked such resources. This result was confirmed in a clinical trial by Ward, Bendel, and Lange (1982).

Furthermore, outcome was significantly related to the quality of the environmental resources. Bromet and Moos (1977) found that among married patients, a more positive family milieu (higher cohesion, lower conflict) was associated with a better than expected treatment outcome. Among working patients, a more positively perceived work environment (higher level of involvement, higher peer cohesion) was associated with better than expected posttreatment performance, but *only* among patients lacking marital support. These results confirm the therapeutic importance of the family milieu. They also suggest that, if cohesion is high, peers in the work environment can have a similar influence on the drinking career of the *unmarried* alcoholic.

Bromet and Moos (1977) invoke the buffer hypothesis to explain these results. They assume that families and work environments moderate the impact of adverse life-events. In a review of the literature on this hypothesis, Thoits (1982) suggests a reciprocal relationship between psychological health, social support, and undesirable life-events. Harmonious individuals may possess strong support systems and be able to ward off undesirable events, while those who are disturbed may have lost or have little social support and may generate, or fail to prevent, undesirable events. Among other effects of support (see Stewart 1989), reinforcement of sobriety and social control of drinking should be emphasized (Room 1989).

The environmental resources available to an alcoholic patient may also include 'community support networks' (Moos, Cronkite, and Finney 1982), ranging from friends and neighbours to religious organizations and mutual self-help groups. Vaillant (1983b, 1984) has shown that community settings may be particularly helpful for the socially unstable alcoholic, who cannot draw on family and work resources. When a sample of 100 male alcoholic patients were followed for eight years, Vaillant found 29 men who had stayed abstinent in the community for at least three years. Half of these remitted alcoholics had attended 300 or more AA meetings. This was true of only one of the 37 men who continued to abuse alcohol.

Of course, the question presents itself whether there is a causal association between frequent AA attendance and remission from alcoholism. Maybe AA attendance is merely a manifestation of good social adjustment prior to treatment or a result of sobriety. Vaillant examined the significance of premorbid factors known to affect prognosis. He found that whereas social stability predicted stable remission, social *instability* predicted heavy use of AA. Thus, socially stable alcoholics tended to become abstinent without AA. But if socially unstable alcoholics were to recover, AA attendance seemed to be an important condition.

The conjecture that drinkers who choose to attend AA regularly tend to have a more problematic life style than nonattenders was corroborated by McLatchie and Lomp (1988a). To be sure, non-experimental data cannot prove a causal relationship between frequent AA attendance and remission, but Vaillant's findings are far more convincing than if a prospective design had not been employed.

His result contradicts the rather gloomy view of the effectiveness of AA which was taken by prior reviewers of alcoholism treatment (Baekeland *et al.* 1975; Orford and Edwards 1977; Miller and Hester 1980). Vaillant believes that the discrepancy derives from the difference between a short-term and a long-term view. Occasional visits to AA meetings may be ineffectual, whereas regular AA attendance is associated with maintenance of abstinence. This conclusion is consistent with that of Pettinati *et al.* (1982*a*) in a meticulously planned four-year follow-up of a clinical sample and with Edwards and his colleagues' (1987) observation at a ten-year follow-up that highly dependent patients with 'good outcome' very often attributed this to high AA attendance. Similarly, in a recent ten-year follow-up, Cross *et al.* (1990) found that involvement in AA was the only statistically significant predictor of sobriety among independent variables including age, sex, history of drug involvement, history of social problems, and the physician's prognosis.

The studies by Bromet and Moos (1977) and Vaillant (1983*b*) both emphasize the importance of long-term social support for remission from alcoholism. They also suggest that different environmental resources may be available to different alcoholics. Of these resources, the family seems to have the greatest influence. For unmarried alcoholics the work environment may serve an equivalent purpose. For alcoholics without stable family or work environments, a community network such as Alcoholics Anonymous or a religious group (Galanter 1981, 1982, 1983) may serve as an important provider of social support.

10.4   A social treatment approach

From a behavioural standpoint AA can be construed as a self-help group which undertakes to replace the alcoholic's usual alcohol-laden milieu with an alcohol-free environment that provides peer reinforcement for abstinence and peer punishment for continued drinking (Nathan and Lansky 1978*b*). Through AA, alcoholics can find warm, supportive, and accepting social contacts whose continued availability is contingent only on earnest efforts to remain abstinent. In addition, the alcoholic's family can learn through Al-Anon and Alateen to deal more effectively with maladaptive drinking.

Alcoholics Anonymous prevents feelings of indebtedness due to insufficient opportunities to reciprocate help and reassurance. A review by Gottlieb (1983) suggests that reciprocity should play an important role in the design of programmes that attempt to enlarge the fund of social support to which people have access.

AA's limited but nonetheless real success has prompted researchers to explore social treatment approaches drawing on the environmental resources available to the alcoholic. In the most successful of these efforts, Nathan Azrin and colleagues (Hunt and Azrin 1973; Miller 1975; Azrin 1976; Azrin *et al.* 1982; Mallams *et al.* 1982; Sisson and Azrin 1986) developed a community-based treatment with the aim of managing the reinforcement contingencies operating on the alcoholic in his or her natural environment.

Initially, this *community reinforcement approach* was studied on two occasions (Hunt and Azrin 1973; Azrin 1976) with altogether 34 male patients, who had suffered withdrawal symptoms and had an extensive record of alcoholism. Subjects were selected to the treatment being studied or the comparison condition by means of a matched-groups experimental design. The comparison groups received standard hospital milieu therapy with counselling on the hazards of continued drinking and information about AA.

The treatment groups received community-reinforcement counselling along with the standard hospital treatment. On the first occasion (Hunt and Azrin 1973), an experienced behavioural clinician helped each patient find employment, improve family and marital relations, enhance social skills, and engage in non-alcohol related social activities. On the second occasion (Azrin 1976), group counselling and peer-advisor procedures reduced counselling time from 50 hours to 30 hours per patient. In addition, supervised use of Antabuse was introduced to inhibit impulsive drinking.

The general approach was to rearrange the alcoholic's social environment in such a way that other reinforcing activities competed with drinking behaviour. In order to be effective, reinforcers had to be valued, regularly occurring, and varied in nature. Furthermore, the newly developed 'natural' reinforcers (e.g. a good job, the wife's sustained attention, access to a social club) were contingent on continued sobriety. Postponement of reinforcers as a result of alcohol intake was immediate. Moreover, since time-out from reinforcement was directly related to his own behaviour, it was possible for the alcoholic to predict and influence events.

On both occasions described above, treatment groups and comparison groups were followed up at six months after discharge from the hospital. On the second occasion, the treatment group was re-interviewed after two years.

At the six-month follow-up, the community-reinforcement groups had spent significantly less time drinking, unemployed, away from home, or institutionalized than the groups receiving only standard hospital treatment. The results of the two-year follow-up were even more encouraging. Alcoholics in the community-reinforcement group continued to abstain from drinking at least 90 per cent of the time. Alcoholics in the matched comparison group, on the other hand, drank during at least 50 per cent of the three months, on average, they spent outside an institution during the first six months after discharge. Considering this poor prognosis, we can reasonably assume that the stable improvement of the community-reinforcement subjects was a result of the special treatment they had been given.

Subjects in treatment groups often reported at follow-up that they were now more satisfied with their life. Often postponement of reinforcers did not occur since drinking never occurred. However, the patients all stated that time-out would occur if they did take a drink and, according to Hunt and Azrin (1973), 'this knowledge of the consequence seemed to be the deterrent' (p. 101).

Later Azrin *et al.* (1982) randomly assigned 43 outpatient alcoholics to one of the three treatment conditions: traditional Antabuse treatment, supervised Antabuse treatment, and supervised Antabuse combined with the community reinforcement approach. Counselling time was reduced to five or six hours per patient. During the sixth month of follow-up, the clients receiving traditional treatment were no longer taking Antabuse as prescribed, and were drinking about half of the days. Clients in the supervised Antabuse programme had been actively encouraged to view the person observing their Antabuse ingestion (spouse, roommate, employer, friend) as a helper rather than a 'watchdog'. These clients were taking Antabuse about two-thirds of the days, and drank about one-fourth of the month. Finally, the clients receiving supervised Antabuse combined with the community reinforcement approach were taking Antabuse about 80 per cent of the days, and drank less than one day per month.

This ranking in order of effectiveness may seem obvious enough. However, a closer inspection of the data revealed a significant interaction between the clients' marital status, their treatment condition, and their drinking at the sixth month (Table 10.1). Among married clients, supervised Antabuse was sufficient to produce nearly complete abstinence. These clients usually obtained jobs and re-established satisfying marital and social relationships with no assistance from the counsellor. Among single clients, on the other hand, the supervised Antabuse programme had little effect alone, whereas the addition of community reinforcement produced nearly complete abstinence. This observation confirms the importance of a job or a community network for the recovery of the unmarried alcoholic.

Table 10.1 Outcomes of traditional Antabuse, supervised Antabuse, and supervised Antabuse combined with Azrin's community reinforcement approach (CRA), in relation to marital status

	Abstinent days in per cent	
	Singles	Couples
Traditional Antabuse	23	58
Supervised Antabuse	27	100
Supervised Antabuse combined with CRA	94	100

In still another controlled trial, Sisson and Azrin (1986) counselled family members of alcoholic persons in the use of reinforcement procedures to reduce drinking and to motivate the drinker to seek treatment. The reinforcement training resulted in a 50 per cent reduction of drinking in the alcoholic before he was counselled directly. Once the alcoholic entered counselling, drinking decreased further to an average of less than one day per month. None of the clients in the comparison group changed their drinking pattern appreciably. Hence, this study replicated the effectiveness of the community reinforcement approach.

However, preliminary results of an outpatient study by Hester, Miller, and their co-workers (1990) in a different population and geographic location did not replicate Azrin's findings. Neither was the community reinforcement approach more effective than traditional disease-oriented treatment at the six-month follow-up, nor did marital status differentially predict response to treatment modes. However, since it is unclear whether the community reinforcers were made contingent on continued sobriety, the validity of these findings is difficult to judge.

Azrin's (1978) research strategy was, firstly, to develop an effective treatment, and secondly, to analyse the relative contributions of different therapeutic components. To be sure, further replications are needed. In addition to the study by Hester, Miller, *et al.* (1990), a major replication by Longabaugh (personal communication, Sept, 1990), Brown University, is under way. Small sample sizes, short follow-up intervals, inadequate data on severity of dependence, experiences drawn from only a few treatment settings, etc., limit the generalisability of Azrin's results. On the whole, however, the community reinforcement approach is promising (see Chapter 3). Yet, except for its supervised Antabuse ingredient (cf. Brewer 1987; ACP 1989; Heather 1989*b*; Wright and Moore 1990), it has been little known and seldom used.

Azrin's success indicates that treatment programmes should involve, more than hitherto, persons in the alcoholic's natural social environment, who remain in a position to influence his or her behaviour even after termination of treatment. It further suggests that therapy should directly address the alcoholic's inability to control his drinking alone, i.e. it should support him in the governance of the self (cf. Mack 1981; Khantzian and Mack 1989; Section 10.2 above).

10.5 Alcoholism—a social career?

Although the conception of alcoholism as 'merely' a symptom of social disruption is outdated, there is emerging evidence for a social model emphasizing (a) the availability of alcohol and the constraints upon its use, and (b) the cultural values, attitudes and mores that regulate the use of alcohol. This model is readily compatible with, and easily integrated into, other models which have been presented above, such as an ecological disease model, a social-learning framework, and recent psychodynamic formulations.

However, the concept of heavy drinking as a social career, or an outcome of aberrant learning processes, must be supplemented by a perspective which draws attention to the drinker's changing reactivity to alcohol and the disabling consequences to personality resulting from excessive drinking (Section 6.2). Over time, excessive drinking is likely to become less mouldable and more independent of other people's reactions. It tends to be robbed of some, but not all, of that normal 'plasticity' (Edwards 1974) which we expect of social behaviour.

Studies by Vaillant (1983b) and Edwards and his co-workers (1987) support this view. Informal efforts to control drinking may effectively influence the behaviour of the less dependent drinker. The rehabilitation and healing of the highly dependent drinker, however, seems to require a more fundamental psychological shift including a reappraisal of the interdependence of self and others. Furthermore, specific skills, such as those prescribed by Sisson and Azrin (1986) or Al-Anon (a self-help organization for spouses of alcoholics), may be useful in modifying the behaviour of the highly dependent drinker, who is less responsive to the kinds of control that are effective in influencing other people and other behaviours than habitual drinking.

Personal or psychological variables may also moderate the impact of the social environment. Longabaugh and Beattie (1985) have developed a preliminary but comprehensive prognostic model for what kinds of patients with what kinds of social environments will differentially respond to which kinds of treatment intervention. One of their hypotheses is that the greater a person's *social investment*, the greater force the social environment will have upon the person's alcoholism as well as on his or her psychological health. Another hypothesis is that persons with low social investment will react differently from persons with high social investment to individually versus relationally focused treatment. Both of these hypotheses were confirmed by Longabaugh and his co-workers (in press). However, a large dropout rate (55 per cent), a questionable directionality of the relationships obtained, a less effective relationally focused treatment, and other factors preclude more specific generalizations.

The research presented above further indicates that the social environment is a highly complex concept. Different environmental resources—such as a stable family, a cohesive work environment, or a community support network—may be available to different alcoholics. Moreover, the ability of all these agents to support sobriety is strengthened or undermined by the drinking level of the population as a whole.

Studies at both the societal level (Skog 1980, 1985) and the individual level (Caudill and Marlatt 1975; Reid 1978; Collins and Marlatt 1981) have suggested that the drinking habits of each individual to a large extent are determined by the drinking habits of others. Individuals with a family history of problem drinking seem to rely even more than other people on the environment to determine appropriate drinking behaviour (Chipperfield and Vogel-Sprott 1988). In their study on the relationship between the mean consumption level in a population and the prevalence of heavy drinkers, Bruun and his colleagues (1975) reminded us of the fact that:

a person with latent tendencies towards heavy alcohol use is less likely to have his drinking fostered in a low-consumption culture, since the majority of his friends will be moderate consumers whose behaviour will counteract such tendencies. By contrast, in a high-consumption culture where drinking is integrated into daily life, social control of the individual's level of drinking, if exercised at all, will not be nearly so effective, and much greater scope will be given the potential heavy drinker to manifest this behaviour. (p. 36)

Indeed, so long as control policies do not tighten up the legal or economic constraints on access to alcohol, and as long as the social norms regarding drinking are maintained, no major decrease in the prevalence of alcoholism is to be expected—no matter how many millions are invested in treatment!

11 A biopsychosocial perspective

In 1977, Pattison, Sobell, and Sobell observed that research on alcoholism treatment was in the midst of a 'paradigmatic' change. It was becoming increasingly difficult to fit the growing body of data into traditional models and concepts. Most researchers were beginning to adopt a multivariant approach according to which alcohol dependence is maintained by a complex interaction of biological, psychological, and social antecedents and consequences. This conception of alcoholism raised the question: What alcohol syndromes at which stage of their development and in what kinds of patients respond under what conditions in what short- and long-range ways to what measures by whom? (Pattison 1966, 1979).

So far, however, no alternative theoretical model has been able to gain general acceptance on the basis not only of its empirical underpinning, but also of its logic, persuasiveness, elegance, and utility. Furthermore, the introduction of new treatment approaches and preventive strategies is not keeping up with the advances in scientific knowledge (Pattison 1977; Miller 1988).

Here I will examine two theoretical models that look upon alcohol dependence in a biopsychosocial perspective. The first model, elaborated by Benjamin Kissin (1977c) and others, combines an individual and a socio-cultural focus. The second model, which synthesizes viewpoints by Mansell Pattison *et al.* (1977), Griffith Edwards (1977), and others, emphasizes the multivariant and dynamic nature of alcohol problems.

11.1 The biopsychosocial equation

Kissin (1977c) attempted to reconcile conflicting views regarding the role of psychological and socio-cultural forces in the development of alcoholism. He introduced a general principle, called 'the psychosocial equation', which runs as follows: 'the general level of psychopathology in a given alcoholic population increases inversely to the prevalence of alcoholism in that subculture' (p. 16).

For example, Kissin pointed out, there are very few Jewish alcoholics. The Jewish tradition (see Glad 1947; Snyder 1958, 1962) prescribes the ceremonial use of alcohol but strongly condemns becoming intoxicated. A study of the Jewish minority in the United States (Glassner and Berg 1980) shows that social controls of drinking behaviour have been sustained despite cultural assimilation and secularization.

The few Jewish alcoholics that do exist, however, appear to show more psychopathology than, for example, American alcoholics of Irish descent

(Schmidt and Popham 1976). This does not rule out the possibility that Irish alcoholics may have severe psychopathology. However, according to Kissin (1977c), the percentage of individuals with psychopathology not produced by alcoholism is relatively small among alcoholic men of Irish and Scandinavian descent. The same, he adds, is true for other subcultures with a high prevalence of alcoholism, such as advertising executives, bartenders, and ghetto residents.

Similar tendencies were observed almost thirty years ago by Jellinek (1960, 1962) in a comparison between drinking patterns in different countries. According to Jellinek, the majority of French alcoholics exhibited no conspicuous signs of psychological vulnerability. In the United States, Sweden, Denmark, Holland, and England during the 1950s, by contrast, the majority of alcoholics were said to exhibit psychological deviations. How can this predominance of low vulnerability on the one side and high vulnerability on the other side be explained, Jellinek asked.

He noticed that alcohol researchers in Anglo-Saxon countries during the fifties often regarded alcoholism as a symptom of an underlying psychiatric problem—a point of view that was opposed by most French students of alcoholism. The latter attributed alcoholism entirely to 'habit', social attitudes, and economic factors. Since in France approximately one-third of the electorate were partly or entirely dependent upon the production, processing, and distribution of alcoholic beverages (mainly wine), it is small wonder that French psychiatrists regarded industrial and trade interests as the decisive factors in the genesis of alcoholism. Jellinek (1960) wrote:

Nothing can provoke greater dissent on the part of French physicians and others interested in alcoholism than the contention that pre-alcoholic maladjustments lead to the heavy use of alcoholic beverages. Suggestions of pre-alcoholic neurotic character or other marked psychological deviations (let alone the terms psychopathy with its many different meanings) meet with strong rejection. (p. 27)

Jellinek thought that the French antagonism to the Anglo-Saxon ideas was to some extent justified, given the high overall consumption of alcohol in wine-growing countries. But at the same time he felt that the symptomatic concept had a certain validity in the United States, England, and other countries that had relatively low alcohol consumption in the fifties. According to Jellinek's calculations, a good one-third of the adult population of Anglo-Saxon countries rejected the use of alcohol in any quantity, and the remaining two-thirds disapproved of heavy drinking.

Jellinek's attempt at a theoretical synthesis could be called the *biopsychosocial equation*. He regards the risk of alcoholism as being a function of the society's degree of acceptance of high alcohol consumption and the individual's psychological or biological vulnerability (cf. Skog 1989). In societies that do not readily accept a high daily consumption of alcohol, the individuals at risk are primarily those who, on account of psychological vulnerability, are tempted to defy social standards. But in societies where a majority of the population accepts heavy drinking, anyone with the slightest psychological or biological vulnerability will be at risk of developing alcoholism.

Kissin's (1977c) hypothesis concerning Jewish and Irish alcoholics, like Jellinek's (1960) interpretation of alcoholism in France and Anglo-Saxon countries, may be regarded as potentially fruitful speculation. However, obtaining a satisfactory answer to the question of how alcohol dependence develops and is maintained requires more than good guesses based on anecdotal evidence. Theories of alcoholism must be confronted with the results of prospective, longitudinal studies.

Such studies have shown that boys with antisocial personality traits run a higher risk of becoming alcoholics than others (see Section 8.1 above). The deviant behaviour pattern of these *psychologically vulnerable* boys is most readily apparent in school, where the problems are manifest in the form of truancy, repeated complaints concerning discipline, or frequent fights with other students. Since these warning signals also mean a higher risk of drug abuse and social maladjustment (e.g. Sarnecki and Sollenhag 1985), teachers, school administrators, and others should keep an eye on them so that preventive action can be taken.

Often *biological vulnerability* is inherited. Twin and adoption studies have confirmed Vaillant and Milofsky's (1982b) observation that boys whose biological fathers are alcoholics run a higher risk of developing alcoholism than sons of non-alcoholics (Goodwin 1985). Goodwin calls for information campaigns to alert adolescents with alcoholism in the family of their increased risk of becoming alcoholics. Since knowledge of genetic factors is seldom complete, he urges all parents to be alert to the following warning signals based on clinical experience: secretive drinking, the capacity to drink large quantities of alcohol without much effect, and oversensitivity toward any comment by an adult concerning drinking practices.

However, this risk analysis must not overshadow the fact that many alcoholics, perhaps most, do not have any familial alcoholism. Even fewer have had serious behavioural problems in school. The biopsychosocial equation predicts that if *society's acceptance of high alcohol consumption* is great enough, virtually anyone can become an alcoholic. In Vaillant and Milofsky's (1982b) study, the boys' subcultural affiliation was of major importance for the prevalence of adult alcoholism. Yet the subject group came from the same part of the same city and was followed up during the same period after the second world war, when alcohol consumption in the United States had not yet recovered after the sharp decline during the Prohibition Era (Moore and Gerstein 1981). In a broader cross-cultural and historical perspective, society's alcohol acceptance, as manifested in both the availability of alcohol and the social norms that regulate its use, emerges as crucial for the risk of developing alcohol abuse and alcoholism (Bruun *et al.* 1975; Mäkelä *et al.* 1981; Colón *et al.* 1982; Moskowitz 1989).

11.2   Multivariant and dynamic

Pattison, Sobell, and Sobell (1977) synthesized contemporary research findings into a multivariant conception of alcohol dependence and its treatment. They formulated a number of propositions aimed at identifying basic conceptual elements and clarifying their interrelationships. According to Pattison and his colleagues, their model should be regarded as a set of working hypotheses that have not yet been adequately tested and verified. The propositions read as follows:

1. Alcohol dependence summarizes a variety of syndromes defined by drinking patterns and the adverse physical, psychological, and/or social consequences of such drinking. These syndromes, jointly denoted as 'alcohol dependence', are best considered as a serious health problem.

At present, there is no factual basis upon which to categorize alcohol problems unequivocally as either purely biological or purely psychological phenomena, and there are compelling arguments against making such a simple dichotomy. On the other hand, there is ample evidence that alcohol problems can affect the physical and/or mental well-being of individuals and that persons suffering from alcohol problems are often in need of a variety of interdisciplinary services.

2. An individual's pattern of use of alcohol can be considered as lying on a continuum, ranging from nonpathological to severely pathological.

3. Any person who uses alcohol can develop a syndrome of alcohol dependence. A variety of factors may contribute to differential susceptibility to alcohol problems; however, these factors in and of themselves do not produce alcohol dependence.

4. The development of alcohol problems follows variable patterns over time and does not necessarily proceed inexorably to severe fatal stages.

A given set of alcohol problems may progress or reverse through either naturalistic or treatment processes.

5. Recovery from alcohol dependence bears no necessary relation to abstinence, although such a concurrence is frequently the case.

6. The consumption of a small amount of alcohol by an individual once labeled as 'alcoholic' does not initiate either physical dependence or a physiological need for more alcohol by that individual.

7. Continued drinking of large doses of alcohol over an extended period of time is likely to initiate a process of physical dependence which will eventually be manifested as an alcohol withdrawal syndrome.

8. The population of persons with alcohol problems is multivariant. Correspondingly, treatment services should be diverse, emphasizing the development of a variety of services, with determination of which treatments, delivered in which contexts, are most effective for which persons and which types of problems.

9. Alcohol problems are typically interrelated with other life problems, especially when alcohol dependence is long established.

Treatment needs should be uniquely assessed for each individual and should address all areas of alcohol-related life and health problems. Similarly, treatment outcome evaluation should measure other areas of life functioning in addition to measuring changes in drinking behaviour. Treatment goals should be realistic and consider the individual's potential for change. Degrees of improvement must be recognized as a beneficial outcome.

10. An emphasis should be placed on dealing with alcohol problems in the environment in which they occur.

This is because of the strong relationships which have been demonstrated between drinking behaviors and environmental variables.

11. Treatment services should be designed to provide for a continuity of care throughout the lengthy process of recovery from alcohol problems. (pp. 4–5)

The thrust of these propositions is directed at the classical disease concept. In fact, they can be viewed as antitheses to the fundamental themes which, according to Pattison *et al.* (1977), are held by the advocates of this concept (p. 50 above).

The previous presentation, however, points rather toward the need for a *synthesis* between the disease model and other theoretical orientations that are widely accepted today, such as the learning model and the social model. Edwards and his colleagues at the Addiction Research Unit in London have shown that it is possible to selectively adopt components from both biological and psychosocial conceptions of alcoholism. Bejerot (1972*a*, 1975, 1977), Kissin (1977*b*; Kissin and Hanson 1982), van Dijk (1972, 1977), and others have developed comprehensive perspectives of a similar kind.

All of these researchers regard alcoholism as a syndrome with a multifactorial aetiology. They believe that a combination of biological, psychological, and social influences contributes to its development. The dynamics of the addictive cycle are assumed to be the result of mechanisms or 'vicious circles' (van Dijk 1977) on all three levels which, by acting simultaneously or in sequence, determine the nature and development of the dependence syndrome. Kissin and Hanson (1982) propose that this point of view be termed the *bio-psychosocial perspective*. The term 'biological' is used here in its more popular sense, as a synonym for 'physiological'.

The biopsychosocial approach is becoming increasingly accepted in psychiatry, especially in the study of psychosomatic diseases (e.g. Fabrega 1979; Leigh and Reiser 1980). But even though different disciplines recognize the value of each other's contributions, they generally do little to explore possible *interactions* between causal agents at different levels. Each discipline tends to regard its own explanations as being primary, while influences of other kinds are assigned a secondary role as 'residual factors' that might accelerate or retard the addictive cycle (Kissin and Hanson 1982; Nathan 1990).

It would take us too far afield here to examine in detail current attempts to integrate theories from various scientific disciplines into a unified perspective for the study of alcoholism. Instead I will use some of the propositions put forward by Pattison, Sobell, and Sobell (1977) to identify major issues that must be addressed in such a perspective. These propositions are repeated below, accompanied by comments on how they must be refined and developed in order that the theoretical model will not be merely *multivariant* but also *dynamic*, that is, capable of describing how the interaction between biological, psychological, and social influences changes from one phase of addiction to another.

Proposition 1: '*Alcohol dependence summarizes a variety of syndromes defined by drinking patterns and the adverse physical, psychological, and/or social consequences of such drinking.*'

Pattison and the Sobells do not distinguish here the medical, psychological, and social complications of drinking from the actual state of dependence or the abnormal desire to take alcohol. This shows that they have not freed themselves entirely of the traditional concept of alcoholism, which was codified in a widely quoted WHO definition (1952) as follows:

Alcoholics are those excessive drinkers whose dependence upon alcohol has attained such a degree that it shows a noticeable mental disturbance or an interference with their bodily and mental health, their inter-personal relations, and their smooth social and economic functioning; or who show the prodromal signs of such developments. (p. 16)

This definition proved to be so vague and ambiguous that it served merely to create confusion. In the most recent versions of the International Classification of Diseases, WHO (1977, 1989*a*) uses the term alcohol-dependence syndrome, differentiating between this state of dependence and alcohol-related disabilities. This refinement of definitions has proved to be exceedingly fruitful. Current attempts to assess the degree of alcohol dependence hold the promise of reproducible research findings and more successful intervention strategies (see Chapter 22; Section 24.1).

Proposition 2: '*An individual's pattern of use of alcohol can be considered as lying on a continuum, ranging from nonpathological to severely pathological.*'

In a comment on this proposition, Pattison and the Sobells maintain that there is no natural dichotomy between alcoholic and non-alcoholic. We are dealing rather with a continuous spectrum of drinking patterns that may result in different combinations of deleterious consequences. If this reasoning is correct, it could be concluded that even alcohol-dependence syndrome is a completely arbitrary designation. Yet a number of phenomena such as a narrowing of the drinking repertoire, the salience of drink-seeking behaviour, a subjective awareness of compulsion to drink, etc., occur sufficiently often in combination to warrant the guess that we are dealing with a specific condition. Edwards (1980) says:

We try today to catch its image descriptively in terms of the dependence syndrome while others before us have certainly been trying to perceive its outline in terms of 'alcoholism as disease'. We are guessing though that somewhere in that landscape there is a real beast to be described rather than an arbitrary cut on a continuum, a label, an abominable and mythical medicalisation. (p. 309)

Kissin (1977c) borrows the language of the traditional models and explains that at some stage, alcoholism stops being a 'symptom' and becomes a 'disease'. Regardless of what may have driven the individual to drink in the first place, it is now the individual's physical and psychological dependence on alcohol that drive him to continue to drink.

Van Dijk (1977) considers psychological and social 'vicious circles' to be of crucial importance in the initial phase of alcoholism. Later, he says, pharmacological and cerebral 'vicious circles' play an increasingly important part, altering the nature of the drinking.

Bejerot (1972a, 1975, 1977) refers to the German nineteenth century philosopher Friedrich Hegel and maintains that the development of dependence entails a dialectic change whereby a certain quality (occasional abuse) under certain circumstances, via successive quantitative increments (repeated abuse), changes over to a *new quality* (dependence). According to Bejerot, the established dependence becomes a force in itself and follows its own laws. It is primarily distinguished by the fact that craving for alcohol assumes the character of a basic drive which dominates the individual and his way of life.

The concept of a qualitative change in the transition from occasional abuse to dependence does not necessarily contradict the notion that people's drinking patterns vary along a continuum. It just has to be kept in mind that among drinkers there is an alcohol-dependent subgroup whose prognosis differs from that of other drinkers. However, the severity of the alcohol dependence also varies, and thereby the alcoholic's responsiveness to controls other than those of biology or conditioning.

The distinction between complications of drinking and the state of dependence itself has facilitated the identification of different phases in the addictive cycle. Even very sophisticated multivariant models for describing and explaining alcohol problems often neglect to take into account the altered character of alcohol abuse with time, which is central to the identification of alcohol dependence as a specific condition. If the time dimension and an understanding of the particular driving forces that characterize the state of dependence are absent, there is a risk that one will see only a scale of greys, but not the 'real beast' which, according to Edwards (1980) and other experienced clinicians and researchers, is out there hiding in the landscape.

Proposition 4: '*The development of alcohol problems follows variable patterns over time and does not necessarily proceed inexorably to severe fatal stages. A given set of alcohol problems may progress or reverse through either naturalistic or treatment processes.*'

It is true, as Pattison and the Sobells propose here, that drinking problems develop in different ways. They do not have to grow steadily worse. But here again, it is important for the sake of conceptual clarity to differentiate between the state of dependence itself and complications of drinking. Many people with alcohol-related disabilities are in no way abnormally dependent on alcohol. Their freedom to increase or decrease their consumption of alcohol is influenced by personal factors and their environment. When a dependence manifests itself, their freedom of choice is restricted. But the borderlines are never absolute; even a severely dependent person can, to some extent, adjust his drinking to avoid getting into trouble. The full explanation as to why some people's drinking problems regress while others continue or grow worse must be sought in psychological and social factors as well as in factors related to the state of dependence itself and its severity (Clark 1976; Vaillant 1980*b*, 1983*b*; Vaillant and Milofsky 1982*a*). The need for a synthesis between social, behavioural, and biological aspects of alcohol problems once again becomes apparent.

Proposition 5: '*Recovery from alcohol dependence bears no necessary relation to abstinence, although such a concurrence is frequently the case.*'

The relationship between remission and abstinence is one of the most hotly debated issues in the outcome literature. Pattison and the Sobells suggest that remission in some cases is synonymous with abstinence, in other cases not. It is likely that distinguishing the dependence syndrome from other alcohol problems can help to untangle the concepts and clarify the relationships. Edwards (1977) has developed the idea that the dependence can reach such a degree of severity that a return to social drinking is highly unlikely. Depending on how alcoholism is defined, there could even be a grain of empirical (non-tautological) truth in the old claim that alcoholics who have resumed control over their drinking were not really alcoholics to start with. These persons may have sustained major disabilities as a result of heavy drinking (i.e. been 'alcoholics' according to the all-embracing criteria of the traditional definition) without having developed an advanced compulsive drinking pattern ('alcoholism' in the sense of severe alcohol dependence).

Up to now treatment research has not delved into the finer distinctions between alcoholics who exhibit dependence symptoms. However, in addition to clinical evidence, occasional research findings (see Chapter 22) support Edwards' (1977) hypothesis about the relationship between severe dependence and the need for abstinence. These findings further underscore the importance of the dependence concept and of the psychobiological aspect for a full understanding of the nature of alcoholism.

Thus, the criticism levelled at the disease concept should not fool us into throwing out the baby with the bath water. On the contrary, the interaction between medical aspects of the addictive cycle on the one hand and social and behavioural aspects on the other would appear to be one of the most promising fields of research for the future.

Part III

Systems of treatment

The classical disease model fostered a tendency to give all patients diagnosed as alcoholics the same treatment. According to the conception outlined in the preceding chapter, however, alcohol dependence is a multivariant phenomenon associated not only with physiological processes but also with psychological factors and social influences. A therapist must take into consideration the difficulty involved in changing behaviour patterns that have evolved over a lifetime. Furthermore, he or she must be aware that the treatment method, the therapeutic relationship, and the treatment setting impose specific role demands on the client. These expectations may not fit the alcoholic's social, cultural, and psychological make-up. If the demands of the treatment and his set of characteristics are incompatible, the result may be a failure.

Key words in contemporary alcoholism treatment are multimodal, multidisciplinary, and continuity of care (Kissin 1977c). That is, multimodal and multidisciplinary when it comes to types of settings, treatment modalities, and professional skills, and continuity and co-ordination between treatment interventions. Adopting a multivariant conception of alcoholism and new strategies in alcoholism treatment research will open up possibilities for a differentiation of therapies so that more individualized treatment can be offered to patients.

Part III examines the implications of the matching concept as a challenge to outcome research and alcoholism treatment. The question of which treatment modalities are appropriate for different types of alcoholics has not yet been adequately explored. The differential treatment of alcoholism that is presented below is therefore based—in good Hippocratic tradition—on a blend of science and proven experience. The treatment systems that are introduced connect and develop concepts that already exist among administrators and therapists. Part III concludes with an account of the first reported attempt to match patients and treatments on a large scale.

12 Matching and the systems approach

Until fairly recently, outcome research took a unitary view of alcoholism. This view proposes that there is one population of alcoholics, to be treated by one best approach, resulting in one therapeutic outcome—abstinence. The findings presented in the preceding chapters indicate that this is not a fruitful approach. Therefore, nihilistic conclusions on the value of differential alcoholism treatment are not justified, despite the fact that a large number of studies have failed to prove that a variation of treatment approach has any significant effect on the drinking behaviour of alcoholics (Section 3.1).

Advocates of a multivariant conception of alcohol dependence (e.g. Pattison 1966–82; Pattison *et al.* 1977; Kissin 1977*c*; Glaser 1980) have raised at least three methodological objections to the conclusion that all therapeutic modalities are of equal value. These objections are examined at the beginning of Chapter 12. In the latter part of the chapter, the systems approach is introduced as an application of the matching concept to alcoholism treatment.

12.1 Potentials and criteria

In the first place, the conclusion that one modality is as good as another can be contested by pointing out that most earlier reports of outcome research failed to take into account the prognosis or *rehabilitation potential* of specific alcoholic populations. Pattison (1976) mentions the skid-row alcoholics as an example of a population with a low potential, where only a five per cent success rate can be expected if the criterion is socialization into a sober and productive life. No treatment approach has any great prospects of 'succeeding' with this population in an absolute sense. By contrast, alcoholic employees surrounded by supervisors and peers who can bring social pressures to bear on their drinking behaviour have a high rehabilitation potential. Hence job-based alcoholism programmes often report that about 70 per cent of the employees recovered from their alcoholism (Trice and Sonnenstuhl 1988).

If consideration is not given to the varying psychological, cultural, and social potentials for rehabilitation, the treatment of severely problematic populations will be doomed in advance. But the effectiveness of a treatment programme cannot be measured by an absolute standard. Since the population of alcoholics and problem drinkers is heterogeneous, a 'recovery rate' will only be meaningful in relation to a given subpopulation with a known prognosis. This requires a control group or at least—as suggested by Costello (1980)—a rough prognosis based on previous experience.

One might expect that at least homeless or skid-row alcoholics would constitute a homogeneous group, since living at missions and shelters has been preceded by a considerable social selection. Indeed, the main impression of the surveys that have been carried out in Sweden is that the homeless alcoholic population consists of individuals with essentially the same type of problems. However, Norman (1979), in his evaluation of a rehabilitation programme in Stockholm, found that the pretreatment social adjustment of homeless alcoholics significantly influenced their prognosis seven to eight years after admission to the programme. Persons for whom staying at a shelter entailed poorer social adjustment than before, and individuals who were relatively well-adjusted (despite severe difficulties in coping with employment or social relations), had a more favourable prognosis than those who had never adjusted to a way of life that is regarded as being normal.

This observation is at variance with the common hypothesis (e.g. Talbott and Gillen 1978) that the existence of a homeless alcoholic has such a severe impact on the individual's life that any difference in rehabilitation potential will be evened out. It does, however, agree well with a multivariant view of alcoholism, according to which drinking behaviour serves different purposes for different individuals in different situations. It is also in perfect harmony with a recent US Institute of Medicine review (IOM 1988), which distinguished between the episodically, the temporarily, and the chronically homeless, each with different needs and prospects.

Another shortcoming in the treatment outcome research is that, until rather recently, it regarded abstinence as the only *criterion of successful treatment*. Other aspects of rehabilitation were considered irrelevant if the alcoholic did not give up drinking entirely. Complete abstention from alcohol was considered to be an absolute prerequisite for improvements in other respects as well. As a consequence, treatment outcome was interpreted more pessimistically than would otherwise have been warranted.

From social, medical, psychiatric, and other points of view, abstinence is a desirable goal for a person who has developed a severe dependence on alcohol. But in the treatment of chronic homeless alcoholics in particular, this treatment goal has seldom been a realistic one. Not many older, socially inept alcoholics with decades of previous heavy drinking are able to maintain abstinence indefinitely—at least not in a society with readily available alcoholic beverages and widespread attitudes favouring drinking. But this does not mean that a reduction of the alcohol consumption and specific improvements in other life areas cannot be achieved, even in the most down-and-out population of alcoholics.

Norman (1979), for example, found that homeless alcoholics, while being provided support in an alcohol-free living environment, drank less, worked more, had a more stable residence, and got into conflicts with their social environment less often than before or after their stay in the programme. This improvement should not be mistaken for rehabilitation. But it seems, nevertheless, to be an important treatment goal in itself for a substantial portion of the homeless alcoholics.

12.2 Spontaneous remission

The third critique of the earlier outcome research is the most essential, as it has to do with the *basic assumptions* (see Section 4.3) of the research. When two or more therapeutic modalities produce almost the same outcomes, this can be interpreted in at least three ways. The outcome can be assumed to be either the result of spontaneous remission, the effect of non-specific (i.e. common) therapeutic factors, or the consequence of a client–treatment interaction. Research on the treatment of alcoholism has, like psychosocial treatment research in general, only recently begun to systematically explore these alternative possibilities. This exploration may facilitate a realistic assessment of the actual and potential effects of alcoholism treatment.

According to the *spontaneous remission* interpretation, no existing treatment approach produces results that differ from the expected rate of 'spontaneous' remission, i.e. a long-term improvement in drinking behaviour due to causes other than the treatment. Several studies have observed that many individuals with severe alcohol problems spontaneously reduce their alcohol consumption in late middle age (Åmark 1951; Drew 1968; Cahalan 1970; Nordström and Berglund 1987*a*). Kendell and Staton (1966), Smart (1975), and Vaillant (1983*b*, p. 123) have examined the scientific evidence for 'spontaneous remission'. They conclude, however, that although the phenomenon undoubtedly exists, the rate of remission within an alcoholic population is probably not more than *a few per cent per year*. Roughly the same conclusions can be drawn from general population surveys that have identified alcoholics and later reinterviewed them (Clark and Cahalan 1976; Roizen, Cahalan, and Shanks 1978; Öjesjö 1981). However, there are few studies of what happens to alcoholics who have not been given any form of treatment.

One sometimes comes across figures indicating that 'spontaneous remission' occurs at the rate of on average one-fifth of a population of alcoholics annually (e.g. Miller and Hester 1980). According to Emrick (1975), the rate of 'spontaneous remission' after six months or longer is no less than 42 per cent. These high figures can probably be explained by the confusion of a temporary improvement between periods of heavy drinking with long-term 'spontaneous remission'. 'Remission' caused by natural fluctuations of the drinking pattern (see Watson and Pucel 1985) is, however, more to be regarded as the artefact of a *statistical regression* (Campbell and Stanley 1963, p. 10 ff.) than as an indicator of recovery. Another reason for the high rate of 'spontaneous remitters' in certain studies may be a definition of alcoholism that includes problem drinkers without severe symptoms of dependence (see Saunders and Kershaw 1979; Öjesjö 1981).

In follow-up studies that extend over a longer span of time, for example five years or more as recommended by Chafetz (1965), Bjerver (1972), Vaillant (1983*b*), and others, it is debatable whether one can or should distinguish 'spontaneous remission' from *effects of treatment*. Firstly, it is very complicated to carry out controlled studies when treating severely alcohol-dependent persons. Alcoholics who have been assigned to control groups cannot be forbidden to seek treatment elsewhere. An alcoholic with constant relapses will probably be given a growing number of treatments (although mostly only of complications of his drinking) as time goes on. This makes it increasingly difficult to use improvements in a control group as a measure of 'spontaneous remission'.

Secondly, it is difficult even in a treatment population to separate 'spontaneous remission' from the effects of treatment. Saunders and Kershaw (1979) interviewed 3600 persons to investigate drinking behaviour and problems in a community. They found that in five out of seven detected cases of alcoholics that had recovered following treatment, the episode of treatment coincided with the development of new or improved significant relationships or a major job change, such as the termination of alcohol-related employment. In three of these cases, the individual had been exposed to specialist services several times before without any improvement. Their last experience of treatment was successful, but coincided with a change in life circumstances of a type that is usually associated with 'spontaneous remission'. It is possible that the change in life circumstances was decisive, but that it would not have occurred without a preceding intervention.

Saunders and Kershaw recognize that the number of remitters was too small to permit generalizations. However, the authors do point out the need to examine more closely and, if possible, ameliorate the environment and the interpersonal milieu of alcoholics in treatment.

Vaillant (1980*b*, 1983*b*; Vaillant and Milofsky 1982*a*) has, in a large longitudinal study of paths to recovery in alcoholism, arrived at similar results. He thinks that the term 'spontaneous' is inadequate. What actually happens in the attainment of stable remission can best be described as a profound behaviour change, mediated by forces that can be identified and understood by social scientists and harnessed by health professionals. Vaillant refers to Orford and Edwards (1977), who wrote that: 'in alcoholism treatment, research should increasingly embrace the closer study of "natural" forces which can be captured and exploited by planned therapeutic intervention' (p. 3).

Realization of the importance of 'natural' forces should not lead us to abandon attempts to improve existing treatment approaches. The appropriate conclusion is instead that the models of therapy should consider the interaction between treatment and such life experiences that are masked by the generic term 'spontaneous remission' (cf. Moos and Finney 1983). Azrin's community reinforcement approach (Chapter 10.4 above), for example, was recently described as a successful attempt to look upon the 'natural deterrents of alcoholism' as an opportunity for learning more about treatment (IOM 1990, Ch. 6).

Edwards (1989), in reviewing a ten-year follow-up, regarded it as 'absurdly medico-centric' to assume that treatment influences are so paramount that every other influence in the interactive field can be discounted. Rather, the treatment experience is 'at best a timely nudge or whisper in a long life course' (p. 20). It should, therefore, be placed within the enormously important totality of the ebb and flow of what happens to that person's life.

As a matter of fact treatment can accurately be conceived as a means of facilitating 'spontaneous' remission. The imitation of nature's efforts in the therapeutic management of disease was at the core of Hippocratism in antiquity and in the Renaissance. The 16th-century French physician Ambroise Paré, the father of modern surgery, is supposed to have said, following a successful operation: 'I dressed him, God healed him.' A similar Hippocratic humility is warranted in the treatment of alcoholism. Treatment or social control focusing on a person's drinking behaviour does not change his or her life. But by supporting a sober way of life, even if only temporary, these measures create a *scope for change* (Saliba 1982) which allows other psychological and social motives than the dependence on alcohol to prevail.

12.3   The non-specific hypothesis

The apparent equivalence of treatment outcomes has also been attributed to placebos or non-specific factors, i.e. active ingredients that are common to a variety of treatment methods (cf. Emrick 1975). However, the attribution of therapeutic influence to *specific* or *non-specific* factors is often arbitrary and misleading. Certain components of treatment that are designated as non-specific, for example a programme's credibility to the client and the expectations for improvement that it generates, are in no way uniformly present in any specific treatment (e.g. Wilkins 1979). Moreover, the ingredients referred to as crucial for one form of treatment, e.g. the duration of treatment, may be regarded as non-specific factors for another therapeutic modality.

Often, referring to ingredients as non-specific simply means that attempts to tie them to an existing theory have failed. The term non-specific factors may then include a nebulous set of as yet unexplored therapeutic influences. It becomes a catch-all for the many concrete variables that deserve to be explored and incorporated into a more comprehensive conceptual framework. In other words, categorizing treatment factors as non-specific tend to obscure the fact that current conceptualizations of the therapeutic change process are at an early stage of development.

Strupp (1986; Butler and Strupp 1986) proposed that the division of therapeutic influences into specific and non-specific should be abandoned. Like Chertok and Stengers (1988), he questioned the method of isolating and separating 'ingredients' as a way of reducing the multitude of events and interactions to be observed. Psychosocial treatment is not a medical technology, and research will never produce a 'psychotherapy antibiotic'. Unlike drugs, he contended, techniques of psychosocial treatment have no meaning apart from their interpersonal context.

However, this position is also fraught with difficulties (Omer 1989). Despite much unproductive controversy, the relative weight of commonalities and differences between techniques remains an important question. Furthermore, any conceptualization involves simplification. The confusion surrounding the specific/non-specific dichotomy stems rather from its either/or aspect, which suggests that non-specific factors can be applied without any accompanying specific technique. Today, however, a promising integration of specific and non-specific concepts is evolving.

Kazdin (1979) criticized the indiscriminate use of the term non-specific treatment factors. He encouraged investigators to identify more specifically the precise variables and interactions that are included. Wilkins (1984) made the same suggestion in an analysis of the placebo concept. In fact, one of the main thrusts of current treatment research is the effort to 'make the non-specific specific' so that these factors can be deliberately used in the context of specific interventions (Omer and London 1988).

A number of investigators (e.g. Frank 1973; Bandura 1977; Bootzin and Lick 1979; Eysenck 1980; Goldfried and Padawer 1982; Leitner 1982; Jones 1983; Karasu 1986; Orlinsky and Howard 1986; Omer 1987; Omer and London 1989) are now exploring the possibility of enhancing the effects of diverse therapies through a better understanding of components that have previously been termed non-specific factors or placebos.

Annis and Davis (1988), for example, used Bandura's theory of self-efficacy to guide the development of a relapse prevention model for the treatment of alcoholics. Moreover, Chapter 25 below elaborates on effective strategies of alcoholism treatment that are not tied to any specific orientation. These strategies are arrived at by an inductive process, which is based on empirical findings regarding therapeutic outcomes and the effects of client–treatment interaction.

12.4   The matching hypothesis

A third explanation of why different treatment methods produce about the same results, is that they are based on the false assumption that the population of alcoholics is homogeneous (the uniformity assumption myth; see Kiesler 1966). The varying potentials for rehabilitation of different individuals have been discussed above (Section 12.1). This concept is fruitful in making comparisons between populations in treatment. But it becomes misleading if taken too literally, since it gives the impression that all treatment methods affect all individuals in a similar manner. One might uncritically assume that individuals with good rehabilitation potentials are responsive to all kinds of treatment, while the opposite is true for individuals with poor rehabilitation potentials.

However, there may be not only *quantitative* but also *qualitative* differences between individuals' potentials for rehabilitation. Different forms of intervention can activate individual resources and conflicts of different kinds and thereby affect individuals with the same general rehabilitation potential in different ways. For example, individuals of type (a) might improve in programme (A) and deteriorate in programme (B), while individuals of type (b) will improve in programme (B) and deteriorate in programme (A). If individuals of types (a) and (b) are treated as a uniform group, successes (the combinations (A) − (a) and (B) − (b)) and failures ((A) − (b) and (B) − (a)) will even each other out so that it looks as if the programmes were interchangeable

Table 12.1 Hypothetical effects of interaction between type of client and form of intervention (+, improvement; −, deterioration).

Type of patient	Programme A	Programme B
a	+	−
b	−	+
a + b	±0	±0

(see Table 12.1). The consequence will be an unwarranted impression that a variation of the treatment would not affect its result.

An effect of such interaction is illustrated by Orford, Oppenheimer, and Edwards (1986; Section 22.2 below) in a study of the two-year outcomes for a sample of 100 married male alcoholics who had been randomly assigned to either a single day's assessment and advice or a fairly intensive outpatient treatment. Treatment outcomes were divided into three categories, which are discussed separately. Accumulated results can be arrived at by a reanalysis of their data. Here, outcome categories are quantified as a rank order, where 'good' outcome is given one point, 'equivocal' outcome two points, and 'bad' outcome three points.

Compared across sub-groups of alcoholics, brief counselling gave as good results as intensive treatment, with the former regime scoring 1.90 and the latter 1.88. A closer inspection, however, reveals an interesting interaction between type of client, treatment modality, and outcome (Fig. 12.1). Gamma alcoholics were more likely to benefit from intensive outpatient treatment, while other alcoholics (primarily Alpha, i.e. problem drinkers without physical dependence on alcohol) were more likely to benefit from a single counselling session. That is, Gamma alcoholics offered intensive treatment had good drinking outcomes (an average score of 1.38), while those given only assessment and advice had poor outcomes (2.57). By contrast, non-Gamma alcoholics given counselling only had rather good outcomes (1.71), whereas those offered intensive treatment scored below the average (2.19).

The results reported above seem to support the naive notion that 'more severely ill' patients do better with intensive treatment and worse with brief counselling. This conclusion is premature, though. Firstly, no effect of a

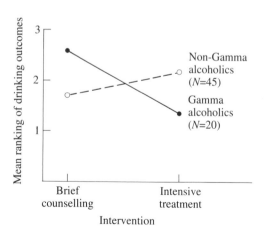

Fig. 12.1 Interaction between degree of alcohol dependence (Gamma vs. non-Gamma), intensity of treatment, and drinking outcome.

client–treatment interaction was observed at the 12-month follow-up of the same sample (Edwards, Orford, *et al.* 1977*a*), although similar criteria were used for classifying alcoholics. Secondly, Orford and his colleagues' (1976) finding has not been replicated by other studies comparing interventions of varying intensity. The lack of internal consistency and external validation makes any policy based on this study problematic. It has been used here rather to exemplify an important methodological issue.

Another example is afforded by a double-blind, placebo-controlled trial of lithium therapy with alcoholic patients (Merry *et al.* 1976; Reynolds, Merry, and Coppen 1977; Coppen 1980). All patients, whether depressed or not, were randomly assigned to either a placebo condition or to treatment with lithium carbonate. One of the outcome criteria was the number of drinking days over a period that averaged 42 weeks after discharge.

Patients who received lithium spent less than half as many days drinking compared to those who received the placebo. It is tempting from such mean data to conclude, as other investigators have done, that 'lithium may be a powerful ally in prevention of periodic or chronic drinking problems' (Kline *et al.* 1974, p. 21). However, a reanalysis by Glaser (1980) revealed a clinically significant interaction between type of patient, treatment modality, and outcome. Depressed patients on lithium greatly reduced (37 fold!) the number of days spent drinking, while non-depressed patients who received lithium actually spent *more* days drinking than otherwise. Thus the favourable average outcome with lithium therapy could be entirely explained by its effects on depressed alcoholics. According to this study then, the use of lithium without due consideration for individual differences would be potentially harmful for non-depressed alcoholics.

The presentation above, however, has no other purpose than illustrating the potential significance of client–treatment interactions. The dropout rate of 46 per cent is alone sufficient to disqualify the study. Moreover, the effect of compliance has to be taken into account (Clark and Fawcett 1989). Liskow and Goodwin (1987) are perfectly justified in concluding that the value of lithium in the treatment of depressed and non-depressed alcoholics has yet to be determined.

Studies of the same kind as those described in this section, but based on a firmer empirical foundation, are examined in Parts III and IV of this book. They suggest that by carefully matching clients and interventions it will be possible to reduce the risk of doing harm, to improve treatment outcomes, and to refute the conclusion that all therapies are equivalent. The philosophy underlying the matching hypothesis was formulated by Gordon Paul in 1967 in a widely quoted passage:

The . . . question posed, 'Does psychotherapy work?', is virtually meaningless. . . . the range of individual differences within standard diagnostic categories remains so diversified as to render meaningless any questions or statements about individuals who become so labelled. . . . the question towards which all outcome research should ultimately be directed is the following: *What* treatment, by *whom*, is most effective for *this* individual with that specific problem, and under *which* set of circumstances? (p. 111)

In the present economic climate, the question '. . . and at what cost?' (Wilson and Rachman 1983, p. 61) is usually added.

The matching hypothesis has proved to be fruitful within disciplines bordering on psychosocial treatment research, such as medicine (Fries 1976), education (Hunt 1971; Cunningham 1975; Solomon and Kendall 1976; Cronbach and Snow 1977; Miller 1981; Dunn 1984) and criminology (Warren 1969; Annis and Chan 1983).

12.5   Monolithic and shotgun approaches

Pattison (1966–82) maintained that the failure to distinguish differences in outcome among treatments for alcoholism has promoted two intervention strategies, both of which are contrary to a consistent matching procedure. One is the *competitive monolithic* approach, in which a certain brand of therapy is offered as 'the' way to treat all alcoholics, with the implicit assumption that other treaments are, if not harmful, at least ineffective. The other is the *shotgun* approach, in which every client is subjected to a wide variety of different treatments, in the hope that 'something will take'.

The 'competitive monolithic' or, as it is also known, the 'monopolistic' approach involves a rallying to 'the only effective way'. This often fosters an antiscientific opposition to rigorous empirical follow-up of treatment interventions (Babow 1975). Another unfortunate consequence is that neither treatment staff nor community agencies assume overall responsibility for alcoholism treatment and for a co-ordination of available resources. In this climate of opinion, those alcoholics who do not fit into the dominant pattern of services are the ones who suffer. They risk being classified as 'poorly motivated' or 'unco-operative'. In a travesty of an old adage, we could put it this way: 'The right man in the right place—others need not apply!'

Einstein, Wolfson, and Gecht (1970) investigated how American alcoholism treatment professionals viewed their work and what they considered important and relevant in the treatment of alcoholism. The respondents were a number of physicians, psychologists, nurses, and social workers. The major conclusion of the study was that a variety of problem drinkers were perceived as being not so different from each other. They were taken care of by professionals who preferred to treat problem drinkers striving to become abstinent. The respondents were mainly concerned about how long and how frequently their patients had been drinking to excess. They were not particularly interested in finding out how much alcohol their patients had consumed.

The availability of inpatient treatment resources was considered to be the most important treatment-related factor. Group therapy and reliance on AA were the most common treatment modalities. The impression of a simplistic and stereotyped approach is confirmed by Rathod (1977):

Many treatment organisations over-emphasise the role of a particular facility—inpatient treatment for example—over all others, even though research might have shown that outpatient or day care facilities can be equally effective. The same applies to the treatment modalities used; group psychotherapy seems to stand supreme in the modes of treatment, even though it has never been proved or disproved that this necessarily is the best type of treatment to offer alcoholic patients. (p. 309)

Pemper (1976) identified six psychological and social dimensions that have been found to be related to problem drinking: attitude toward drinking, environmental support for heavy drinking, impulsivity and non-conformity, alienation and maladjustment, looseness of social controls, and unfavourable expectations. These dimensions were used in a questionnaire sent to psychiatrists, psychologists, and social workers to determine what they considered to be of greatest importance for the improvement of the patient.

It turned out that the professionals were only interested in those changes that has to do with the patients' attitude toward drinking. Other aspects of the alcoholics' life were regarded as irrelevant, or at least as not being affected by a treatment programme. Yet a changed attitude toward drinking by itself seems unlikely to be sufficient to bring about the changes in patterns of vocational, family, and interpersonal maladjustment that are often necessary for a stable remission. Pemper (1976) commented: 'If the professionals' perceptions are accurate and representative, it is possible that the questionable value and efficacy of alcohol treatment programs is related to this limited focus of treatment' (pp. 648–9).

The 'shotgun' approach, which allows each alcoholic to sample all the treatment modalities available, may at first glance appear the opposite of the rigidity and narrow-mindedness described above. However, both approaches are distinguished by the absence of a deliberate and systematic pairing of patients and interventions. Many researchers (e.g. Levinson and Sereny 1969) have warned of the dangers of 'too much' treatment. It is not true that if a little treatment is good, a lot of treatment is always better. Nor is it true that since most treatment modalities do some good, no one will be harmed by a mix of different therapies. A situation where the alcoholic wanders from one agency to the next, and where he is exposed to lots of treatments without any connection, fosters confusion and insecurity. As noted by Kissin (1977c), 'the patient, taken care of by everybody, may end up being taken care of by no one' (p. 45).

In a review of outcome research, Costello (1975a, 1975b) found that short-term treatment programmes without either documented principles of selection or continuity of care, exhibited the lowest rate of success in terms of sobriety or drinking with no associated problems as well as the largest per cent reported dead or lost to the follow-up.

12.6   The systems approach

The unsystematic nature of treatment for alcohol problems has been an international phenomenon. Surveys of the organization of alcoholism treatment in, for example, Alaska (Miller *et al.* 1974), Pennsylvania (Glaser *et al.* 1978*a*), and Washington State (Pattison, Coe, and Rhodes 1969; Pattison, Coe, and Doerr 1973) have all documented a glaring lack of planning and purposefulness. Holder and Stratas (1972), who studied programmes for alcoholics in North Carolina, described the general situation as follows:

Historically the public response to the alcoholic or problem drinker or to the collective problem called 'alcoholism' has been partial and segmented. . . . To view this situation through 'systems eyes' reveals a cluttered, disjointed, overlapping, uncoordinated, and ineffective set of public and private programs that are opportunistic and responsive primarily to an immediate crisis or community tension. Lacking is a purposeful and continuing system that approaches the problem both at the micro (individual drinker) and macro (community) levels, that is able to bring together current resources and activities effectively and that is responsive to changes in the population served. (p. 64)

The *systems approach* (Pattison 1966–82; Nathan *et al.* 1968; Ward and Faillace 1970; Holder and Stratas 1972; Glaser *et al.* 1978, 1984, 1985; Galanter and Sperber 1982) applies the matching hypothesis to the administration of a multi-programme treatment network. This approach is based on the notion that the treatment resources will be best utilized if individual programmes clearly define the population of alcoholics they believe they can expertly help, the goals that are reasonable for this group, and the methods that are most appropriate to achieve these goals.

A *system* is defined as follows in *The Oxford English Dictionary*:

A set or assemblage of things connected, associated, or interdependent, so as to form a complex unity; a whole composed of parts in orderly arrangement according to some scheme or plan; rarely applied to a simple or small assemblage of things (nearly = 'group' or 'set'.) (Vol. 17, 2nd edn, p. 496)

A systems approach in alcoholism treatment assumes that there is a complementary relationship between different treatment programmes. The whole must be more than the sum of its parts and must be modified when individual parts (population characteristics, treatment facilities, therapeutic techniques, etc.) and external circumstances (e.g. alcohol control policies) change. The perspective is often broadened to include co-operation with community agencies, such as health care settings, social agencies, educational institutions, occupational settings, and the criminal justice system. The scope and structure of the system may vary according to local conditions.

The establishment of a treatment system does not entail the replacing of existing programmes with entirely new ones. Nor does it mean that the same therapeutic philosophy is to be adopted by all programmes. The purpose is instead to incorporate them in a dynamic whole without the individual programmes having to compromise their individuality. What is important is that they contribute towards satisfying the specific treatment needs of a specific alcoholic population. By concentrating primarily on the outcome, the stage is set for free competition between different therapeutic concepts and philosophies (Magaro *et al.* 1978). However, the systems approach requires specified goals, recurrent evaluation, and modification as needed in parts of the integrated system.

The following chapters of Part III investigate different aspects of the systems approach. Chapter 13 examines the conditions for a consistent matching procedure. A deliberate assignment of patients to treatment methods is already taking place in many facilities. Information on the patients is usually combined in an informal manner, often during a staff conference. This 'clinical' method has, however, proved to be rather unreliable as a basis for treatment decisions, especially when both subjective judgements and objective facts must be taken into consideration. Matching in the sense of a deliberate and consistent selection of treatment seems to require 'statistical' methods of prediction.

Mansell Pattison's conceptual model is introduced in Chapter 14. Pattison was one of the first to penetrate the question of how to select optimal treatment for alcoholics. He investigated the impairments of different treatment populations and proposed that needs for improvement should be considered in terms of specific 'life health' areas.

Chapter 15 presents the Core–Shell Treatment System, a pioneering project which was in operation from 1975 through 1981. The system was developed by Frederick Glaser at the Addiction Research Foundation in Toronto. It presupposed a close interaction between treatment and research. Even though it has not yet been tested fully, its structure and planned mode of operation may provide an idea of the practical implications of the matching hypothesis and of the feasibility of employing the systems approach to alcoholism treatment.

Chapter 16 describes the Penn-VA Project, a research and treatment approach developed and tested by Thomas McLellan and his colleagues at the University of Pennsylvania and the Veterans Administration in Philadelphia. The model incorporates many of those prerequisites for successful differentiation of treatment that are emphasized in previous chapters. For example, an instrument for assessment and outcome determination (Addiction Severity Index, ASI) was devised that is both reliable (Chapter 13) and comprehensive (Chapter 14). With the aid of assessment, matching, and outcome monitoring, McLellan was able to modify a network of four treatment units for alcoholics so that it produced better outcomes despite unchanged resources. This project illustrates how outcome information can be used to modify the functioning of treatment as envisaged by the core–shell model (Chapter 15). Finally, the results accentuate the importance of attending to psychological patient characteristics, in addition to the usual demographic and clinical variables (cf. Part IV).

Recently, a committee of the US Institute of Medicine (IOM 1990) designated the systems approach 'the cornerstone' of its vision of the probable evolution of treatment for people with alcohol problems. The committee concluded that 'there is no single treatment approach that is effective for all persons with alcohol problems' (p. 147), and therefore recommended that presently existing treatment programmes should be integrated into carefully planned systems. It is this generic approach that the committee found compelling, rather than any specific design. However, the presence of the following elements were viewed as critical:

(1) a collaborative effort between community agencies and the specialized treatment sector;

(2) comprehensive assessment prior to treatment;

(3) matching to optimal treatment;

(4) continuity of care;

(5) determining treatment outcome; and

(6) the feedback of outcome information in order to modify guidelines for matching.

These components are not at present to be found in most treatment settings. However, the committee identified them to a variable degree in a dozen programmes that have existed, are currently viable, or are planned for the future. Among these are the Penn-VA Project, the Core-Shell System (CSS), and two systems of which one has adapted practices of the CSS (Brookfield Clinics) and the other is as an outgrowth of the CSS (Ontario Assessment and Referral System; Section 15.7 below). In the committee's examples, comprehensive assessment, matching, and outcome determination were most frequently present. Feedback occupied a middle ground, and was more often planned than implemented. The community component and the continuity assurance were the two elements least in evidence.

The committee proposed that these previous and current efforts could serve as prototypes for a series of demonstration projects intended to define effective system approaches that could be transferred to the treatment field in general. It was recognized that:

this is both a major and a novel undertaking, even though its continuity with the current thrust in the field is quite clear. It is a formidable task. But an undertaking of appropriate magnitude is required if the challenge of alcohol problems is to be met. (IOM 1990, p. 340)

13   Clinical versus statistical prediction

The systems approach requires a consistent selection of appropriate interventions for alcoholics. This in turn necessitates the ability to predict, with some probability of success, which treatment will be of most benefit for the individual patient. Client variables that appear to be useful in this context are presented in Chapters 16 to 22. The question of how these variables should be applied in alcoholism treatment brings up one of the oldest methodological issues in clinical psychology: the relationship between *clinical* and *statistical* methods of prediction.

Clinical methods of prediction require the participation of professionals, e.g. psychologists, doctors, or social workers. The problem can consequently be reformulated into the question: 'What role should be played by psychologists and other clinicians in the selection of treatment for alcohol problems?' This question, which is fundamental no matter what treatment system is to be applied, merits closer examination.

In the US during the second world war, Sarbin (1943) and other researchers posed the question: 'How can the services of the experienced psychiatrist or psychologist be used to achieve better predictions than any clerk could make by statistical means with the aid of clinical data?' The statistical analysis produced a baseline that could be successfully improved upon by the judgement of the experienced clinician—or so it was thought.

The findings, however, did not support the superiority of the clinical method. In a classic study, Paul Meehl (1954) summarized the results of some twenty investigations that systematically compared clinical and statistical methods of prediction. In all these studies, the prediction based on an actuarial formula produced a result that was better or at least as good as the one obtained by the clinical judge.

The statistical method classified patients by combining demographic, clinical, and psychological data in a purely mechanical manner. The prediction was then obtained from a statistical table, usually based on an empirically derived, linear regression equation incorporating client variables and the behaviour to be predicted.

With the clinical method, doctors or psychologists formulated a hypothesis about the psychological structure and dynamics of the individual, generally at a staff conference and on the basis of subjective impressions and objective information of a demographic, clinical, and psychological nature. The personality hypothesis or 'diagnosis', along with expectations as to external events, finally served as the basis for a prediction.

Meehl's book aroused heated debate and gave rise to a large number of studies of whether clinical assessments really are inferior to much simpler statistical methods of prediction. However, ten years after the publication of his pioneering work, Meehl (1965) found that of the approximately fifty empirical studies that had been conducted in the meantime, only one favoured clinical prediction. The rest of the research literature supported, broadened, and refined the conclusions he had previously arrived at. The results had been repeated in criminology, education, medicine, and industrial psychology as well as in various fields of clinical psychology (e.g. prediction of stayability and outcome in psychotherapy, recovery from psychosis, response to electric shock treatment, formal psychiatric nosology, personality description, etc.). Meehl (1965) summarized: 'It would be difficult to mention any other domain of psychological controversy in which such uniformity of research outcome as this would be evident in the literature' (p. 27). A closer examination by Goldberg (1968) showed that the exception to the superiority of the statistical method which Meehl thought he had found did not hold up. Since then, attempts to find evidence in favour of the clinical method of prediction seem to have ceased.

Jack Sawyer (1966) carried out a sophisticated analysis of the previous research literature. He pointed out that a fair comparison between clinical and statistical methods should study each procedure at its best. Even if the doctor, the psychologist, and the social worker were found to make poor predictions, this should not disqualify these professionals as clinical observers and 'measuring instruments'. The quality of a prediction is dependent on both the way of collecting and the mode of combining data, as well as on the interaction between these two methods. A conclusive judgement on the relative merits of the clinical and statistical methods of treatment selection must consequently take into account both of these aspects.

Sawyer introduced the term *mechanical* as a substitute for 'statistical'. The former term is applicable to both collection and combination of data without the participation of a clinician. Sawyer noted that data on patients can be collected in three ways (clinical, mechanical, or both) and combined in two ways (clinical or mechanical). These distinctions permit a classification of prediction methods into six main categories, plus two more that describe 'syntheses' of prediction methods. The identifying names and examples are not exhaustive. They only suggest typical procedures in each category.

1. *Pure clinical*: *clinically* collected data, *clinically* combined. Here the psychologist (doctor, social worker) predicts the patient's behaviour on the basis of an interview or other direct observation, without having access to any test results or other objective information.

2. *Trait ratings*: *clinically* collected data, *mechanically* combined. The psychologist collects data in the same way as in the pure clinical method.

He then assesses the patient along a number of prespecified personality dimensions. But instead of predicting future behaviour himself, he uses statistical tables or some other mechanical device to combine the information.

3. *Profile interpretation*: *mechanically* collected data, *clinically* combined. The psychologist uses a set of test scores or other objective information to make a prediction, based on clinical experience, about a patient he has not seen. A typical example of this method is the interpretation of unknown persons' MMPI profiles (MMPI = Minnesota Multiphasic Personality Inventory; see Section 19.4).

4. *Pure statistical*: *mechanically* collected data, *mechanically* combined. The patient fills in, say, a form with biographical information and a psychological test that can be administered with no or minimal clinical participation. Data on variables that have previously been found to be correlated with the outcome to be predicted are then combined mechanically, for example with the aid of a multiple regression equation.

5. *Clinical composite*: *both kinds* of data, *clinically* combined. The psychologist makes his or her prediction by integrating the results obtained from, for example, a clinical interview, observations, psychological tests, and biographical information. This is assumed to be the most common method in clinical practice.

6. *Mechanical composite*: *both kinds* of data, *mechanically* combined. Like the clinical composite method, this method uses data collected by both modes (clinical and mechanical), but integrates them mechanically.

7. *Clinical synthesis*. The prediction is produced *clinically* by using all available data together with a prediction previously derived *mechanically* on the basis of these data. A 'sophisticated clinical' approach of this type has been suggested by a number of psychologists (e.g. Holt 1958) as a fair compromise in the discussion of clinical versus statistical methods of prediction.

8. *Mechanical synthesis*. The prediction is produced *mechanically* by using a prediction previously derived *clinically* on the basis of these data.

There are, of course, reasonable arguments for and against each of these prediction methods. But what is needed, according to Sawyer (1966), is a systematic, empirical comparison. Hence he analysed 45 studies that had predicted outcome in behavioural terms rather than establishing a diagnosis or a personality structure. Many of the studies examined reported on more than two methods of prediction, giving Sawyer a total of 75 comparisons on which to base his analysis.

Table 13.1 Summary of conclusions from 45 studies comparing predictions based on clinical versus mechanical modes of collecting and combining data

| Mode of data collection | Mode of data combination | | | |
	Clinical	%	Mechanical	%
Clinical	1. Pure clinical	20[a]	2. Trait ratings	43
Mechanical	3. Profile interpretation	38	4. Pure statistical	63
Both	5. Clinical composite	26	6. Mechanical composite	75
Either or both[b]	7. Clinical synthesis	50	8. Mechanical synthesis	75

[a]The percentage is a measure of the efficacy of the mode. It indicates the percentage of comparisons in which the method surpassed, plus one-half the percentage of comparisons in which it equalled, the method with which it was compared.
[b]Plus, for the clinical synthesis, the prediction by Method 2, 4, or 6; or, for the mechanical synthesis, the prediction by Method 1, 3, or 5.

The clearest comparison of the studied methods is presented in Table 13.1. Here, each method is classified according to how the data were collected (lines) and combined (columns). The percentages comprise summary measures of the efficacy of each method. The standard is the percentage of the comparisons in which the method was superior, plus one-half the percentage of the comparisons in which it was equal to the method it was compared with. The comparisons on which the table was based exhibited a remarkable degree of agreement. Sawyer did not discover a single pair of methods for which one study found one method to be better while another found the other method to be better.

The results reported in the table can be summarized in the following points:

1. A comparison between the results in the two columns shows that, regardless of the mode of data collection, the mechanical mode of combining the data is superior, by margins of 23, 25, 49, and 25 per cent respectively.

2. A comparison between the first line and the others shows that, within each mode of data combination, the clinical mode of collection by itself provides an inferior basis for making predictions, by margins ranging from 6 to 32 per cent.

3. The difference in results between modes of combination is influenced (with a single exception) very little by the mode of collection, and vice versa. This gives little reason to prefer particular modes of data combination for particular modes of collection, even though the choice of methods in these 45 studies in fact shows that such preferences are strongly held.

4. The one exception to this low interaction between mode of collection, mode of combination, and result is the clinical composite. The result here

is about 24 per cent lower than the other seven values would give reason to expect. Table 13.1 warrants the conclusion that when the combination is mechanical, it is better to have both clinically and mechanically collected data; but when the combination is clinical, having both kinds of data is little better than having only clinically collected data and *not as good* as having only mechanically collected data.

5. The clinical synthesis, where the psychologist is aware of the prediction made mechanically, produces better results than clinical predictions made without this extra information. However, the mechanical composite prediction by itself produces better results than all clinical predictions and is *not* improved by knowledge of the clinical prediction. In other words, neither the 'sophisticated clinical' nor the mechanical synthesis appears promising.

In summary, Sawyer's review of the literature confirms Meehl's (1954) conclusion that the mechanical mode of *combining* data on patients is always better than or equal to the clinical mode. Moreover, the study shows that this conclusion is valid regardless of how the data have been collected (clinically, mechanically, or by both modes).

The choice of an appropriate method for *collecting* data on patients is more complicated. The most successful method of prediction according to Table 13.1—the mechanical composite—utilizes information collected both clinically and mechanically. (So does the mechanical synthesis, which predicts as well but requires more data.)

The question of what role psychologists and other clinical practitioners should play in the selection of treatment for alcoholics can thus be given a preliminary answer. The psychologist (doctor, social worker) may contribute most by carrying out valid and reliable assessments that can be combined with the results of simple psychological tests, biographical information and other data collected by persons without special clinical skills. The actual combination of data into a prediction used in treatment selection, however, should be done by statistical means, particularly if the data are of a composite nature.

More recent studies have confirmed the assertion that a linear regression equation provides better predictions than one or more human judges can accomplish by intuition. This is true even if the weights of the prediction variables are chosen randomly, except for sign (Dawes and Corrigan 1974).

Human judges who combine individual data not only assign prediction variables invalid weights (Dawes and Corrigan 1974); they also apply their weights inconsistently. A statistical model of a clinical judge, reconstructed on the basis of the weights he or she has previously applied, will outperform the human judge due to improved reliability alone (Goldberg 1970).

There is an extensive body of experimental research on how people combine data from different sources of information for the purpose of making predictions (see Nisbett and Ross 1980; Kahneman, Slovic, and Tversky 1982; Sjöberg 1982). Besides fatigue, boredom, stress, poor memory, and similar factors, most of us fall into a number of traps that systematically undermine our cognitive powers. Vivid, concrete data on individual cases, for example, have often been found to make a greater impact than evidentially superior but dull and abstract data on group tendencies. This phenomenon may explain the finding that clinical judges who have access only to mechanically collected patient data tend to make much better predictions than judges who can also utilize information collected by clinical methods (interview, observation).

The human judge's greatest weakness seems to be that he does not take sufficient account of how common the various outcomes are (Nisbett and Ross 1980; Kahneman *et al.* 1982). The following examples illustrate how this tendency can manifest itself in alcoholism treatment:

1. Therapist A is convinced that his insight-oriented approach is successful with socially stable, well-motivated alcoholics. But these clients have good prospects with other treatment as well, or without any intervention at all. The insight-oriented therapy may, in fact, delay improvement that would have taken place without it (see Chapter 8).

2. According to treatment orientation B, it is not possible to help an alcoholic successfully until he has 'hit bottom'. However, it can always be predicted that a person will change for the better after he has 'hit bottom'. Firstly, a change for the worse would mean that he actually had not yet experienced the lowest point in his life. Secondly, particular success with clients that have rapidly deteriorated may actually be an effect of natural fluctuation, which in statistics is known as 'regression towards the mean'.

3. The board members of rehabilitation unit C, to which older, severely disabled alcoholics are sent, feel that the programme has a miserable record. But the board members should keep in mind that institutions that accept the severest group of alcoholics always exhibit poor results, even if they do as well or even better than other institutions for the same clientele (cf. Campbell and Erlebacher 1970).

The research on clinical versus statistical prediction has important implications for clinical psychology (Wiggins 1973) and for alcoholism treatment (Skinner 1981*a*). It shows that the study of interaction effects is of more than just academic interest. The discovery of simple, objective indications for the selection of treatment approach can be of great practical value, especially for routine decisions such as recommendation of abstinence versus controlled drinking, referral to inpatient versus outpatient treatment, and choice between programmes with different degrees of structure and directiveness (see Chapter 24).

The scientific basis required for an appropriate choice of treatment is currently often lacking. The clinical decision-makers have only their own experience and theoretical orientation to fall back on. In the absence of empirical studies, they have to guess which client characteristics are related to the prognosis in specific treatment programmes. However, a number of studies (Wiggins and Hoffman 1968; Goldberg 1970) have shown that it is possible to improve the reliability of the predictions by devising a statistical model based on observations of how one or more experienced clinicians combine information on their clients. With models of this kind, the predictions will be more consistent and not as influenced by variations in the clinician's mood and concentration.

Some substantiated prognostic indicators are well established in treatment selection for alcohol problems. For example, an experienced therapist discourage alcoholics with acute liver damage from any attempt at controlled drinking. However, the chances of making correct predictions are greatly reduced when the interaction effects—as is usual (see Section 23.4)—are complex and when the predictors are not only clinical but also demographic and psychological. Under these circumstances, a deliberate and consistent pairing of clients and interventions must probably be achieved statistically, with computer support or the aid of some other mechanical device to combine data.

However, research can discover clinically useful interactions only by analysing, systematizing, and refining the qualitative knowing gained from clinical experience. Accordingly, psychologists and other clinical practitioners have an important role to play in treatment research. They can serve as full-fledged partners in the scientific process by formulating testable hypotheses about how patient characteristics and treatment dimensions interact to bring about a successful result. A promising approach is the *deviant case analysis* (Ross 1963, 1981; Garfield 1981*a*; Barlow, Hayes, and Nelson 1984, Ch. 12), i.e. detailed case studies of individuals whose treatment outcomes run counter to what would be expected in view of their rehabilitation potential.

The formulation of hypotheses about interaction is essential not only for the selection of therapeutic mode, as illustrated above. It is also of major significance for the more intuitive adjustments that are constantly required by the therapist during the course of treatment (cf. Hunt 1980; Hunt and Gow 1984).

14 Pattison's treatment profiles

In a series of articles and books, Mansell Pattison has advocated a systems approach to alcoholism treatment (Pattison 1974, 1976, 1978, 1979, 1982*a*, 1982*b*, 1982*c*; Pattison *et al.* 1969, 1973, 1977). He maintains that the main problem in alcoholism treatment today is neither a lack of treatment centres, a lack of effective treatment methods, nor a lack of interested, committed, and determined staff. There is also a body of clinical and experimental research. What is lacking, however, is a systematic utilization of the resources and the knowledge that exist.

The systems approach is described as a multivariant approach that seeks to examine and exploit knowledge on the interaction between different levels and components of a total social system. As has been shown above (Chapter 11), Pattison subscribes to the view that there are different kinds of alcoholics who should be treated with different methods for the purpose of achieving different outcomes. This view implies that it is not possible to talk about treatment outcomes in general. Treatment outcomes must: be analysed in their individual constituents; be related to characteristics of the patient population; and be related to characteristic features of the setting and the treatment method. Instead of formulating global treatment goals, Pattison recommends the establishment of specific *treatment profiles*, which describe selection of treatment methods and goals in terms of specific target areas.

Long-term treatment planning must focus on multiple areas of life function. Improvement in drinking behaviour does not automatically lead to success in other areas. And conversely, a treatment plan that ignores drinking as a problem in itself is likely to fail. Pattison proposes that goals and evaluation criteria should be considered in terms of total *life health*, including: drinking health, emotional health, vocational health, interpersonal health, and physical health.

In a couple of essays on treatment philosophy, Pattison (1967, 1969) maintains that the therapist should strive to enhance the patient's capacities to deal with his society rather than merely make the patient conform to society. Social control, restrictions, legal sanctions, etc. are justified to the extent that they help the alcoholic take responsibility for himself and his life. Life health can, in this perspective, be interpreted as an individual's access to those personal and environmental resources that will enable him to cope.

Pattison's first stage in treatment planning is an analysis of what functions drinking behaviour fulfils for the individual in different situations (cf. Chapter 9). The second stage consists of an assessment of the alcoholic's personal and environmental resources. In the third stage, the person is asked about

his subjective needs. Finally, the therapist and client carry out an evaluation
of which changes are both *possible* and personally *desirable.*

An assessment of the patients' life health prior to treatment often reveals
that they function well in certain areas, while their function is severely
impaired in other areas. There may be little need or room for improvement
in some life areas. This is especially true for many 'hidden' alcoholics, who
manage to cope with problems in their life despite uncontrolled drinking.
In contrast, homeless alcoholics tend to have severe dysfunction in all areas
of life health.

In order to plan the treatment carefully, it is necessary to specify the target
areas of life health in which improvement can be expected, the degree of
dysfunction in each area, and the degree of improvement that can reasonably
be anticipated. This procedure results in a differential prognosis for each
individual and each area of life health.

To illustrate the principles of differential treatment, Pattison refers to a
study conducted in collaboration with Ronald Coe and Hans Doerr in 1973.
The study compared alcoholic populations from four treatment facilities:

(1) an aversion-conditioning private medical hospital;

(2) an outpatient clinic offering psychiatric and social work counselling;

(3) a halfway house with an emphasis on peer-group support; and

(4) a police farm work centre providing alcoholics with shelter and structure.

Pattison and his co-workers found that the patients in these programmes had
different definitions of their alcoholism and aimed at different treatment goals
(see Table 14.1).

Alcoholism treatment apparently meant quite a different thing to each of
the four alcoholic populations. Pattison (1974) concluded that alcoholics seek
a type of treatment that is congruent with their particular perception of
alcoholism. Thus, it is not chance alone that determines what programme

Table 14.1 Patients' conception of alcoholism and treatment goal in four programmes

	Aversion hospital	Outpatient clinic	Halfway house	Police farm
Conception of alcoholism	Medical allergy	Neurotic symptom	Life problem	Secondary nuisance
Treatment goal	Abstinence	Resolution of personal conflicts	A new style of life adaption	A time of 'drying out' and relief

an alcoholic ends up in. Some people, for example, regard their drinking as a spiritual problem that can be cured only by spiritual restoration or salvation. The assumption that these alcoholics will benefit from a spiritual programme is indirectly supported by Rosenbaum, Friedlander, and Kaplan's (1956) observation that deeply religious patients are not very receptive to conventional psychotherapy. Other alcoholics seek vocational and social training, while still others look for medical or psychiatric help.

Rehabilitation is a social enterprise, and its outcome is dependent on a set of cultural values and attitudes. For this reason, Pattison does not believe in one 'best' treatment approach. A systems approach must embrace a number of perspectives on alcoholism, with the various programmes and goals these perspectives dictate (cf. Emrick 1975).

Table 14.2 presents a differential assessment of disability in different life health areas for each of Pattison, Coe, and Doerr's (1973) four alcoholic populations. As is evident from the numerical profiles, each population's problems have a characteristic pattern. The profiles that describe the degree of expected change also differ considerably. In other words, the populations present differential treatment profiles. The population at the *aversion hospital* can be regarded as 'hidden' alcoholics. They function well in most areas and can therefore not expect any great changes as a result of treatment. The improvement that can be hoped for is almost exclusively in the drinking area.

The population that visited the *outpatient clinic* have greater initial disabilities. They can thus be expected to exhibit greater improvements within a number of life health areas. Since the population's disabilities are not particularly severe, however, the treatment cannot bring about any dramatic changes.

The population at the *halfway house* have severe disabilities within almost all life health areas; but these alcoholics have also a high potential for rehabilitation. They are the classic alcoholics whose once successful lives have been ruined due to their alcoholism. The alcoholics in this population can be expected to exhibit the most dramatic improvement.

The population found at the *police farm* are the homeless and the socially inept alcoholics. They also have severe disabilities within all life health areas, but unlike the clients at the halfway house, they have no previous history of successful socialization. They have very poor prospects for rehabilitation, and no great improvements can be expected as a result of care and custody.

It should be added that recent research findings (Chapter 8) suggest that severe alcohol dependence is a contra-indication for the type of psycho-therapeutic approach that Pattison associated with the outpatient clinic. The objection is valid regardless of how the alcoholic himself perceives his alcoholism. An outpatient clinic looking upon alcoholism as a symptom must thus, in order to have any justification, carefully screen its candidates by assessing their degree of alcohol dependence.

Table 14.2 Differential assessment of disability and expected improvement for four alcoholic populations

Life health area	Aversion hospital		Outpatient clinic		Halfway house		Police farm	
	Disability on admission	Predicted degree of improvement	Disability on admission	Predicted degree of improvement	Disability on admission	Predicted degree of improvement	Disability on admission	Predicted degree of improvement
Drinking	4[a]	4[b]	4	4	4	4	4	2
Emotional	1	1	3	3	4	4	4	1
Interpersonal	1	1	2	2	4	4	4	1
Vocational	0	0	1	1	4	4	4	1
Physical	1	1	0	0	2	2	4	3

[a]Disability is rated on a scale of 0–4, with 0 = no disability, and 4 = highest disability.
[b]Degree of improvement is rated on a scale of 0–4, with 0 = no improvement, and 4 = greatest degree of improvement.
N.B. The figure is a *relative change index* (see e.g. Stallings and Oncken 1977), not a measure of how clients are expected to function in a particular area.

Pattison's descriptions of patients' potential for rehabilitation are based more on clinical experience than on scientific findings. Bromet *et al.* (1977), however, confirmed the assumption that different programmes promote different rehabilitation patterns quite similar to those described above.

Finney and Moos (1979; Section 18.3), on the other hand, found a greater distribution of patients with the same type of disabilities across different treatment facilities than had been reported by Pattison and his co-workers (Pattison *et al.* 1969, 1973). Availability and chance seemed to play a significant role in the 'choice' of treatment programme (see also Gibbs 1980). For example, alcoholics who had never been successfully adapted to society and had very low prospects of ever becoming so, were found in large numbers in the therapy-oriented halfway house and the hospital-based programme as well as in the Salvation Army facility for homeless alcoholics. Conversely, more than half of the patients at the Salvation Army facility probably had resources to benefit from a more intensive social and psychological rehabilitation.

15   The Core–Shell System

During the years 1975 to 1981 a unique research and treatment organization, the Core–Shell Treatment System (CSS), was evaluated at the Addiction Research Foundation of Ontario (ARF) in Toronto, Canada. An attempt was made to design, test, and implement a systems approach within the framework of ARF's Clinical Institute. The Institute is a treatment facility incorporating several programmes in outpatient and inpatient treatment which admitted about 2400 new clients per year. The project director was the American psychiatrist Frederick Glaser, who has described the background, structure, and function of the CSS in a number of articles and reports (Glaser 1977, 1980, 1984d, 1990; Glaser et al. 1978, 1984, 1985).

15.1   The background

Since the beginnings in 1949, researchers at Ontario's Addiction Research Foundation have investigated numerous aspects of alcohol dependence: the epidemiology of alcoholism, the biochemistry and physiology of dependence, medical sequelæ of abuse, the efficacy of preventive public policy measures, etc. However, it was not until the 1970s, with the establishment of the Clinical Institute and a general review of ARF's activities, that treatment research was given a prominent place in the research programme.

The deliberations concerning treatment research became heavily influenced by two phenomena: the emerging multivariant approach in research on alcohol dependence (see Chapter 11 above) and in psychotherapy research (Section 4.1); and Edwards and Orford's controlled trial of 'treatment' and 'advice' (see Sections 15.3, 22.1). A desire to study the outcome of differential treatment was formulated. An organizational model was sought which would not only assign several thousand clients annually to various kinds of treatment; all clients should also be potential research subjects, so that large samples for testing of hypotheses could be generated. Such a model required a more refined division of labour than is usual in alcoholism treatment.

The answer was the CSS. The experience from the pilot phase with this programme is, according to Glaser et al. (1985), highly encouraging. The systems approach was not only feasible; it was also received very positively by clients and treatment staff. It was found, for example, that the attrition rate between initial contact and entry into treatment was significantly reduced. Despite this and other favourable preliminary results, the systems approach was not incorporated as a permanent framework for treatment and treatment research at the Clinical Institute. The system has, however, inspired other projects currently in progress (Sections 15.6, 15.7) as well as the treatment systems vision recently elaborated by a committee of the US Institute of Medicine (IOM 1990).

15.2 The core and the shell

The core–shell model is based on the hypothesis that a successful treatment system must contain four components: *primary care, assessment, research,* and *specific interventions.* These components can be further subdivided into those that are required for *all* clients seeking treatment and those that are required only for *some* clients. Each client is considered to need help from one person, who assumes overall responsibility for his care, provides continuity, and co-ordinates interventions (primary care). The assumption that alcoholics constitute a heterogeneous population means that it is necessary to specify each client's resources, needs, social situation, life style, etc. (assessment). Furthermore, the record should be so detailed that every client is an eligible subject for outcome research, though practical considerations prevent the follow-up of more than a representative random sample (research). Finally, some—but not all—clients will require specialized treatment (specific intervention).

Primary care, assessment, and research are thus essential components in the treatment of all clients, while secondary care (specific interventions) is considered necessary for some, but not all clients. Moreover, it is the system as a whole, not each treatment programme, that has to be effective for all kinds of clients. The individual programmes need only demonstrate that their specific interventions are effective for one particular client population.

These considerations explain the structure of the CSS (Fig. 15.1). As the name indicates, it is an organization of treatment resources with a *core* and a *shell.* The three universally required components are grouped together in the centre of the diagram and constitute the core programme. They are surrounded by a shell consisting of specialized programmes. All clients enter the system through the core. This constitutes a radical departure from the standard practice whereby the client is admitted directly to a specific treatment programme. This latter practice has many disadvantages. While the client's suitability for the particular programme may be discussed at an intake interview, there is usually no systematic assessment of the benefits the client may derive from alternative programmes, nor are any referrals made. Consequently, clients often begin treatments that may be quite inappropriate to their actual needs. According to Glaser and his co-workers, this may explain why many clients prematurely terminate treatment, why programmes have poor success, and why treatment staff often become discouraged.

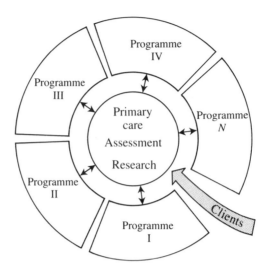

Fig. 15.1   The Core–Shell Treatment System.

But it is not only the choice of specific intervention, where such is called for, that is facilitated by an entry through the core. Continuity of care is assured by the fact that each client who enters the system makes initial contact with a *primary care worker*. This person, who may be a nurse or a paraprofessional, assumes overall responsibility for the management of the client's care. He or she also maintains contact by visits, telephone calls, etc. In a project patterned after the CSS, Glaser and Hubbard (1985) recommend that primary care workers also should be trained in relapse prevention techniques.

Finally, a comprehensive assessment prior to treatment creates excellent conditions for outcome research. The follow-up can be performed by a central cadre without any ties to individual treatment programmes, so they can be relatively objective. Both the continuity of care and the systematic outcome monitoring are features displayed by few large-scale treatment organizations.

15.3   Primary care

The first question that must be answered when a client comes into contact with the core–shell programme is whether there is a need for sobering-up, detoxification, or care for emergency sequelæ of drinking. When any immediate problems have been resolved, the client meets his primary care worker. He then undergoes an individual assessment, which is carried out at a special unit by personnel hired and trained for the purpose. Clients who are unwilling to be assessed (they were less than 15 per cent) and clients who do not require more intensive care are offered continued primary care contact alone. In analogy

Table 15.1 Primary care and secondary care

Dimension	Primary care	Secondary care
Aim	Care	Cure
Orientation	General	Special
Structure	Simple	Complex
Hazardousness	Less hazardous	More hazardous
Cost	Less expensive	More expensive

to the Hippocratic conception of medicine as a co-operative art, treatment is regarded as a question of preventing relapse, with the option of intensive intervention for those who do not respond to minimal intervention alone.

According to Glaser (1984*b*), *primary care* and *secondary care* differ in five basic respects: aim, orientation, structural organization, level of hazardousness, and cost (see Table 15.1). With its emphasis on a relationship that goes on over a prolonged period of time, the CSS exhibits similarities with certain paraprofessional organizations such as AA, with its 'buddy' system and reinforcement of sobriety. Doctors, psychologists, and social workers who receive outpatient alcoholics for formal treatment are not, however, providing primary care in the CSS's definition.

The ethics committee of the Addiction Research Foundation in Toronto shared Glaser's and his co-workers' conviction that it is irresponsible to assign someone to an intensive programme (in the shell) without a prior assessment of his or her potential to benefit from that particular programme. It has, Glaser maintains, been recognized since antiquity that the more powerful a given therapeutic intervention (surgical procedure, drug use, etc.) is, the greater the hazards associated with it are.

The hazards of psychosocial treatment have been slower to be recognized. In the field of alcoholism, Blumberg *et al.* (1973), for example, pointed out that treatment programmes which reject many clients at an early stage due to unrealistic demands are probably worse than no treatment at all. Spradley (1970) and Straus (1974) have, in research on subcultures, shown that too permissive care is not harmless either, since it probably helps maintain and reinforce the social dependency of certain alcoholics.

Glaser finds support in outcome research for a restrictive use of intensive interventions. Edwards and his co-workers (1977a) found that a comparatively expensive and elaborate 'average package of care' given to all alcoholics does not, on average, produce better results than a counselling session (see Section 22.1). In a discussion of the implications of this result, Edwards and Orford (1977) maintained that: 'what can fairly be concluded from the sum of the research literature, including these findings, is that the approach to alcoholism treatment should in general include less intervention than has been the fashion' (p. 344).

There is no valid evidence for the view that most alcoholics should be provided intensive care, the two researchers claimed. Individualized advice that reinforces the client's sense of self-responsibility and self-direction can often produce similar or better results. According to Edwards and Orford (1977), recovery from alcoholism is more a question of problem-solving and decision-making than of 'treatment' in the medical sense. One should thus resist the temptation to rapidly escalate the intensity of treatment if advice does not produce immediate results. Advice and other less intensive measures should, however, not completely replace services of the type that have previously been standard, Edwards and Orford added.

Later on, Miller and Hester's (1980) review of 650 articles on the effects of alcoholism treatment led to a similar conclusion:

The consistent finding that extensive and intensive interventions are no more effective in general than more minimal treatments suggests that it would be unwise policy to routinely provide multimodal, long-term, or broad-spectrum treatment for *all* clients. Rather, both minimal and more intensive alternatives should be available, with the latter used selectively. (pp. 108–10)

As a suitable solution, Miller and Hester recommended a systems approach with the same components as the CSS.

15.4   Individual assessment

Glaser (1984*a*) rejects the spontaneous response that individual assessment in the sense of the systems approach is already standard practice in alcoholism treatment. According to Glaser, assessment today rarely goes further than establishing that the individual is actually seeking help for his alcoholism, thus providing evidence of 'motivation', or completing a form containing demographic data and perhaps a brief, two-line 'statement of the problem'. There is nothing in the surveys I have referred to above (Sections 12.5, 12.6) to contradict this gloomy picture.

This discussion may give the impression that the Clinical Institute had specific treatment methods and selection criteria at its disposal which differed significantly from the customary ones. Such was not the case. The pilot project in Toronto made use of eighteen already existing, conventional-type inpatient and outpatient treatment options. In the absence of validated matching methods, the system relied on a combination of (a) simple and objective indications developed in collaboration between system administrators and staff of the treatment programmes, and (b) patient preferences.

All patients were given an outline of salient features of each intervention. They were also asked to rank a number of goals that treatment personnel had said to be of central importance in their particular programmes. As objective criteria for relaxation training, for example, different scales that measure intelligence and stress level were used. Although every second client expressed interest in the treatment, the eligibility criteria indicated that only one of three would benefit from it. Similarly, half of all clients were interested in individual therapy, but only one of four fulfilled the requirement of at least average intelligence and moderate social stability.

Glaser and his co-workers found that the largest single client group were those who either wished to have only primary care or, after individual assessment, were judged not to benefit from other interventions (24 per cent of the men, 16 per cent of the women). More than two specialized interventions were justified for only 28 per cent of the clients. This is a significant result in a situation characterized by scarce resources for care and treatment. Glaser quotes Hiatt (1975), who pointed out that the US—like, presumably, the entire Western world—is approaching a point where marginal gains to the individual are becoming a threat to the welfare of the society as a whole.

The most important difference between the CSS's eligibility criteria and those used in other treatment organizations is that the former were *explicit*. Because the criteria and methods of assessment are specified in advance, they are accessible to critical examination. If the indications for a given intervention should fail to predict a positive outcome, they can readily be changed. Although not directly referred to by Glaser, research on clinical versus statistical prediction (Chapter 13) is relevant here. Explicit eligibility criteria have often proved to be a prerequisite for reliable prediction. Despite numerous studies that have tried to prove the opposite, prediction based on implicit criteria and clinical intuition have thus far never surpassed statistical forecasts based on clearly defined and empirically derived prognostic indicators.

Glaser (1984*a*) recommends a far-reaching standardization of the individual assessment. With standardized data, the computer can be employed as an aid in coordinating the large quantities of information that are necessary for rational treatment planning and continuous evaluation research (see Skinner and Allen 1983; Gazda 1984).

15.5   Treatment research

The treatment system presented here is constructed in a way that provides an infrastructure for research and development. Glaser and his co-workers (1985) admit that the system in itself does not answer the many complicated questions that remain concerning the efficacy of different interventions. But it does provide a means by which these questions can be addressed in a fruitful and precise manner. And it particularly facilitates research involving the matching hypothesis, i.e. projects that investigate the interaction between patient, treatment, and outcome.

Since all interventions are preceded by individual assessment, a good basis is created for experimental research designs with pretreatment and post-treatment data. All patients, even in control groups, are guaranteed primary care. The continuous contact with a primary care worker facilitates follow-up. In addition, a special *follow-up unit* would assist in the evaluation studies, which means that it would not be necessary to assemble and train a new follow-up team for each individual research project. The CSS's services were planned to be available to any investigator whose project met the rigorous standards set by the scientific, ethical, and administrative management.

With these favourable conditions for continuous evaluation, Glaser believes that the treatment system can be self-regulating. It will be possible to ensure that resources for intensive intervention are utilized by those who need them most, and that treatment is adapted to the patients. Instead of providing a multitude of facilities for the same type of patient (see Section 12.5), an attempt can be made to develop programmes for those clients who are not receiving effective service from the treatment system.

15.6 Implementation

Experience tells us that we should be wary of making too much of initial treatment success. Glaser (1984*a*, p. 91) notes that the division of labour, which is a fundamental part of the systems approach, can make certain tasks (in particular the assessment of clients) monotonous. A problem that is specific to the systems approach is the bottleneck (Glaser 1984*d*). Research on interaction effects does not permit any clear-cut conclusions on what constitutes valid indications for different kinds of treatment. According to Ogborne (1984), some researchers at the Addiction Research Foundation also felt that the system restricted their freedom too much.

Campbell (1984) warned in another context against an intimate association between research and administrative decision-making. 'The more any quantitative social indicator is used for social decision-making, the more subject it will be to corrupting pressures introducing bias and invalidity', he concluded (p. 26). Here he touches upon a problem which may be, in fact, the Achilles' heel of the CSS and every rationally managed treatment organization.

As indicated above, the Clinical Institute chose to organize their treatment and research in a more traditional manner after the pilot project was concluded. Instead of investing in a large project, they preferred, partially due to limited resources, to opt for a variety of smaller projects. It has been characteristic of the organization to lay the groundwork and then retreat, allowing others to further develop its ideas. A project modelled on the CSS currently exists in the US (Brookfield Clinics in Detroit). A major project, very much like the original system, was planned by Glaser and Hubbard (1985) for the province of Alberta, Canada (Northern Addiction Centre). It is expected to open in 1992 (IOM 1990, p. 338).

All of the above reasons may have been of importance when the management at the Clinical Institute decided to abandon the CSS. But Frederick Glaser (personal communication 1983) suspected that the decision was also based on less rational considerations:

> From another perspective, I would hazard the guess that the degree of subjugation of individual wills to the good of the whole which is inevitably required by a systematic approach was simply too great to be tolerated at that point in the history of our organization. At least in this particular area . . . a systems approach was ahead of its time. Yet I continue to feel it is the most reasonable and the most effective approach, and that its time is now fast approaching.

With the recent IOM (1990) endorsement of treatment systems, we may be on the verge of the era envisaged by Glaser.

However, the treatment organization at the Clinical Institute did retain some key features of the CSS (Ogborne 1984). Specifically, the organization preserved a system of primary care workers who make initial contact with patients and help them deal with practical problems and acute crisis situations. The primary care workers also provide case-management and follow-up of treatment interventions. For some patients, the support provided by primary care is all they need.

The Clinical Institute has also allocated central resources for assessment, referral, and follow-up. This service makes it easier for formally approved research projects to get help with selecting appropriate patients and administering tests and follow-up interviews. In addition, the data on all patients are now stored in computerized form and can conveniently be retrieved for various research purposes.

15.7   Regional systems

Ogborne maintained in 1979 that the organizational principles of the CSS could easily be moved out into the community. They do not necessarily have to operate within the walls of a specialized hospital for alcoholics such as the Clinical Institute. He supported this claim by referring to a number of independent programmes of a similar kind that had been developed in community settings (Pittel and Hofer 1974; Dukta et al. 1976; Rosenbaum et al. 1977).

This paper was immediately rebutted by Evans (1979), who maintained that Ogborne had underestimated the difficulties resulting from current administrative and funding arrangements. Treatment programmes need a certain minimum of clients in order to survive. From this viewpoint, it can be most rational for the individual programme to accept all applicants, or to select the most 'motivated' clients, rather than to ask self-critically which alcoholics the programme can best serve and which should be referred to another programme. In other words, the programme's natural urge to survive may promote inefficiency. A systems approach therefore requires, according to Evans (1979), more than simply investigations of treatment outcomes. The evaluation of treatment systems must include sociological studies of how organizations are maintained and changed.

Ogborne apparently listened to the criticism. In collaboration with Rush, he has developed and described an ARF assessment/referral system at the provincial level, which combines ideas of the CSS with a broader social perspective (Ogborne and Rush 1983). With reference to Aiken *et al.* (1975), the writers distinguish between three levels of service delivery: the client level, the agency level, and the funding level.

The *client level* includes individual assessment, which is common to all programmes connected to the system. This assessment leads to a referral to appropriate treatment for the client's most urgent problems. A team of experts at ARF in Toronto recently completed work on a multidimensional diagnostic instrument (ASIST 1989) intended to facilitate the choice of intervention. A case-manager is attached to each client at the time of assessment and continues to support and advise the client, follows up the treatment interventions and assists in crises.

Ogborne and Dwyer (1986) evaluated 20 regional assessment/referral services for alcohol abusers in the province of Ontario. Some of these services already were committed to goals which the writers considered essential at the client level:

1. Providing a comprehensive assessment to substance abusers with a view to making referrals to agencies in the community, and a clear demonstration that client needs and not assessment worker preferences determine referral recommendations (in a previous survey of community agencies, Rush, Brook, and Graham (1982) found a bias in favour of within-professional referral).

2. Providing or mobilizing on-going care for assessed clients.

3. Using uniform assessment procedures and instruments.

4. Monitoring clients, at least during the period when the initial referral recommendation is to be carried out.

5. Making constructive use of assessment and outcome data to generate empirically justified referral recommendations or service development proposals.

Efforts at the *agency level* could well be served by the establishment of coalitions of community agencies, according to Ogborne and Rush (1983).

Such coalitions process information at the 'systems level', and representatives of different agencies are given an opportunity to identify and prioritize treatment needs in the community. Sometimes new treatment services are developed through a mutual pooling of staff resources. In other instances, these collaborative efforts among the agencies result in joint proposals for additional funds for new services. Alternative models at the agency level in Ontario have been examined and evaluated by Dwyer and Ogborne (1984).

The allocation of funds for treatment services takes place at what Ogborne and Rush call the *funding level*. Here, efforts are needed to get different government agencies (e.g. health, social welfare, and corrections) to coordinate their services for alcoholics. Unclear or conflicting goals at this level will hamper collaboration at the other levels.

In a 1986 survey (Ogborne and Rush 1990), assessment/referral services were viewed very favourable by community professionals. They attracted 10 per cent of all clients seen within Ontario's addiction treatment system. However, only a very small proportion of admission to residential or outpatient services were referred from assessment services. With current Canadian funding arrangements, Ogborne and Rush note, there are no incentives for making treatment contingent upon the results of an independent assessment.

16 The Penn-VA Project

The University of Pennsylvania in Philadelphia, USA, is a well-known centre for psychotherapy research. Two large projects have recently been directed, both of which were examining how interaction between client characteristics and treatment factors influence outcome. The Penn Psychotherapy Project is one of them (see Chapter 24). It was studying the effects of psychotherapy on non-psychotic patients in outpatient psychiatric treatment. The second project was examining outpatient and inpatient treatment of alcohol and drug abusers. This research and development effort is known as the *Penn-VA Project* (The Pennsylvania Veterans Administration Project; see overview by O'Brien *et al.* 1988). Head of the work being done on patient–treatment matching was the psychologist *Thomas McLellan*. He has, in collaboration with Lester Luborsky, Charles O'Brien, George Woody, Keith Druley, and others, described the results achieved in a series of reports (McLellan *et al.* 1980*a*, 1980*b*, 1980*c*, 1981*a*, 1981*b*, 1981*c*, 1981*d*, 1982, 1983*a*, 1983*b*, 1983*c*, 1985*a*, 1986).

The approach employed by this research team is innovative and sophisticated. It is characterized by a fruitful interaction between researchers and programme staff (cf. Ogborne 1988). McLellan and his colleagues' research can be described as an extension of Kissin's and Pattison's multivariant approach to alcoholism treatment (Chapter 20) insofar as they have studied how a combination of social and psychological client resources influence the outcome of various kinds of treatment.

Kissin's and Pattison's preliminary theses on how clients and interventions should be co-ordinated have had some influence on the treatment of alcoholism, at least in the US. McLellan's more well-founded conclusions will probably have at least as much impact. But the significance of the Penn-VA research lies not only in the multifactorial interaction effects that have been identified. Perhaps even more important is the model developed to establish indications for various programmes. This model provides a standard example of how the matching hypothesis and a systems approach may prove fruitful to outcome research and facilitate the tailoring of treatment to the particular needs of each patient.

16.1 Is treatment effective?

With their project, McLellan and his colleagues addressed three central questions in outcome research: Is treatment more effective than no treatment?

Are some types of treatment more effective than others? Do certain types of clients do better in certain types of treatment?

The question of whether treatment of alcoholics is effective at all was dealt with in a separate study (McLellan *et al.* 1982). The study group consisted of 554 male alcoholics who were admitted to the Coatesville and Philadelphia Veterans Administration (VA) Medical Centers during 1978, and who remained in treatment for at least five days. Seventeen per cent of the alcoholics admitted to the Medical Centers had dropped out of treatment within five days and were thus not eligible for the study. McLellan and his colleagues were able to follow up 83 per cent of the subjects six months after admission to treatment. Thus, complete data were available for 460 alcoholics. The patients at the VA clinics in Coatesville and Philadelphia were considered to be slightly older, better educated, and more socially stable than other alcoholics in the metropolitan area (McLellan *et al.* 1981c).

The study group was distributed among three inpatient programmes and one outpatient programme. There is no evidence that any of the programmes was more effective for all alcoholics than the others. The researchers were, however, able to discover specific effects for subgroups of alcoholics. These effects, as well as the characteristics of the programmes, are described in Sections 16.3 and 16.4. The following discussion is restricted to certain general results with regard to all treatment programmes and the patient group as a whole.

The patients spent an average of about 50 days in treatment. The standard deviation (SD) was 17 days. During the treatment period, patients received individual therapy on average 26 times (SD = 7) and group therapy on average 24 times (SD = 7). The proportion of irregular discharges (dropouts) was about one third.

Individual assessment at admission and follow-up was performed by independent researchers who had nothing to do with the treatment. Standardized information on the patients was collected by means of the Addiction Severity Index (ASI), a multidimensional diagnostic and evaluative instrument (see Section 16.2). ASI evaluates the severity of the patients' problems as regards medical condition, employment, alcohol use, drug use, illegal activity, family and social relations, and psychiatric condition.

Table 16.1 compares the severity of patients' problems during the 30-day periods prior to admission and prior to follow-up six months later. Higher ratings indicate more severe problems. The absolute values are not very informative. What is interesting are the changes from admission to follow-up. The table shows that the most significant improvements ($p < 0.01$) occurred in regard to alcohol use, employment, and interpersonal relations. The medical condition of patients seems to have changed very little.

These improvements are not, however, necessarily a result of the treatment employed. Natural fluctuation of the drinking pattern ('regression towards the mean') and life experiences that have nothing to do with the treatment

Table 16.1 Change in 460 alcoholics from admission to follow-up six months later

Problem area[a]	Admission	Follow-up
Medical	13.6	12.8
Employment	10.3**	− 3.6**
Alcohol use	38.4**	16.2**
Drug use	4.0*	1.9*
Legal	2.2	1.1
Family/social	10.9**	4.3**
Psychiatric	13.1*	9.5*

*$p < 0.05$; **$p < 0.01$.
[a]Problem severity was rated during 30 days before admission and before follow-up six months later. Higher scores indicate greater severity.

itself could theoretically explain the observed changes. An experimental researcher takes these 'external' factors into account by the use of a control group that receives no or minimal treatment. However, such an approach may be questionable on ethical grounds and is often impractical to implement. On the other hand, it is impossible to draw any conclusions on the effects of treatment without, as in the experimental model, taking into account various nontreatment influences. This is a dilemma that every evaluator of treatment has to face (cf. p. 22, 173 f.).

Certain studies, such as the Rand reports (Armor *et al.* 1978, Polich *et al.* 1981), have attacked the problem by comparing patients with varying duration of treatment. McLellan and his co-workers (1982) similarly considered comparing the group that stayed in treatment with those patients who dropped out of the programmes during the first five days. However, an examination of these dropout patients indicated that they generally had more severe problems at admission and clearly worse prognoses than the treatment group. A comparison between the two groups after six months would therefore be misleading.

McLellan's research team chose a different solution to the evaluator's dilemma. They selected a comparison group consisting of all patients from the larger sample who received treatment for more than five but fewer than 15 days, and who had a favourable discharge. These criteria defined a short-term (ST) treatment group comprising 98 of the 460 alcoholics in the study group.

A comparison between the ST group and the long-term (LT) group showed that there were no significant differences between the patients with regard to age, education, or ethnic distribution. In fact, ST patients had significantly fewer previous treatments ($p < 0.05$) and significantly lower severity ($p < 0.05$) in the family and social problem area. ST and LT patients had been assigned to the programmes in the same manner and in the same proportion. The proportion of favourable discharges was also the same. Therefore McLellan and his colleagues (1982) argue that a comparison between the ST and LT groups will provide a conservative and adequate estimate of the effects of treatment.

Table 16.2 presents comparisons *within* both the ST and LT groups with regard to problem severity at admission to treatment and at follow-up after six months. The LT patients show a greater number of significant improvements at a generally higher level of significance than do the ST patients. However, the ST patients also show significant improvement in several areas.

In *between-group* comparisons, the researchers took into account age, race, number of previous treatments, and pretreatment problem severity. Table 16.2 (last column) shows that the LT group had significantly better outcome than the ST group with regard to employment, alcohol use, drug use, illegal activity, and psychiatric condition, despite some significant improvements by the ST alcoholics from admission to follow-up. Medical condition and family or social relations, on the other hand, did not improve more in the LT group than in the ST group.

The McLellan group maintains that these results, together with some other findings (including Armor *et al.* 1978), support the notion that treatment of alcoholics produces 'significant, pervasive, and sustained positive changes'. Unfortunately, this conclusion is hardly tenable. A serious objection concerns the brief follow-up interval, a one-month period only three to five months after the termination of treatment (six months after admission to treatment). Such a short-term perspective does not permit any conclusion about the

Table 16.2 Comparisons within and between groups of alcoholics with varying duration of treatment

	Within-group comparisons				
	Long-term treatment ($N = 362$)		Short-term treatment ($N = 98$)		Between-treatment
Problem area[a]	Admission	Follow-up	Admission	Follow-up	comparisons[b]
Medical	14.0	12.2	12.8	13.0	—
Employment	10.3**	− 4.3*	10.1*	− 2.7*	$p < 0.01$
Alcohol use	37.1**	14.2**	39.9**	20.6**	$p < 0.01$
Drug use	3.6**	0.5**	5.0	2.8	$p < 0.05$
Legal	2.4*	0.6*	2.0	1.6	$p < 0.05$
Family/social	11.6*	6.0*	7.4*	3.8*	—
Psychiatric	13.4*	8.6*	12.5	11.7	$p < 0.01$

*$p < 0.05$; **$p < 0.01$
[a]Problem severity was rated during 30 days before admission and before follow-up six months later.
[b]With statistical controls for age, race, number of previous treatments periods, and pretreatment problem severity.

stability of treatment results. On the basis of outcome research presented in Section 3.1 above, it was concluded that temporary improvement can normally be expected during the year after treatment, but that more enduring effects of treatment have not been demonstrated.

The difference in outcome between a treatment group and a control group has been found to decrease as a function of time. This makes the Penn-VA team's comparison between ST and LT groups somewhat dubious. The follow-up interval after termination of treatment was roughly 50 per cent longer for the ST group than for the LT group. With large samples, even small differences can give rise to significant p values (Bakan 1970). Since the follow-up intervals differed so much, the comparison between the ST and LT groups (Table 16.2) becomes extremely difficult to interpret. What appears to be significant and pervasive improvement as a consequence of fairly mainstream treatment can just as well be a methodological artefact caused by the short follow-up interval in the LT group.

However, even with a prolonged and uniform follow-up interval the problem of compliancy would remain. Although the ST and LT groups were similar in many important respects, commitment to programme goals or approval of the treatment orientation may have been greater among those who stayed for more than two weeks. This interpretation is strongly suggested by experimental comparisons showing that programmes of a few weeks to a few months duration have no better outcome than a period of brief inpatient stay (p. 26 above).

In summary, the evidence marshalled by McLellan and his colleagues (1982) on behalf of the general effectiveness of alcoholism treatment is not very convincing. In contrast, the value of their diagnostic and evaluative instrument is great enough to warrant a separate examination.

16.2   The Addiction Severity Index

The Addiction Severity Index (ASI) is a structured clinical interview developed by McLellan and his colleagues (1980*a*, 1980*b*; 1985*b*) to fill the need for a multidimensional diagnostic and evaluative instrument in the field of alcohol and drug abuse. The research group at the Philadelphia VA started by examining more than 70 admission surveys, questionnaires, and indexes used to assess various dimensions of alcoholics' functioning. They criticized most of these instruments for only concentrating on information regarding the patient's drinking pattern (e.g. the widely used Michigan Alcoholism Screening Test, MAST; Selzer 1971). Marital and occupational resources have, for example, proved to be of vital importance for the rehabilitation potential of alcoholics (Bromet and Moos 1977; Cronkite and Moos 1980). Yet many instruments lack items that shed light on the patient's resources in these respects.

According to McLellan *et al.* (1980*a*, 1980*b*), even the more comprehensive instruments are so influenced by a particular orientation, for example a psychological perspective, that the overall picture they provide is biased. Information on patients is considered relevant only to the extent that it can be interpreted within the cherished conceptual framework. This bias may go so far that an alcohol-oriented questionnaire will have no items concerning drug abuse. In addition, many comprehensive interviews were judged to be difficult to summarize from different clinical aspects and to quantify for research purposes. Others make no attempt to separate objective information from subjective reports. Finally, the instruments are often lengthy and difficult to administer.

The design of the ASI is based on the premise that alcohol abuse and those problems which are associated with such behaviour must be considered together. The questionnaire provides a multidimensional description of problems that is reminiscent of Pattison's treatment profiles (Chapter 14). As previously mentioned, the Penn-VA researchers differentiate seven clinically relevant problem areas: medical status, employment/support status, alcohol use, drug use, legal status, family/social relationships, and psychiatric status.

Two aspects of the ASI are deserving of special attention. In the first place, the severity of problems within each area is defined as 'need for additional treatment'. The authors (McLellan *et al.* 1980*a*, 1980*b*) illustrate the implications of this definition by using the example of a patient who has very poor eyesight, which has been corrected by glasses. This patient would still be considered to have a severe vision problem if severity were defined as 'deviation from optimal function'. But from the perspective of the ASI, the problem is negligible since no additional treatment would be required. This operational definition of severity relates directly to the primary mission of health care: the delivery of treatment.

Another important aspect of the ASI concerns the relationship between the problem areas. Each area is judged as objectively and comprehensively as possible, without reference to other areas. Items that concern medical health, for example, seek to ascertain in an unbiased manner the current state of health and past medical history of the patient. In other words, they are not solely concerned with health problems that are clearly alcohol-related. In this way filtering of information through a given treatment philosophy can be avoided.

Information on the severity of patients' problems is collected and presented in a standardized way, providing the basis for a *reliable* and *valid* evaluation (see Chapter 13). The assessment within each area is based in part on objective information regarding the number, extent, and duration of problems, and in part on the patient's subjective rating of the severity and importance of problems during the previous month. After objective information has been collected, the interviewer makes a quantitative severity rating. This rating is then modified based on the patient's own perception of his problems.

The interview takes about 45 minutes to administer. The interview and the scoring can be carried out by a non-professional after a brief period of training. In McLellan's project, the alcoholics are only given the ASI after they have remained in treatment for at least five days, to protect validity and to avoid assessment of patients who will not be followed up.

The assessment of, for example, psychiatric severity is based on the patient's previous and current symptoms of anxiety, depression, confusion, paranoia, trouble controlling violent behaviour, etc. The rating does not take into account problems in other areas, for example alcohol or drug abuse, family-related problems such as divorce or a family that is heavily involved in abuse, or work-related problems such as unemployment or casual work.

The psychiatric severity rating, as well as other severity ratings, have proved to be reliable and valid. McLellan et al. (1980b; 1985a) report an inter-rater reliability for the severity ratings of around 0.90, and a test-retest reliability of the same magnitude, even when the initial interview and the reinterview were performed by different persons.

Comparisons between the psychiatric severity rating and results of psychological tests (Health–Sickness Rating Scale, Schedule of Affective Disorders and Schizophrenia, Maudsley Neuroticism Scale, Beck Depression Inventory, Hopkins Symptom Checklist, and a measure of cognitive impairment) produced correlation coefficients of 0.60 or higher (McLellan et al. 1983a). The correlation between the ASI psychiatric severity rating and the intelligence quotient was, however, low (0.13). In summary, the psychiatric severity scale provides a valid global estimate of the extent to which the patient suffers from psychological disorders.

The ASI was used by the Veterans Administration Medical Center in Philadelphia as a basis for the planning of treatment (McLellan, personal communication 1984). Severity ratings were used for matching alcoholics to clinics (Section 16.4) and for identifying treatment needs within each clinic. Problems rated at five or more on the ten-point severity scale are considered to warrant special treatment.

Severity ratings are not, however, used as an evaluation criterion. Composite scores have been developed for this purpose (McLellan et al. 1985b), composed of those items from each problem area that are capable of showing change. The follow-up interview asks for the problem severity during the past month. It is normally conducted by telephone and takes about 20 minutes. McLellan's programme in Philadelphia, which admitted around 1250 patients per year, employed two half-time students for the admission interviews, while conduct of the follow-up interviews rotated between all researchers in the project (McLellan, personal communication 1984).

The diagnostic and evaluative instrument described above gave McLellan and his colleagues (1981c) a means to examine (a) the relationship between the severity of alcohol abuse and severity of problems in other areas,

Table 16.3 Pretreatment correlations of problem severity measures

	Employment	Alcohol use	Drug use	Legal	Family/ social	Psychiatric
Medical	0.11	0.15	0.01	0.00	0.07	0.10
Employment		0.17**	0.03	0.00	0.02	0.10
Alcohol use			−0.09	−0.01	0.11	0.07
Drug use				0.73**	0.12	0.04
Legal					0.04	0.15
Family/social						0.33**

**$p < 0.01$

and (b) the relationship between improvement in drinking behaviour and improvements in other areas. The subject group consisted of 460 alcoholics who were admitted for treatment during 1978 and followed up six months later (see Section 16.1). The dropout rate was 17 per cent.

Table 16.3 presents pretreatment correlations between severity measures in the ASI problem areas. The correlation coefficients are quite low. The significant relationships (between alcohol abuse and problems with employment/ support, between drug abuse and legal status, and between psychiatric status and family problems) are scarcely surprising. What is more notable are the low correlations between alcohol abuse and problems in other areas.

Table 16.4 describes the relationships between change scores from admission to follow-up on each problem severity measure. Once again, the correlation coefficients are strikingly low. This is particularly true of the relationships between changed drinking behaviour and changes in other areas. An improvement of psychiatric status is the only change that shows any relationship with improvements in most other areas, including drinking behaviour.

Table 16.4 Correlation between change scores on problem severity measures from admission to follow-up six months later

	Employment	Alcohol use	Drug use	Legal	Family/ social	Psychiatric
Medical	0.06	0.07	0.04	0.02	0.07	0.23**
Employment		0.16**	−0.03	−0.06	0.09	0.19**
Alcohol use			0.04	0.03	0.21**	0.21**
Drug use				0.13	0.02	−0.01
Legal					0.01	0.11
Family/social						0.29**

**$p < 0.01$

These low inter-correlations may seem perplexing. Many evaluations have, after all, showed general improvements in legal status, employment, and social relationships following treatment for alcoholism. McLellan and his co-authors (1981c) maintain, however, that the improvements from admission to follow-up that have been observed in previous studies (e.g. Emrick 1974) represent average changes in a subject group. These results do not necessarily mean that most patients presented with most problems and were improved in most areas. They can just as well be a result of the fact that different groups of patients with different problems aside from alcohol dependence showed changes of different kinds. The careful observations made by the Penn-VA researchers with the aid of the Addiction Severity Index support the latter interpretation (McLellan et al. 1980b, 1981c).

The research group emphasizes, however, the fact that the interval from admission to follow-up was only six months, which maximizes short-term effects of treatment. It is quite possible, they point out, that stable improvement in the employment, family, and legal problem areas may require a continued control of drinking behaviour. More recent studies by Pettinati et al. (1982a) and Fink et al. (1987) support the suggestion that the correlation between severity of alcohol abuse and severity of problems in other areas is greater with a longer follow-up period. Pettinati and his co-workers found that over a four-year follow-up period a decreasing proportion of patients were able to drink and still function well in other areas. Fink and his co-workers observed between two follow-ups, 12 months and 24 months after treatment, the same tendency, especially regarding the relationship between drinking behaviour and physical health, psychological health, and readmission for treatment.

But even if changed drinking behaviour is a *necessary* condition, it is not always a *sufficient* condition for improvement in other areas. Moreover, the relationship between alcohol consumption and problem severity in certain other areas is probably reciprocal (Chapters 8, 10). Finney and his co-workers (1980), for example, have shown how the family situation and other environmental influences promote or counteract a stable remission of alcoholism.

The Addiction Severity Index has proved to be quite useful in making individualized treatment plans, predicting treatment response, and assessing outcome of treatment. It has been widely applied and is even recommended for use in cross-cultural research (Hendriks et al. 1989). However, the validity of the instrument can probably be further improved. This is particularly true of the problem severity measure in the area of alcohol use. The usefulness of this measure would most likely increase if it were tied to WHO's concept of dependence and to attempts to assess the degree of alcohol dependence (Chapter 7).

16.3 The role of psychiatric severity

McLellan and his colleagues have used the ASI to examine whether the outcome of treatment can be improved by a deliberate and consistent pairing of clients and interventions. The subject group, 460 alcoholics at the Coatesville and Philadelphia Veterans Administration Medical Centers, have been described above (Section 16.1). After admission for alcoholism treatment at either hospital, patients were assigned to one of four rehabilitation programmes on the basis of personal request, the clinical judgement of the admitting staff, administrative considerations (e.g. bed census), and simple chance.

Following are brief descriptions of the programmes:

1. *The alcohol clinic.* This is a 60-day therapeutic community based on the principles of Alcoholics Anonymous (AA) as well as notions derived from psychoanalysis and transactional analysis. The staff conducts small-group therapy four times weekly.

2. *The research clinic.* This is an extension of a research programme designed to examine and treat alcoholism in an environment with periodic access to alcohol in limited quantities. Group and individual therapy are offered daily during the six-week treatment cycle (see Thornton *et al.* 1979). The programme is not intended to teach controlled drinking. After termination of treatment, patients are referred to AA.

3. *The combined clinic.* This is a 45-day programme that delivers intensive milieu therapy as well as some individual therapy and educational material to both alcoholics and drug addicts. Treatment is based on the principles of AA and Narcotics Anonymous. The programme was originally set up to save money by co-ordinating the resources of different treatment units (LaPorte, MacGahan, and McLellan 1979).

4. *The outpatient clinic.* This is a variable-length treatment programme that concentrates on the medical, psychological, and social problems of outpatient alcoholics. Therapeutic goals include alcohol abstinence through referral to AA and the alleviation of medical and psychological problems associated with alcoholism.

The research group's (McLellan *et al.* 1981*d*, 1983*a*) initial examination of the evaluation, which took place six months after admission, indicated hardly any significant interaction between patient characteristics, programme type, and outcome regardless of criterion (medical, employment, alcohol use, drug use, legal, family/social, psychiatric). The outcome measures had been adjusted statistically prior to interaction analysis for variations with regard to age, race, education, number of previous treatment periods, problem severity within each area prior to treatment, treatment duration, and type of discharge (favourable/irregular). This initial result seemed to confirm the findings presented by previous major studies in the field (e.g. Armor et al. 1978).

However, McLellan and his colleagues found a highly significant ($p < 0.001$) relationship between the ASI psychiatric severity score on admission and the treatment outcome six months later. Significant relationships were seen on five of the seven outcome measures of the ASI. Severe psychiatric problems led in general to poor outcome of treatment. The psychiatric severity measure alone accounted for an average of 12 per cent of the total outcome variance across the seven criteria.

The patients' severity of employment/support difficulties showed the next-highest correlation with the treatment outcome six months after admission. This predictor was significantly correlated ($p < 0.01$) with three of the seven outcome measures. The remaining admission severity scores were usually well correlated with the corresponding measure at follow-up, but not with other outcome measures.

Psychiatric severity was of such importance for treatment outcome that the researchers decided to divide the sample into a *low*, a *middle* and a *high* group, based on their psychiatric severity scores on admission. It was assumed that different patient groups might exhibit qualitatively different interaction patterns. The division into subgroups was made on purely statistical grounds. The sample mean on the psychiatric severity scale, plus/minus one standard deviation, differentiated the middle group. This group included 60 per cent of the alcoholics. Individuals who had psychiatric severity scores less than or greater than one SD from the mean of the middle group were classified as belonging to the low group (22 per cent of the alcoholics) and the high group (18 per cent), respectively.

Table 16.5 presents results of a study by McLellan et al. (1981a) in which 131 alcoholics were asked whether they had experienced significant periods of depression, anxiety, suicidal thoughts, hallucinations, or cognitive confusion (trouble thinking, remembering, concentrating) which did not occur while under the influence of alcohol. Patients in the low group generally had no symptoms of psychiatric problems or had slight problems of anxiety or minor depression in their past. Patients in the middle group had, for example, recent symptoms of depression, anxiety, or cognitive confusion, but no clear history of recurrent symptoms. Patients in the high group generally reported repeated periods of intensive anxiety, suicidal thoughts, clear thought disorder, or cognitive confusion.

The division into subgroups revealed significant relationships that had been masked in the initial analysis of results for the subject group as a whole (McLellan et al. 1983a). The low group, i.e. patients with no or insignificant psychiatric symptoms on admission, showed significant improvement and

Table 16.5 Alcoholics in low, middle, and high psychiatric severity groups who had experienced significant periods of symptoms

| | Severity group | | |
| | Low (N=26) % | Middle (N=82) % | High (N=23) % |
Symptoms			
Depression	15	63	90
Anxiety	11	57	100
Suicidal thoughts	3	29	50
Suicide attempts	3	14	31
Hallucinations	—	4	68
Cognitive problems	7	41	59

the best outcome across virtually all criteria six months later, regardless of which treatment programme they entered. According to the Penn-VA researchers, the characteristics of this group is suggestive of the small group of patients described in the first Rand report (Armor *et al.* 1978) who were able to return to 'social drinking' (without symptoms of dependence), and of those patients in the study by Edwards and Orford (Edwards, Orford *et al.* 1977*a*) who seemed to benefit from 'advice' alone.

Alcoholics with severe psychiatric problems (the high group) showed little improvement and uniformly poor results regardless of which treatment they entered. The authors did not feel that any of the programmes available at the Coatesville and Philadelphia Veterans Administration Medical Centers were very effective with these patients. One particular difficulty is the fact that the psychiatric problems of this group are not generally ameliorated by alcohol abstinence alone.

However, McLellan *et al.* (1981*a*) assert that inpatient alcoholism treatment nevertheless has a place as a first step in the extended treatment of alcoholics with severe psychiatric problems. In the experience of the authors, purely psychiatric programmes are notoriously ineffective in dealing with these alcoholics, who are unable to control their drinking long enough to allow an adequate diagnosis to be made and appropriate medication to be administered. A month or two of alcoholism rehabilitation can improve the general status of these patients enough to permit conventional psychiatric treatment in an inpatient or outpatient setting.

When the high and the low psychiatric severity groups (who together made up 40 per cent of the subject group) had been excluded, several significant *interaction effects* emerged (McLellan *et al.* 1983*a*). Patients in the middle group with greater than average employment or family problems showed, for example, worse outcomes in the outpatient programme than in other programmes. This finding was consistent with the authors' clinical experience. The outpatient clinic often seemed to be able to deal effectively with severe alcohol abuse and even with medical or legal problems. Patients with fairly severe psychiatric problems, in combination with employment and family problems, on the other hand, seemed to do better in inpatient treatment.

Moreover, the research group found that two of the inpatient programmes, the alcohol clinic and the research clinic, achieved poor outcomes with those patients in the middle group that had severe legal problems. However, such problems did not appear to be a contra-indication for the other treatment programmes at the Coatesville and Philadelphia Veterans Administration Medical Centers. McLellan (personal communication 1984) described these patients as 'sociopaths' and guessed that they were unable to cope with the less structured approach at the alcohol and research clinics.

It should be emphasized that all of the patients studied had been admitted to treatment for a primary problem of alcoholism (McLellan *et al.* 1981*a*). Even patients in the group with severe psychiatric problems had been judged to be in sufficiently good condition to be able to benefit from alcoholism treatment. They also stayed as long in treatment and had as high a proportion of favourable discharges as other patients. Furthermore, the sample only included patients who had remained in a rehabilitation programme for at least five days, which in the authors' experience means that patients with extreme psychiatric problems had been eliminated through early dropout.

These research findings underscore the importance of paying attention to *psychiatric/psychological* predictors and indications for alcoholism treatment programmes. McLellan and his co-workers (1983*a*) point out that previous studies have concentrated excessively on demographic variables and measures of the alcohol problem itself. This is thought to explain why efforts to predict treatment outcome have been so ineffective. However, the research conducted by the University of Pennsylvania in collaboration with the Coatesville and Philadelphia VA is innovative in still another respect. For the first time in alcoholism treatment research, retrospective analyses of interaction have been followed up by a documented prospective study of matching.

16.4 Matching—a prospective study

The subjects in the prospective study of patient–treatment matching were 238 male alcoholics admitted for treatment at the Coatesville and Philadelphia Veterans Administration Medical Centers during 1980. Forty-nine of the men (21 per cent) dropped out within five days and were thereby excluded from the sample. Of the remaining 189 alcohol patients, McLellan and his co-workers (1983*b*, 1983*c*) were able to follow up 178 (94 per cent) six months after admission.

After five days of detoxification and stabilization, patients were assigned to one of the four rehabilitation programmes that had been studied two years earlier (see previous section). In the meantime, a couple of directors and some other personnel had been changed. Some programmes had moved to different quarters. However, no programme had changed its treatment orientation or its programme length.

Matching of patients to programmes was accomplished by a decision-tree model (Table 16.6). The assignment criteria were the patients' problem severity ratings on admission, graduated from 0 to 9 on the seven scales of the Addiction Severity Index. The psychiatric severity rating on the ASI was used at an initial stage to assign patients to a low (0 to 2 on the severity scale), a middle (3 to 6), or a high (7 to 9) severity group. These intervals had been derived by the retrospective study (Section 16.3).

At the second stage in the decision-making, the severity of patients' other problems was rated on the ASI, and each individual was assigned to the most appropriate programme. Table 16.6 describes the criteria that were used. Specific components within the three psychiatric severity groups are ranked according to their weight in the decision strategy. The selection criteria are based on the results of the preceding retrospective study. (The minor

Table 16.6 Decision hierarchy with criteria for assignment of 179 alcoholics to appropriate treatment programmes

If psychiatric severity is low (0–1), and . . .
  . . . employment severity is greater than 6, then choose any of the inpatient clinics, but not the outpatient clinic.[a]
Otherwise, choose the oupatient clinic.
Matched: 31 of 47 (66%); mismatched: 16 of 47 (34%).

If psychiatric severity is middle (2–5), and . . .
  . . . legal severity is greater than 4, then choose the combined clinic or the outpatient clinic, but not the research clinic or the alcohol clinic.
  . . . employment severity is greater than 4, then choose any of the inpatient clinics, but not the outpatient clinic.
  . . . family severity is greater than 5, then choose the research clinic or the alcohol clinic, but not the combined clinic or the outpatient clinic.
Otherwise, choose the outpatient clinic.
Matched: 49 of 83 (60%); mismatched: 34 of 83 (40%).

If psychiatric severity is high (6–9) . . .
  . . . try to transfer the patient to a psychiatric ward. None of the above clinics is able to offer these patients appropriate treatment.
Matched: 0 of 49 (0%); mismatched: 49 of 49 (100%).

[a]For description of the treatment programmes, see Section 16.3.

deviations from the previous conclusions that occur in the decision hierarchy can be ignored here.)

None of the patients was denied continued treatment. But for different reasons, only 62 per cent of the patients were 'matched' to appropriate treatments in the manner prescribed by the model (Table 16.6). The major ground for not matching was lack of bed availability or a treatment slot in the appropriate programme (approx. 27 per cent). Approximately 13 per cent of the 'mismatches' were due to the patient's refusal or inability to accept assignment to the programme, while about seven per cent were due to simple assignment errors or clinical overriding of the decision strategy. It is important to note that the staff members in each of the programmes were unaware of which patients were 'matched' and which were 'mismatched'.

In the following analysis, McLellan and his colleagues (1983c) compared the during-treatment and six-month follow-up performance of (a) those patients who were treated in the programme which was predicted to be best for them (*matched patients*) and (b) those patients who were treated in a programme other than the one which was predicted to be best for them (*mismatched patients*). Given the facts that pretreatment problem severity of the two groups was essentially the same, that treatment programmes were the same for all patients, and that treatment staff were unaware of which patients belonged to which group, any better performance by the matched patients was taken as evidence that the matching procedure was effective.

As can be seen in Table 16.6, high psychiatric severity patients were considered to be mismatched in all programmes. As a consequence, the mismatched group included a high proportion of severely impaired persons which could distort the result of the comparison with matched patients. The Penn-VA researchers therefore eliminated all high severity patients from the data prior to the main analysis.

Table 16.7 shows the during-treatment performance of the low and middle psychiatric severity groups. The results indicate that the matched patients were significantly more motivated ($p < 0.01$), stayed in treatment longer ($p < 0.05$), and had a higher proportion of favourable discharges ($p < 0.05$) than their mismatched counterparts. (A more detailed analysis indicated that it was mainly in the outpatient programme that the length of stay and the type of discharge were affected by the matching procedure.)

Table 16.8 compares the status six months after admission of matched and mismatched patients belonging to the low and middle severity groups. The comparisons between matched and mismatched patients (last column) have been adjusted statistically for differences with regard to age, race, number of previous treatments, and pretreatment severity within each ASI problem area. The matched patients showed significantly ($p < 0.05$) better outcomes than their mismatched counterparts with respect to medical condition, employment, drug use, legal status, and family/social relations. Six of the seven follow-up comparisons showed better outcome for the matched patients.

Table 16.7 During-treatment performance of matched and mismatched alcoholics, excluding those with severe psychiatric problems

Criterion	Matched (N = 80)	Mismatched (N = 50)
Motivation		
Resistant to treatment	25%*	36%*
Motivated for treatment	61%**	46%**
Length of treatment	60 days*	52 days*
Discharge		
Favourable discharge	63%*	46%*
Irregular discharge	33%	45%
Considered appropriate for the programme by treatment staff[a]	86%	82%

*$p < 0.05$; **$p < 0.01$.
[a] A printer's error (transposed percentages) in the source has been corrected after personal communication with McLellan, 1984.

Drinking behaviour was slightly more improved in the *mis*matched group, but the difference is not statistically significant.

McLellan and his co-workers (1983c) found positive effects of matching both in the low and middle severity groups and in all of the treatment programmes examined. Thus, the outcomes showed consistency. The results indicate that the factors which were predictive of treatment outcome in the retrospective study in 1978 were again predictive in the prospective study two years later. This was considered noteworthy in view of the poor history of replicated results in treatment outcome research and in view of the changes in the patient population and the programme personnel that took place between the two studies.

According to the authors, the outcome could scarcely be a result of the fact that mismatched patients started treatment with more negative expectations than matched patients. Most of the mismatched patients had chosen their treatment programme themselves. In fact, it was more often the case that matched patients were directed to a programme which they had originally not planned to enter than that mismatched patients ended up in such a programme.

This study is the only prospective study of matching in the treatment of alcoholism that has been published. All studies that are presented in Part IV below are retrospective. In view of this, the evidence given for the fruitfulness of the matching hypothesis and the efficacy of the systems approach hold particular promise.

Table 16.8 Follow-up performance of matched and mismatched alcoholics, excluding those with severe psychiatric problems

Problem area[a]	Matched ($N = 80$)	Mismatched ($N = 50$)	Between-group comparisons[b]
Medical	275	350	$p < 0.05$
Employment	357	437	$p < 0.01$
Alcohol use	217	186	—
Drug use	11	33	$p < 0.05$
Legal	24	101	$p < 0.01$
Family/social	210	263	$p < 0.05$
Psychiatric	121	134	—

[a]Problem severity was rated during 30 days before admission and before follow-up six months later. Higher scores indicate greater severity.
[b]With statistical control for age, race, number of previous treatments, and pretreatment problem severity.

By evaluating a system of treatment units, and not just individual programmes, the Penn-VA researchers showed that alcoholism treatment can be made more effective without requiring additional personnel, equipment, or facilities. Unlike many other cost-saving measures, the matching process was generally well accepted by both patients and staff. Patients were assigned to treatments that had the best record of dealing with their particular problems, and treatment staff received the type of patients with whom they had had the most success. O'Brien, Woody, and McLellan (1983) argue that there is now evidence indicating that in the long run flexible, multimodality treatment systems are the most cost-effective approach to the treatment of substance abuse.

The researchers at the Philadelphia VA believed that their success can mainly be explained by the fact that they took into account psychiatric severity in deciding which programme was most appropriate for a particular patient. A global estimate of psychiatric impairment turned out to be the best general outcome predictor in the study. This finding was replicated by McLellan *et al.* (1986) in a study of two alcoholism treatment centres with different populations including adolescents, females, and patients from higher socioeconomic strata. Pretreatment psychiatric severity has also proved to be a robust predictor of outcome in drug abuse treatment (McLellan *et al.* 1983*a*, 1983*c*; Woody *et al.* 1983) and outpatient psychotherapy (Mintz, Luborsky, and Cristoph 1979). The Penn-VA researchers recommended that this factor always be taken into account in the selection of psychosocial treatment.

According to McLellan and his co-workers (1983*c*), low severity patients can almost always be assigned to outpatient programmes. This alternative is usually as effective as inpatient treatment, but at a much lower cost. High severity patients, on the other hand, were believed to require some psychiatric treatment as a part of their treatment for alcohol abuse.

Both the findings of the study and the authors' clinical experience indicate that patients with more severe employment or family problems do less well in outpatient treatment. The research group believed that an extended inpatient rehabilitation programme can help these patients to concentrate on their rehabilitation while providing a respite for the patient's family. It is therefore presumed that measures of employment and family problems are also of general importance for treatment selection.

According to the Penn-VA researchers, more specific predictors (e.g. legal status) are not necessarily the most important for other treatment populations, other programmes, or other times. They are expected to change as a result of changes in the programmes or the patient populations. The authors believe, however, that their methodology for research and development is widely useful as an effective and relatively inexpensive method of determining which specific factors affect outcomes with different patient groups and with different kinds of programmes. McLellan and his co-workers (1980c) maintain that

given the many sources of variation in a treatment network, the development of a generalizable evaluation process may be more useful and feasible than an attempt to discover one set of generalizable predictive factors. (p. 194)

One of the cornerstones of the Penn-VA Project is the multidimensional diagnostic and evaluative instrument, the Addiction Severity Index (ASI). With this index, positive effects of matching were revealed that would not have been discovered with a conventional measure of the change in drinking behaviour. The research group did not find any differential impact on the alcohol problem itself.

Since the correlation between alcohol abuse and problems in other areas tends to increase with time (p. 160 above), the gains of matching can be expected to gradually decline. With this in mind, the results appear less encouraging. On the other hand, researchers, administrators, and therapists in alcoholism treatment should get used to the idea that short-term and limited effects are better than no effects at all—especially if they can be achieved without additional resources and without an experimental research design with a control group that receives no or minimal treatment.

Part IV

Studies of interaction

There is a growing interest in the interaction between client, intervention, and outcome in the treatment of alcoholism. However, the discussion has been based on a body of rather unsystematically collected and reported empirical data. Part IV examines reports dealing with the effects of interaction (see also Sections 12.4, 16.3), including important investigations that have arrived at negative results and a few pertinent studies from neighbouring areas of research, such as psychiatry, education, and criminology.

Research on interaction can be classified according to the client characteristics examined. Studies that have arrived at negative results with regard to interaction concentrated, with few exceptions, on a heterogeneous set of demographic and clinical (primarily alcohol abuse) variables. By contrast, researchers who have been able to demonstrate client–treatment interaction studied psychological characteristics (including degree of alcohol dependence), sometimes in combination with demographic variables. Those lines of research that have proven to be fruitful examined personality traits, a combination of social and psychological resources, cognitive styles, and degree of alcohol dependence.

In the following review, different lines of research are arranged according to the order in which they emerged in the field of alcoholism treatment research. Each approach is introduced with the pioneering study. This is followed by a presentation in chronological order of research that has examined similar client attributes. Each study is evaluated, and the most important ones are analysed in sufficient detail to provide the reader with a fairly clear idea of the validity of their conclusions.

Readers who are more interested in the conclusions of this review than in the path taken to arrive at them can skip to Part V, where the results of the interaction studies are summarized and interpreted.

17 Research methodology

Studies of the effects of interaction between client characteristics and treatment dimensions offer no clear-cut answers. Several major studies have arrived at negative results (see Chapter 18). Neither the first Rand report (Armor *et al.* 1978), Smart (1978*b*), Finney and Moos (1979), or Stinson *et al.* (1979) found any evidence to support the assumption that a client's prognosis is affected by the extent to which his or her individual characteristics are matched to the particular orientation of the treatment.

However, three of these studies are non-experimental, which makes it more difficult to discover interaction effects (Skinner 1981*b*). Skinner (1980*b*) pointed out:

> Clearly, if one is to have a fair test of the 'matching hypothesis' then treatment interventions must be appreciably distinct and all client types should be equally represented in each programme. In brief, there is no substitute for a controlled study that involves random assignment of client types to interventions. All short-cuts are problematic. (p. 252)

Nor is a randomized controlled trial unproblematic (Cook and Campbell 1979; IOM 1990). Selective dropout, for example, is a factor to be reckoned with, since some clients may not accept the treatment to which they have been assigned. Emrick (1975) further claimed that patients in alcoholism treatment who receive treatment of a lower intensity or prestige can be demoralized if they find out that there are other treatments that have a better reputation and involve a greater commitment of resources. This control group effect can retard improvement and distort research results. Nevertheless, the experiment is the method that can most convincingly demonstrate the effectiveness of treatment (see p. 22 above).

But experimental clinical research is expensive and time-consuming. In practice, it is therefore often necessary to take 'short-cuts', no matter how problematic they may be (Gottheil, McLellan, and Druley 1981). The limited applicability of the experimental model for the study of treatment outcome does not warrant its rejection in principle, nor does it justify resorting to anecdotal reports or arbitrary evaluation criteria. There are, however, many options between the experiment and the anecdote for innovative, rigorous, and systematic research (cf. Chapter 16).

Campbell and Stanley (1963) proposed that the quasi-experimental approach be used '*where better designs are not feasible*' (p. 34; ital. in orig.), i.e. where the possibility of random assignment to experimental conditions does not exist. The quasi-experimental design, which is the most common in alcoholism treatment research, studies client groups that have been assigned to treatment conditions in a non-random fashion. The effect of other factors than the treatment is statistically controlled for. Since the factors in the treatment situation and their predictive validity are poorly understood, however, this design is inadequate for assessing the effectiveness of alcoholism treatment as compared to no treatment (see Section 3.1). Nevertheless, it can, as in some of the studies examined below, suggest the existence of an interaction between client, treatment, and outcome.

Single-subject experimentation (Kratochwill 1978; Kazdin 1982; Barlow *et al.* 1984; Barlow and Hersen 1984) and case studies (Kazdin 1981) are other valuable auxiliaries to the true experiment. In order for these approaches to provide valid information on rehabilitation effects, an independent follow-up of the client's progress after the conclusion of treatment is naturally necessary. Some authors (Barlow *et al.* 1984; Barlow and Hersen 1984) claim that single-case experimental designs with time-series analysis can very well be used to study interaction effects. It is simply a matter of confronting a sufficient number of clients with the relevant treatment conditions (clinical replication).

Kazdin (1982) pointed out, however, that the result will be unsatisfactory unless it is ultimately possible to distinguish between the effects of client characteristics, treatment dimensions, and possible external factors. Group studies with a control group or statistical controls are more appropriate for research on interaction, since they permit the simultaneous study of one or more independent variables (multivariate analysis). In the present study, conclusions about interaction effects will therefore be based primarily on *experimental* and *quasi-experimental* group studies.

The general purpose of summarizing and evaluating the literature is to 'find the knowledge in the information' (Glass 1976). Science is a cumulative enterprise. To extract useful knowledge, we must compare and systematize the results of individual studies. Treatment outcome research is no exception in this respect.

The traditional procedure in research reviews has been reporting the theoretically relevant studies, reviewing them from a methodological point of view, and then tallying up the number of relevant and methodologically acceptable studies that confirm versus fail to confirm the studied relationship. This method has been called into question, however. Greenwald (1975) has shown that both researchers and editors of scientific publications are prejudiced against results that reject tested hypotheses. Null results of the type 'no effect of treatment' are often left unreported or filed away in a drawer. The 'file drawer problem' (Rosenthal 1979) can in turn lead to an overestimation of the scientific support that exists for current treatment theories (Smith 1980; Kurosawa 1984).

Other researchers have maintained that the method of tallying up the significant relationships found in various studies weakens the inferences being drawn. Light and Smith (1971), for example, pointed out that this procedure, which they called *taking a vote*, disregards the size of the sample. Large samples lead more often than smaller ones to 'statistically significant' effects. Suppose, they said, that we have ten studies available, each with ten subjects. Suppose further that only one of the ten studies shows a statistically significant treatment effect. Using a voting procedure, we would probably conclude that the treatment is ineffective. However, if all 100 subjects were 'pooled' into the equivalent of a single large study, a highly significant treatment effect might have emerged.

Light and Smith's (1971) example should be viewed as hypothetic. Considering the widespread prejudice against results that reject preferred hypotheses (Greenwald 1975), it is unlikely that researchers would carry out nine replications of a study that has yielded almost only negative results, and that editors of scientific publications would print nine reports from studies that—with samples consisting of only ten subjects!—reject the same hypothesis.

However, small samples are often used in treatment outcome research, which in itself predisposes to the conclusion that there are no differences between treatment conditions. Gibbs and Flanagan (1977) were scarcely able to find any stable general prognostic indicators in alcoholism treatment. One reason for the conflicting results may be that the size of the sample in the theoretically relevant studies varied from 24 to 2323! The authors noted that in studies with 99 or fewer subjects, an average of 4.7 significant predictors were reported, while the significant predictors in studies with 100 or more subjects averaged 8.8.

Shapiro and Shapiro (1982) found in a review of 132 evaluations of psychotherapy that the difference in outcome between treatment and control groups was significantly ($p < 0.001$) less in studies with more subjects. This finding may be a consequence of the tendency to only publish statistically significant results ('the file drawer problem') and the fact that effects do not have to be as large in a study with many subjects in order to be significant. With a large sample, effects found to be significant at the 0.05 level are mostly of such a moderate size that they are only of limited clinical relevance.

Consequently, statistically significant effects are neither a *necessary* nor a *sufficient* criterion of the value of a treatment. Myers (1972) remarked that: 'in practice we expect the experimenter to use his brains as well as his F ratios to draw inferences' (p. 169).

Of course, no statistical technique can take the place of an intimate knowledge of the field of research. The statistical significance of a relationship is a rather uninteresting measure for most purposes unless the investigator is well acquainted with the pattern of symptoms, personal characteristics, and social situation of the treatment population studied.

In the present review of interaction effects, the presentation of the design of the relevant studies is more detailed than in previous reviews, which, with one exception (Ogborne 1978), lack a consistent methodological evaluation. The purpose of the detailed, critical account is not only to enable the reader to judge the validity, generalizability, and clinical relevance of the findings; because the field of interactions is high on the agenda of alcoholism treatment research, it may also be of interest in itself to evaluate the designs that have been used.

Where possible, a combination of quantitative and qualitative data has been utilized. But unfortunately, reports on patient–treatment interaction rarely provide more than fragmentary information on the therapeutic process, the context of the intervention, and clients' perception of the treatment received. Taken individually, therefore, the observed effects of interaction are often difficult to interpret.

Since the research literature on interaction between client, intervention, and outcome in alcoholism treatment is very limited, I have, where warranted and possible, broadened the perspective by including examples from research on psychotherapy, education, and corrections. These accounts are intended to identify interesting client factors, important problems, and fruitful research designs.

18 Studies with negative results

18.1 Rand Report I

A study funded by the Rand Corporation (Armor *et al.* 1978; Polich *et al.* 1981) showed that approximately 40 per cent of around 800 male alcoholics, randomly selected from eight programmes in different parts of the USA, were improved four years after they had begun treatment (see also Section 21.2). The Rand study found a weak correlation between the amount of treatment received by a person and his condition at follow-ups 18 months and four years after admission. These findings seem to support the common claim that clients often drop out of treatment before it has had any effect. However, clients were not randomly assigned to conditions with differing amounts of treatment. Therefore, other interpretations are also possible, according to the Rand group (Polich *et al.* 1981, p. 212–3). For example, clients who had a poor initial prognosis or who failed to respond to treatment could have dropped out at an early stage.

No correlation was found to indicate the superiority of a given type of treatment over another (e.g. inpatient versus outpatient treatment). Nor did Rand Report I (Armor *et al.* 1978, pp. 130–51), which presented data from follow-ups six and 18 months after intake, come up with any evidence to indicate that specific client groups were changed in different ways within programmes of different kinds. Client characteristics—both severity of alcoholism symptoms and the client's social stability and socioeconomic status—had a substantial impact in all treatment settings studied: hospital care, intermediate care, and outpatient care alone or in combination with either hospital or intermediate care. However, client factors explained only 10 per cent of the total variance in treatment outcome. Client factors and treatment factors together explained 13 per cent of the total variance.

The uniformity of treatment effects suggests a policy of substituting outpatient programmes for more expensive hospitalization programmes, summarized the Rand researchers. They added—in view of the apparent importance of amount of treatment—that very short-term intervention should be avoided in favour of slightly longer treatment periods.

However, a number of objections can be raised to the Rand reports that limit the validity of the conclusions. There are, for example, several studies that have compared the outcome for clients that have been assigned randomly to treatment programmes of varying duration (Section 3.1). These trials all showed that there was no overall advantage in outcome from longer treatment programmes. Thus, the body of evidence supports the alternative view suggested by the Rand group, namely that the correlation between 'amount' of treatment and remission rates was an effect of biased sampling. For example, socially stable alcoholics may have completed treatment to a higher extent than socially unstable alcoholics.

However, certain subpopulations of alcoholics may benefit differentially from longer programmes. In fact, the results of an inpatient study by Feuerlein and Küfner (1989) indicated 'the necessity of making available treatment of different lengths' (p. 156). But the non-randomized assignment to programmes of varying duration and the inconsistent results prevent more specific conclusions from being drawn.

Reverting to Rand Report I, another argument concerns the absence of interaction. Armor and his co-workers (1978) cautioned that they had used the clients' drinking behaviour as the only evaluation criterion. A broader measure of improvement might have changed the overall picture and perhaps affected the study of interaction between client characteristics, type of treatment, and outcome.

The Rand group also made the questionable assumption that the treatment settings studied did offer qualitatively different types of treatment. Since the details of the various programmes are not described, it is quite possible that their goals and methods were very similar. The setting—hospital, intermediate, or outpatient—may be of subordinate importance for the outcome with clients that differ only in clinical and social respects.

Even if the treatment methods were different, the quasi-experimental design does not rule out the possibility of self-selection resulting in a non-random distribution of clients among different programmes. As a consequence, the influence of client selection may mask the effect of any interaction between client characteristics and type of treatment.

Moreover, the interaction study in Rand Report I included only a few client attributes. Psychological characteristics, expectations, and other subjective factors were not investigated. Finally, Rand Report II (Polich et al. 1981) demonstrated a complex relationship between client characteristics (age, marital status, degree of alcohol dependence), nature of improvement at 18 months (abstinence or 'normal' drinking), and outcome at the four year follow-up. This finding supports the hypothesis that matching clients to treatment goals, at least, may improve the outcome of alcoholism treatment (see Section 22.2).

18.2   Smart

Reginald Smart (1978b) has reported the results of a large-scale evaluative study of about 1100 alcoholics from seven treatment facilities, both inpatient and outpatient, in Ontario. Clients were given thorough interviews and tests both at intake and at follow-up one year after they had begun treatment.

In the processing of data, 186 interactions were examined. These encompass 31 client characteristics (12 demographic variables, 11 scale scores, eight assessments of drinking habits) and six characteristics of the treatment (outpatient versus inpatient, profession of principal therapist, medical assessment, length of treatment period, group therapy versus individual therapy, type of medication). Smart found no statistically significant effects of interaction to indicate that some clients did better with one treatment programme than with another. Together, client characteristics and treatment variables explained only a fraction (six per cent) of the total variance in outcome (change in drinking behaviour).

Smart's study is one of the most comprehensive and detailed investigations of interaction in the treatment of alcoholism. It has, however, the same kind of deficiencies as the Rand reports. The use of group therapy versus individual therapy, for example, does not say much about the treatment content. Glaser (1984c) proposed that psychosocial interventions should instead be classified according to what sort of problem they most appropriately deal with. Such a classification—which was tested in the core-shell system in Toronto (Chapter 15)—emphasizes highly specific attributes of the treatment, thus making the matching hypothesis more relevant.

18.3   Finney and Moos

Finney and Moos (1979) presented a more complete picture of their subjects than the first Rand report (Armor et al. 1978) and Smart (1978b), which studied how single client attributes influence the outcome of treatment. Finney and Moos combined a number of social and psychological background variables in order to achieve a fairly broad description of a manageable number of clinically relevant types of alcoholics. Previous attempts to divide alcoholics into homogeneous subtypes, for example Knight's (1937) distinction between 'essential' and 'reactive' alcoholics, have, according to the authors, been either simplistic or overly concerned with personality differences. Moreover, clients have usually been drawn from a single programme, which is one reason why empirical analyses of the effects of interaction between client type and treatment orientation are so rare in the literature.

Finney and Moos (1979) were able to follow up 429 of 494 alcoholic clients, randomly selected from five inpatient programmes, six months after termination of treatment. Complete background information was obtained on admission for 387 persons (Bromet, Moos et al. 1977), who were thus chosen as subjects for the investigation. There were no statistically significant differences in social or psychological respects between the group followed up and the dropout group.

Statistical cluster analysis was used to group the alcoholics into eight types, six of which were used to study the presence of interaction effects: low social competence and low personal resources, low social competence and medium resources, low social competence and high resources, high social competence and low resources, high social competence and medium resources, and high social competence and high resources.

The five treatment programmes were chosen to represent a broad spectrum in terms of both therapeutic orientation and clientele. They included a private aversion conditioning facility, a private programme with a therapeutic community orientation, a halfway house with an emphasis on individual counselling and group therapy, a public hospital-based programme, and a Salvation Army facility offering milieu therapy and vocational training.

No interaction was found between client type, therapeutic orientation, and outcome in terms of drinking behaviour, alcohol-related disabilities, or social adjustment. The prognosis for the identified alcoholic types seems scarcely to have been influenced by which treatment programme they entered. Clients with different social and psychological characteristics were not, however, evenly distributed among the five programmes. Alcoholics with low social and psychological resources were more often found in the Salvation Army facility, at the public hospital, and in the halfway house, while the high-resource alcoholics were overrepresented at the aversion conditioning clinic and in the therapeutic community.

Finney and Moos are not the only Anglo-Saxon researchers to have found a relatively homogeneous clientele in different alcoholism treatment programmes. Similar results have been described by Schmidt, Smart, and Moss (1968), Pattison, Coe, and Doerr (1973), Edwards, Kyle, and Nicholls (1974), and English and Curtin (1975). Skewed selection of clients to different programmes makes it more difficult to detect any interaction effects. The absence of statistically significant effects of interaction may sometimes stem from the fact that clients who are not suitable for a given type of treatment are screened out from the start or quickly drop out of the programme.

Cronkite and Moos (1978), in a report using the same clinical material as Finney and Moos (1979), have described a statistical path analysis that takes into account *indirect effects* of different variables, i.e. effects that are mediated by other variables. The analysis showed that treatment variables explained a considerably larger proportion of the variance in outcome than would have been expected on the basis of previous research. The effect of treatment variables was as great or greater than (depending on the outcome criterion) the effect accounted for by client characteristics alone. The kind of treatment, however, did not even explain one per cent of the outcome variance, regardless of criterion. Almost all of the effect accounted for by treatment variables was due to variation in treatment experiences (amount of treatment, level of participation in programme activities, length of stay) and in clients' perception of the programme.

However, these treatment variables were closely related to social background characteristics. The indirect effects indicate that high-resource clients are

(a) more motivated to become involved in programme activities and thus receive more treatment, and (b) function better within the programme and thus perceive the environment as being more positive. The effect of such congruence between client characteristics and treatment variables has been underestimated in previous research and attributed to client variables alone, note Cronkite and Moos (1978).

The authors maintain that it is unwise to conclude from the body of research that all patients should be placed in uniform low-cost treatment programmes. The results of their study indicate that it would be sounder to study how the choice of treatment and matching can *indirectly* influence the outcome by having an impact on clients' perceptions of programme activities and their actual participation in such activities.

18.4 Stinson

David Stinson, William Smith, Imat Amidjaya, and Jeffrey Kaplan (1979) compared four systems of care in northern Illinois to get answers to the following questions: Are certain systems of care more effective than others? Are certain systems of care more effective with alcoholics who have specific characteristics?

The four systems of care were obtained by combining two inpatient programmes with two outpatient programmes. The inpatient programmes had a length of four to six weeks. The *intensive incare* programme had a high staff–patient ratio, based on the assumption that intensive staff–patient interaction is of vital importance in rehabilitation. Staff-directed group processes formed the cornerstone of this approach. Treatment interventions included psychotropic medication, individual counselling, family therapy, group therapy, role playing, audiovisual playbacks of therapy sessions, alcoholism education, sociotherapy, vocational counselling, and participation in AA meetings. Aftercare planning began early and received heavy emphasis. Family, friends, employers, and clergy were drawn into the treatment process whenever possible. The entire programme was organized and carried out by a close-knit treatment team.

The *peer-oriented incare* programme had a low staff–patient ratio and operated under the assumption that patient-to-patient interaction plays a critical role in rehabilitation. The newly admitted patient was assigned to a self-governing group of patients, each of which had a professional consultant at its disposal. The patients were encouraged to initiate, implement, and evaluate their own incare management plans. They devoted an average of only 1.26 hours daily to treatment, while the equivalent number of hours in the intensive programme was 3.79.

The *network outcare* programme consisted of an organized set of community services to meet the rehabilitation needs of alcoholics. Detoxification units, halfway houses, specific outpatient and emergency services, etc. were available to the alcoholics. The consortium kept careful track of each patient and made efforts to involve the discharged patient in as many active services as he was judged to require. The *informal outcare* programme had no co-ordinated management and small resources. Patients sought out mental health clinics, AA groups, and the like on their own initiative. The cost per capita was only one-third of that for the network programme.

All adult admissions during one full year with a primary diagnosis of alcoholism were randomly assigned to one of the two incare programmes. No patients were excluded. Patients who remained in the network area for at least one year were designated as the network outcare group. Those who moved to another area without a network were classified as patients in an informal outcare programme. In other words, each patient was treated in one of the following systems of care: intensive incare and network outcare; intensive incare and informal outcare; peer-oriented incare and network outcare; or peer-oriented incare and informal outcare.

The research group compared the outcomes of these systems for 466 alcoholics of both sexes. The four treatment groups were found to be roughly homogeneous in clinical and demographic respects. The follow-up period extended for 18 months after admission. The dropout rate was 14 per cent. The outcome criterion was drinking behaviour and social adjustment. Family members were also interviewed.

As expected, all treatment groups showed a significant improvement from admission to follow-up. However, there were no differences between the four systems on outcome measures—with one exception. In terms of *drinking behaviour* a significantly higher rate of success was achieved with the *peer-oriented incare* programme than with the intensive incare programme.

The proportion of clients whose drinking behaviour was improved 18 months after they had begun treatment was 68 per cent with the peer-oriented programme as compared to 57 per cent with the intensive programme. In a quasi-experimental study with a follow-up period of six months after discharge, Welte *et al.* (1979) arrived at a similar result: severely alcohol-dependent patients improved more with peer-oriented than with medically or psychologically oriented programmes. Stinson *et al.* (1979) speculate that patient responsibility and engagement are greater in peer-oriented programmes. However, the results do not warrant any definite conclusion on the value of peer-orientated versus professional treatment of alcoholics (see also Section 19.3).

Stinson and his co-workers used 13 demographic and clinical characteristics to determine whether certain systems of care were more effective than others with certain types of alcoholics. The variables considered were sex, age, education, marital status, vocational skills, rural–urban origin, father alcoholic, mother alcoholic, years of heavy drinking, years of problem drinking, days of treatment prior to study, pattern of drinking, and longest abstinence. The researchers were not able to find any interaction between patient background, system of care, and outcome that could be used to differentially assign patients to the most appropriate treatment. The authors did not categorically rule out the existence of interaction effects, but they suggested that personality characteristics and individual motivation have to be investigated in order to identify such effects. Stinson and his co-workers' study supports the first Rand report's (Armor *et al.* 1978) and Smart's (1978*b*) conclusion that the outcome of alcoholism treatment is probably not very much influenced by interactions between demographic or clinical characteristics and treatment intensity or modality. The question of what constitutes effective treatment appears to be much more complex and to involve psychological characteristics as well.

Smart (1978*b*) concluded his large study with the following comment:

Most treatment variables . . . were all unimportant. Again these results are similar to those in the Rand study . . . However, the Rand study examined only one treatment variable related to the in-patient/out-patient dimension. The results do not mean, however, that some other combinations of treatment may not interact with these or other patient characteristics. Perhaps if treatment were more clearly defined and fewer patients received combinations of treatments, more differences would be found. Experimental studies where patients are randomly assigned to treatments may also give more positive results. (pp. 74–5)

A research strategy of the type applied by the first Rand study, by Smart, and by Stinson and his co-workers has occasionally been called statistical 'fishing expedition' (e.g. Maher 1978). Those who employ this metaphor probably envision modern trawl-fishing. The studies to be examined in the following chapters can, in contrast, be compared to fly-fishing. A fly-fisherman must know the subtleties of the art, be familiar with the waters as well as the kinds of fish and their habits, and last—but not least—he or she must be equipped with good intuition. That is, anyone trying to identify effects of interaction would be well advised to choose his variables with care and be guided by a reasonable notion of what occurs in the process of treatment.

19 Personality traits

19.1 Wallerstein

Between 1950 and 1952, Robert S. Wallerstein (1956, 1957) directed an alcohol research project at the Winter Veterans Administration Hospital in Topeka, Kansas. This hospital is affiliated with The Menninger Foundation and was the main teaching locus for The Menninger School of Psychiatry. Wallerstein's project has been widely discussed mainly because of the successful results that were achieved with Antabuse treatment. When the study was initiated, this was a new and untried method. Today, however, the study is regarded increasingly as a pioneering effort in the attempt to differentiate treatment by co-ordinating clients and interventions in a deliberate and consistent manner.

The project started at a psychoanalytically oriented treatment unit for alcoholics with a closed-ward setting. The treatment efforts that had been pursued in this and similar treatment programmes had met with such discouraging therapeutic results that serious questions were raised as to whether the programme was really accomplishing anything for the alcoholics and their families.

Wallerstein and his associates decided to create an experimental treatment unit to test the most recent treatment methods. They chose to compare four methods: Antabuse, aversion ('conditioned-reflex') therapy, group hypnotherapy, and milieu therapy. This latter experimental modality was originally intended as a control modality. It proved, however, to have its own inherent therapeutic qualities, despite the fact that there was no specific treatment of the patients' alcoholism. Owing to the lack of alternatives to 'talk therapy', the patients were more or less forced to avail themselves of the standing invitation to individual and group psychotherapy to a greater extent than was done in the other experimental groups.

The project included 178 male patients, who were randomly assigned to the four experimental groups. All patients had volunteered for the programme. They underwent treatment for 60 to 90 days on a single ward with 25 beds and access to individual therapy, occupational therapy, and a recreational programme. All patients attended group therapy once a week, except for the milieu therapy group, which requested permission to meet its group therapist twice a week as a compensation for the absence of a special therapeutic device.

Wallerstein (1957) observed that most evaluational studies had either used a follow-up period that was too short or restricted their interest to complete abstinence, without taking into account the social and psychological adjustment of the patients. He chose to follow up his subjects every other month during a two-year period following discharge. The evaluation criteria included drinking behaviour, social adjustment, psychological well-being, and an assessment of personality dimensions.

The purpose of the study was two-fold. In the first place, Wallerstein wanted to find out if any of the treatment methods is preferable to the others. In the second place, he wanted to find out if there are any special indications that point towards a given treatment method being most appropriate for a given type of patient.

Differential treatment indications presuppose an understanding of the patient, the treatment method, and the interaction between these two components. During the first month after admission, a thorough psychological and medical examination of each individual patient was therefore carried out. The examination included a series of psychiatric interviews and a projective test (the Szondi Test). The examination results were presented at a case conference with the entire psychoanalytically oriented project staff, who made a diagnosis of certain personality traits on the basis of these results. Any personality changes were determined through clinical interviews and personality tests at the follow-up visits.

The first question was answered in the negative: none of the treatment methods was so superior to the others that it could be recommended as the single best method. Treatment with Antabuse did give the best results overall, but certain contra-indications also emerged which showed that Antabuse could be highly inappropriate in certain cases.

The second question gave rise to interesting clues for continued research. In a subsequent reexamination of the results, Wallerstein identified a number of personality dimensions along which patients might be differentiated in terms of suitability for one or another of the specific therapies. There seemed to be an interaction between the 'psychological meanings' of the treatment methods and the psychic 'needs' of the individual patients.

Antabuse treatment entails that the alcoholic submits to a form of external control that inhibits relapses. Wallerstein found that the more compulsive the patient's personality was and the more he could ritualize the Antabuse ceremony itself, the better his prognosis was after discharge from the treatment programme. It did not matter which diagnostic category the patient belonged to otherwise (character disorder, neurosis, psychosis, etc.). Improvement in individual patients was often accompanied by a shift towards increasingly compulsive personality traits. Many patients said that they had to keep themselves busy so that they would not be tempted to stop taking Antabuse and return to drinking.

Many succeeded in maintaining their new-found compulsive defences chiefly due to their close ties to the hospital and the therapist. According to Wallerstein, the Antabuse pill became the daily concrete symbol of a new dependence. Of the nine patients who improved and could be followed up throughout the agreed-upon two-year period, six had relapses at the end of their formal contact with the hospital. In all cases it was their first drinking binge in two years. Wallerstein draws the conclusion that an effective treatment with (and without) Antabuse may require a continuing relationship of indefinite duration.

Some patients were incapable of making the commitment to total abstinence entailed by the Antabuse treatment. In the present study, this group consisted of 'latent schizophrenics' and severely depressive patients, who were said to use alcohol as a kind of self-medication. Of five 'latent schizophrenic' patients, only one was helped to an improved state by Antabuse. The only chronically depressive patient in the Antabuse group became even more depressed than before when he left the hospital in a sober state. He completely lost hope when he became aware of his incapacity to realize his fantasies of how life might have been if only he did not have the bad habit of drinking. After a period of suicidal thoughts, he resumed drinking and returned to his old fantasies of how different life could have been if he had been able to stay sober.

Kissin (1977b) and others have confirmed the observation that Antabuse therapy is seldom successful with depressive patients. It is a reasonable assumption that the rehabilitation of alcoholics with severe mental disturbances requires a combination of treatment for alcoholism and psychiatric treatment (cf. treatment of drug addicts; Woody et al. 1984). Vaillant (1983b, p. 208 ff), who claims that most alcoholics are depressed because they drink and not vice versa, emphasizes that the more severe the alcohol dependence has been, the longer time must be allotted for rehabilitation.

Aversion therapy, says Wallerstein, can best be conceptualized psychologically as representing a punishing agent, directed from the outside, which the individual is powerless to control, but must instead somehow internalize and assimilate. Our attention is therefore drawn to personality dimensions that relate to the individual's characteristic reaction to aggression and his psychologic 'need' for punishment. The empirical data also showed that the strength of the patient's aggressiveness could be used as an indication of his ability to respond effectively to aversion therapy (Table 19.1).

More aggressive patients were significantly less successful than others, regardless of which evaluation criterion was used. They tended to be provoked rather than helped by the threat of punishment. If patients who did not maintain a regular contact during the two-year follow-up period are considered as failures, as recommended by Baekeland et al. (1975), then the

Table 19.1 Outcome of aversion therapy by level of aggression

Level of aggression	Improved	Unimproved	Lost to follow-up
Less aggressive	8	1	11
More aggressive	4	16	10
Total	12	17	21

improvement rate in the less aggressive group is 40 per cent, while the improvement rate in the more aggressive group is only 13 per cent. If only 75 per cent of all patients lost to follow-up are classified as failures, which may be a more realistic procedure (Laundergan 1982), the improvement rates are 54 and 22 per cent respectively.

No such difference between 'less' and 'more' aggressive patients was found in the Antabuse group or in the milieu therapy group. There was, however, a similar, though weaker, tendency in the group treated by *group hypnotherapy*, a technique whose effectiveness in treating alcoholics remains controversial (Stoil 1989). Here the more aggressive group was more difficult to hypnotize and less prone to complete the treatment programme and the follow-up. According to Wallerstein, hypnotherapy posed a threat to the defences of aggressive patients against deep-seated dependency longings, causing *reaction-formation* (i.e. an exaggerated resistance to being influenced by others). The more openly passive-dependent the patients were, the better they responded to hypnotherapy.

The depressed patient responded well to aversion therapy. The perception of punishment can, claims Wallerstein, help alleviate guilt and externalize the aggressive charge. In contrast, very passive or masochistic personality traits appeared to be a contra-indication, since aversion therapy could reinforce these accustomed neurotic reaction patterns. There were, however, too few depressive, masochistic, and passive patients for Wallerstein to draw any conclusions in these respects.

The effect of *milieu therapy*, finally, was not affected by the psychiatric diagnosis of the patients. On the other hand, Wallerstein found a clear relationship between treatment outcome and the patients' relationship to the doctor, the hospital, and the treatment programme. It was found that a general *attachment factor* based on marital status, work adjustment, and sexual adjustment could be used as a prognostic indicator (Table 19.2).

Characteristic of milieu therapy was the fact that the patients had to assume the major responsibility for change. They could not rely on external agents. The ability to form stable, predominantly positive attachments to other people is naturally of great importance in all forms of therapy. But its relative significance was heightened in the milieu programme, owing to the absence of any specific, 'extra' treatment. Those who succeeded with milieu

Table 19.2 Outcome of milieu therapy by attachment factor

Attachment factor	Improved	Unimproved
Positive	10	5
Negative	1	10
Total	11	15

therapy were primarily the small portion of the alcoholics who were able to benefit from conventional psychotherapy. But Wallerstein also recommends milieu therapy for patients who tend to fail in the other treatment programmes.

Wallerstein's hypothesis that an attachment factor influences the outcome of milieu therapy is indirectly supported by a study within the field of educational research. Chan (1975, 1980) has demonstrated a statistically significant relationship between, on the one hand, students' *need for affiliation* and, on the other hand, the probability that they will benefit from small-group studies over individual studies for generating hypotheses, and their tendency to prefer learning in small groups to learning on their own.

Wallerstein (1957) regarded his study of the interaction between personality dimensions, treatment modalities, and outcome as a first step on the road to individualized treatment programmes for alcoholics. However, he did not believe that the study was sufficiently large in scope to say with confidence which of the four programmes offers each patient the best prognosis.

Wallerstein's experimental design has a number of limitations. Therefore great caution is required in interpreting the results. The admission criteria were, to be sure, more generous than at many other American treatment institutions. But the least treatment-motivated group was nevertheless excluded, by virtue of the requirement that patients were to seek admission on a voluntary basis. In addition, only four treatment methods were investigated and, for natural reasons, none of the cognitive or social-learning models that have been tried out during the past decade. Furthermore, the methods were offered in a special way, with special (psychoanalytically oriented) therapists and in a special care setting (a closed-ward programme lasting between two and three months).

The dropout rate during the two-year follow-up period varied from 15 per cent in the Antabuse group to 42 per cent in the group treated with aversion therapy. Those who were lost to follow-up were classified as failures. This method can be criticized in a study with several treatment groups with different dropout rates. Wallerstein does not take into account the possibility that certain improved patients may have broken the contract after discharge because they felt no need to maintain contact with the hospital.

A serious objection to Wallerstein's study and other psychoanalytically oriented studies is the low reliability of personality descriptions based on psychiatric interviews (see Chapter 13). Bloch and his co-workers (1977), for example, had 27 teams, each with three highly experienced psychiatrists, evaluate the severity of the clinical state of some 40 patients. As a basis for this evaluation, they had for each patient a videotaped, loosely structured interview of one hour's duration. The interview revolved around a list of problems prepared by the patient and the patient's responses to a standardized questionnaire intended to measure the psychiatric symptom level. The members of the teams were supposed to rate the severity of the problems of each individual patient along a scale from one to nine. The result was discouraging. Only three of the 27 teams achieved a level of agreement between the members that was significant at the 0.05 level.

Wallerstein did supplement the clinical assessment of the patients with a projective test. But such tests also have low reliability and validity, especially when they are used to identify a whole array of personality traits (Anastasi 1968). Perhaps Wallerstein has put far too much faith in what the noted psychotherapy researcher Morris Parloff, quoted by Bloch *et al.* (1977), called: 'one of the most favourite convictions/myths in the field of psychotherapy, namely, that the well-trained expert clinician is our most finely honed and sensitive research tool' (p. 412).

Moreover, the psychiatric diagnoses were made not before, but during ongoing treatment and on the basis of, among other things, a series of interviews with the psychiatrist on the ward where the trial was being conducted. This constitutes a threat to the validity of the diagnoses, since it is difficult to distinguish between what is an expression of the patient's basic personality and what is a reaction to the treatment. Nor is it improbable that the ward psychiatrist's and the project group's hypotheses as to which patients are suitable for a given programme may have influenced the diagnosis.

Finally, it should be added that Wallerstein's study has great merits as well. These make it interesting as more than just a historical example. The combination of quantitative and qualitative data, of experimental methodology and case studies etc. is a virtue that many modern research manuals (e.g. Patton 1980) subscribe to, but is rarely practised as consistently and creatively as by Wallerstein. The ambition to follow up alcoholics after conclusion of treatment on repeated occasions over such a long period as two years still has few parallels. Studies of interactions including psychological variables are equally rare.

19.2   Annis and Chan

The approach represented by Wallerstein (1957), at once both experimentally and psychologically oriented, is once again being taken up in treatment research. Helen Annis and David Chan (1983) at the Addiction Research Foundation in Toronto have presented a study of interaction between personality traits, treatment method, and results that meets stringent methodological requirements. Although it is a criminological study, the conclusions can be assumed to have a considerably broader range of application.

Annis and Chan state that there is a growing interest within correctional research in how to tailor treatment programmes to specific offender groups. However, there is as yet no agreement on how offenders should be classified. The authors decided to base their classification on the personality dimensions *self-image* and *interpersonal relation pattern*. These dimensions are commonly used in criminological theory, but no one had previously applied them to test for differential treatment effects.

The study group consisted of 150 adult male offenders with alcohol and drug problems sentenced to two years at a minimum security correctional institution. All subjects had volunteered to participate in an intensive, highly confrontational group therapy programme consisting of 224 hours per man over a period of eight weeks (Annis 1979). The study group was randomly assigned to two experimental conditions: 100 persons were assigned to group therapy (the treatment group), while 50 persons received routine institutional care only (control group).

An analysis of the background of the offenders confirmed that the treatment group and the control group were comparable as regards demographic characterstics, type of convictions, and drug use. The mean age of the subjects was 25 years, with a range of 18 to 64 years. Fifty-seven per cent of the men reported a daily alcohol consumption equivalent to at least 12 bottles of beer (seven or more fluid ounces of absolute alcohol); 51 per cent had used marijuana, 41 per cent LSD, 41 per cent amphetamine, 15 per cent heroin, and 12 per cent cocaine.

Two types of offenders, one with a positive and the other with a negative self-image, were identified by means of a hierarchical cluster analysis based on eleven personality measures. Although reconviction, rather than relapse, was the outcome measure, Bohman *et al.* (1982) found that the number of criminal convictions is correlated with the severity of alcohol abuse within alcoholic criminals.

The study arrived at three notable findings:

1. The intensive group therapy programme failed to produce overall lower recidivism rates than did routine institutional care. This finding is consistent with the usual observation that a variation of treatment measures does not have any significant influence on the offenders' criminal career (Sechrest, White, and Brown 1979).

2. The offenders' self-image generally did not influence the probability of recidivism. Persons with a positive self-image returned to crime just as often as persons with a negative self-image. This finding is contrary to a few earlier studies, where a connection was found between self-image and the likelihood of recidivism.

3. Although no significant overall effect of either treatment condition or offender type was observed, there was evidence of a significant effect of inter-action between type of treatment, self-image of offender, and outcome with respect to number of reconvictions ($p < 0.05$) and the severity of the most serious offence ($p < 0.01$) during the year following release (see Fig. 19.1). Offenders with a positive self-image who had participated in the intensive group therapy exhibited fewer reconvictions and less serious offences than offenders in the control group. However, offenders with a negative self-image who had gone

through the intensive group therapy exhibited *more* reconvictions and *more* *serious* offences than offenders who received only routine institutional care.

It should be added that the interaction between self-image and treatment method accounted for only a modest percentage of the outcome variance (11 to 16 per cent), measured in terms of number of reconvictions and severity of offence for a period of one year after release. Nevertheless, the measured interaction effects are superior to the average outcome ascribed by Gallo (1978) to psychologically oriented treatment compared to no treatment at all. At the present-day level of knowledge, every positive result—no matter how modest—is worth further examination.

Annis and Chan draw the conclusion that if confrontational group treatment experiences are to be offered to offenders with alcohol and drug problems, careful selection of candidates would appear to be essential. The success of intensive group therapy seems to require a relatively positive self-image on the part of the participants.

The study illustrates the fact that even professionally administered, psychologically oriented treatment can be associated with risks (cf. Lambert, Bergin, and Collins 1977). The same conclusion has been drawn by Wilbur,

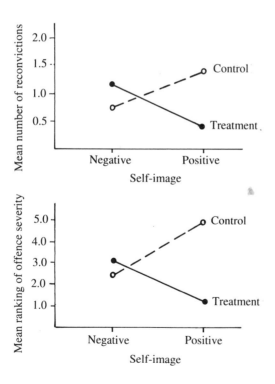

Fig. 19.1 Interaction between self-image, treatment condition, and recidivism.

Salkin, and Birnbaum (1966), Norman and Schulze (1970), and McLellan *et al.* (1984) in studies of the reactions of homeless alcoholics and mentally disturbed drug addicts to programmes that apply the principles of the *therapeutic community.*

19.3   Lyons and Sokolow

The observation that intensive group therapy with a confrontational content tends to have a negative effect on the prognosis for criminal alcohol and drug abusers with a negative self-image (Annis and Chan 1983) probably also has implications for the treatment of female alcoholics, who often have a very poor self-image (McLachlan *et al.* 1979). Joseph Lyons, Lloyd Sokolow, and their colleagues (Sokolow *et al.* 1980; Lyons *et al.* 1982) have presented results that underscore the need for more research in this area.

The research team investigated the outcome for 1340 clients from 17 inpatient treatment programmes in New York State, three and eight months after termination of treatment. They classified the programmes according to dominant treatment orientation: peer group oriented programmes, which are run by recovered alcoholics and paraprofessionals, psychologically oriented programmes, and medically oriented programmes (with prescription of Antabuse and tranquillizers).

The purpose was to study whether the treatment orientation influences different kinds of alcoholism clients in different ways. The clients were classified according to drinking pattern and demographic variables such as age, race, sex, socioeconomic status, and social stability. The criteria of success were abstinence, reduced alcohol consumption, and improved overall life situation.

Analysis of the outcome data revealed that the only demographic variable that significantly interacted with dominant treatment orientation was the sex of the client. Within the group labelled 'alcoholics' (with more severe symptoms than 'behaviourally impaired drinkers'), females did best when treated in medically oriented programmes, while men achieved the best outcome with the peer group oriented programmes.

Lyons *et al.* (1982) guess that the stigmatization to which the female alcoholics are subjected is alleviated by contact with a physician, which is presumed to support the concept of alcoholism being a disease. It is a common observation that female alcoholism is less socially acceptable than male alcoholism. McLachlan and his co-workers (1979) found that female alcoholics had very low self-esteem. It was concluded that treatment must first be aimed at strengthening the women's self-esteem.

In a further analysis of the evaluation data, Sokolow *et al.* (1980) found that an interaction between client sex and the percentage of women in a treatment programme had a statistically significant effect on the drinking outcome. Thus, more women were abstinent when treated in a programme with a lower proportion of women, while men had a more successful outcome when treated in a programme with a higher percentage of women. This finding is interpreted as suggesting that in a programme with fewer women, the attention paid to a female client tends to increase. As a consequence, the self-esteem of the female alcoholic may be enhanced.

Most of the subjects in the programmes studied by Lyons, Sokolow, and their colleagues were men. This fact limits the conclusions that can be drawn from the data. Sokolow *et al.* (1980) assume that a programme with women alone may have a different effect on its clients. This assumption has recently been corroborated by Dahlgren and Willander (1989) in a controlled study of women in an early stage of addiction, with no previous treatment for alcohol problems. These authors found that females treated in a programme with all women had a more successful outcome than women in traditional alcoholism treatment.

It is certainly not possible to draw any definite conclusions from Lyons' or Sokolow's findings. In the first place, the source of the findings is a non-experimental study with follow-up data only on the drinking pattern (alcoholism/behaviourally impaired drinking). In the second place, there was considerable overlap between different treatment orientations. In the third place, the dropout rate after eight months was 33 per cent. And in the fourth place, in a study with more than 1300 persons, the high probability of finding significant correlations in large samples must be taken into consideration (Bakan 1970). Biased selection, weak tendencies without clinical relevance, and similar factors can easily give rise to significant results with such a large group as the one studied by Lyons, Sokolow, and their colleagues.

Nevertheless, the hypothesis advanced concerning sex-specific interaction effects highlights a long-neglected field of research. In a total review of the English-language evaluation literature between 1950 and 1978, Annis (1980) found only 13 reports where the authors explicitly compared the treatment outcome for women and men. Data examining sex differences are specially rare among male authors (Vannicelli and Nash 1984). Thus, there are many opinions concerning the treatment of female alcoholics, but few established facts (see reviews by Annis 1980; Annis and Liban 1980; Vannicelli 1984; Blume 1986).

19.4   Personality typologies

Since no common personality traits of alcoholics were found (Chapter 8), many attempts have been made to identify several subtypes of alcoholics (see reviews by Nerviano and Gross 1983; Hesselbrock 1986; Morey and Skinner 1986). These classification schemes are called *typologies*.

The Minnesota Multiphasic Personality Inventory (MMPI) is the most widely used instrument in studies of alcoholic personalities (Clopton 1978; Graham and Strenger 1988). The instrument has been employed to compare the client make-up of different treatment programmes, to study how clients change over the course of treatment, and to identify relatively distinct personality types among alcoholic clients.

Skinner (1979, 1980*b*) developed a model of psychopathology with which he integrated the results of previous studies based on the MMPI. The model defines three superordinate clinical syndromes: a neurotic type, a psychotic type, and a sociopathic type. None of these personality types differentiate alcoholics from other psychiatric or normal groups. In a review of the MMPI literature Graham and Strenger (1988) identified at least six rather distinct MMPI profile types among alcoholics. In addition to the four profile types reported by Goldstein and Linden (1969), two types suggestive of psychiatric disorder were consistently found. As in Skinner's study, none of these profile types was found to be unique to alcoholics.

Most empirically derived alcoholic typologies have been used for descriptive purposes rather than for theory testing (Meyer, Babor, and Mirkin 1983). Only a few studies have investigated the treatment response of different MMPI personality types. Hypotheses concerning 'ideal' combinations of treatment and alcoholic subtypes based on the MMPI (Thurstin and Alfano 1988) and other inventories (Morey *et al.* 1984) have been formulated. But as yet no such hypothesis has been tested.

At present there is an emerging trend in the classification of alcoholics to reconsider the utility of theoretically derived typologies (Alterman and Tarter 1986; Hesselbrock 1986). Several classification schemes have been tried, including gender differences, psychopathology, and family history. In contrast to earlier theoretical models, recent formulations rest on a strong empirical base obtained largely from adoption, high-risk, and familial studies. Although conclusions based on these formulations should be tempered (Searles 1988), preliminary results suggest that aetiological and therapeutic conceptualizations can be integrated.

The two forms of alcohol abuse described by Cloninger (1987; Cloninger *et al.* 1981, 1988*a*, 1988*b*) comprise one of those typologies that are analytically most sophisticated. These subtypes, based on a series of adoption and family studies in Sweden and the US, can be distinguished in terms of distinct alcohol-related symptoms, personality traits, age of onset, and pattern of inheritance.

One form, type 1 alcoholism, is associated with loss of control, guilt feelings, and fear of dependence on the anti-anxiety effects of alcohol. This form of alcoholism is also called 'milieu-limited', since onset follows heavy drinking that is reinforced by external circumstances, usually in late adulthood (e.g. drinking at lunch or after work at the encouragement of friends).

The second form, type 2 or 'male-limited' alcoholism, is characterized by impulsivity, risk-taking, and a tendency toward antisocial behaviour, such as fighting in bars and drunken driving. This form of alcoholism, which is much less prevalent, usually has an early onset and is associated with a persistent seeking of alcohol for its euphoriant effects. It is strongly influenced by heredity and found exclusively in men.

In a study of successful long-term adjustment of alcoholics, Nordström and Berglund (1986, 1987c; Nordström 1987) investigated the predictive validity of the typology proposed by Cloninger. Fifty-five well adjusted male alcoholics, all having a life-time diagnosis of alcohol dependence, were personally followed up 20 years after their first admission to hospital. Three kinds of outcome drinking patterns were accepted as successful, namely abstinence, social drinking (no abuse days), and stable sporadic abuse (at most three abuse days per month). The stable sporadic abusers reported that drinking was generally confined to Friday or Saturday nights, or to vacations, so as not to interfere with work.

The categorization of the alcoholics into type 1 and type 2 was based on the criteria used by von Knorring et al. (1985a). Nordström and Berglund (1987c) found that patterns of successful adjustment differed between subgroups of alcoholics. The type 1 alcoholics who had improved were more often abstainers or social drinkers, whereas the majority of the type 2 alcoholics with an improved status were stable sporadic abusers. The finding that type 2 alcoholics were not able to become social drinkers or abstain entirely is attributed by Cloninger et al. (1988c) to their seeking of alcohol for its euphoriant effects. However, von Knorring, Palm, and Andersson (1985b) reported abstinence and social drinking in type 2 alcoholics as well.

Those who were stable sporadic abusers generally attributed their adjustment to social pressure and an experience of responsibility (Nordström and Berglund 1986). This finding is interpreted as indicating that the deficient internal control of most prospective sporadic abusers narrows the range of effective therapeutic factors, and that the social network should be integrated in the treatment of these alcoholics.

The finding that stable sporadic abuse is a feasible outcome for type 2 alcoholics and the hypothesis that social network involvement may be instrumental in promoting such an improvement are interesting. Since 'antisocial' alcoholics tend to have the worst outcome in traditional alcoholism treatment (e.g. Poldrugo and Forti 1988), innovative approaches are commendable. However, the clinical utility of emerging, theoretically derived typologies remains to be proven.

19.5 Kadden

So far, little research has been done on the relationship between personality and response to treatment. A recent study by Ronald Kadden, Ned Cooney, Herbert Getter, and Mark Litt (1989) in Connecticut suggests that this line of research may be clinically significant. Kadden and his co-workers investigated aftercare programmes that were considered to be representative of what is currently offered to alcoholics in the USA. Following completion of a three-week inpatient programme, eligible subjects were randomly assigned to either coping-skills training or interactional group therapy.

The coping-skills training was modelled after procedures used in cognitive-behavioural relapse prevention programmes (see Section 9.3) and provided a highly structured group experience. Therapists avoided focusing on interpersonal conflicts or feelings that developed among group members. The goal of the interactional therapy groups, in contrast, was to explore participants' interpersonal relationships and immediate feelings as they occurred in each session. Some structured techniques were used to facilitate the group process, but no specific advice about how to cope with problems was provided.

Of 505 subjects screened for the study, 162 had a diagnosis of alcohol dependence or abuse, completed the inpatient programme, were referred to weekly aftercare group treatment, and met the other criteria for inclusion in the study. The study group was made up of those 96 subjects who also consented to being randomly assigned to type of aftercare and who attended at least three aftercare sessions. Almost everyone in this group had a job, and about half of the subjects were married. Aftercare in both treatment conditions consisted of 26 weekly, one-and-a-half hour group sessions. Each therapy group was led by an experienced therapist who followed a detailed treatment manual. Therapists were supervised by the research staff to ensure a high level of treatment integrity (Yeaton and Sechrest 1981).

Data were obtained for 92 per cent of the subjects immediately after termination of aftercare treatment. The data indicate that overall, and in terms of both drinking behaviour and psychosocial adjustment, coping-skills and interactional treatments produced comparable results over the six months of treatment. This finding is consistent with other studies comparing cognitive-behavioural and interpersonal treatments for alcoholism (e.g. Ito, Donovan, and Hall 1988). Evidence for differential outcomes was found, however, when subjects were separated along the dimensions of *sociopathy* and *global psychopathology*.

Sociopathy was measured by the California Psychological Inventory-Socialization Scale, CPI-So (Megargee 1972). This instrument provides a continuous measure of antisocial behaviour and personality characteristics (e.g. guileful, deceitful, given to excess) that are indicators of sociopathy. A study by Cooney, Kadden, and Litt (1990) indicates that the CPI-So is a valid and easily administered measure of sociopathy in alcoholic patients. Global psychopathology was assessed by the Psychiatric Severity subscale composite score of the Addiction Severity Index (ASI; see Section 16.2), which is based on recent symptoms of anxiety, depression, cognitive confusion, and other psychiatric problems. Kadden *et al.* (1989) showed that sociopathy and global psychopathology were not closely related to each other.

Although other outcomes were examined, only drinking outcomes were related to the interaction between patient characteristics and type of treatment. Kadden and his co-workers found that coping-skills training was more effective for subjects higher in sociopathy and global psychopathology, whereas interactional therapy was more effective for subjects lower in sociopathy. Both treatments appeared equally effective for subjects lower in psychopathology. The authors concluded that their findings are supportive of the general notion of patient–treatment matching and of the importance of sociopathy and psychopathology in this process.

Kadden *et al.* argued that alcoholic patients with significant coexisting psychopathology are likely to find interactional therapy 'too challenging'. Since the interactional therapy relies on the development of good therapeutic relationships, the research group had expected it to be less effective with sociopathic patients who lack the social skills that facilitate the formation of meaningful relationships. Similarly, it is no surprise that patients who are able to form rich and deep relationships benefited from the interactional group therapy. The latter finding is consistent with Wallerstein's (1957) observation that alcoholics who were able to form stable attachments gained from a milieu programme (Section 19.1).

The study by Kadden and his co-workers illustrates the increasing sophistication of studies of alcoholism treatment and patient–treatment interaction. Treatment conditions were well defined, distinctively different, and representative; measures were taken to ensure that treatments were implemented as planned. The choice of prognostic indicators was guided by reasonable hypotheses about which patient characteristics are likely to affect outcome with specific treatments; indicators were measured by reliable and valid instruments. A large sample was used; patients were randomly assigned to treatment conditions; and higher order interaction, i.e. interaction between different combinations of degree of socialization and psychiatric severity, type of treatment, and outcome, were investigated (Section 23.4).

The major weaknesses of the study, also noted by Kadden and his co-workers, are its lack of posttreatment follow-up and its retrospective design. Since data were collected at the end of aftercare treatment, it remains to be seen whether the results are stable after the ongoing group support has been discontinued; this issue will be explored in subsequent reports by the research group. Another necessary step will be to match patients to treatments prospectively, since groups comprising patients who are homogeneous along a critical dimension (e.g. groups consisting of sociopaths only) may have a very different group process and treatment outcome from those of groups made up of a heterogeneous mix of patients (Finney and Moos 1986).

20 Social and psychological resources

20.1 Kissin

Benjamin Kissin and his co-workers (Kissin *et al.* 1968, 1970, 1971; Kissin 1977*b*) were long one of the few research groups conducting in-depth studies of which treatment modalities are most appropriate for different types of patients. In their most widely quoted study, they randomly assigned 458 male alcoholics to one of four groups: (a) outpatient drug therapy, (b) outpatient psychotherapy plus adjunctive drug therapy, (c) inpatient medical, social, and psychological rehabilitation, and (d) no treatment for six months (control group). Patients who rejected drug treatment were offered no alternatives. Those who rejected psychotherapy were offered drug treatment as the only alternative. Those who rejected inpatient rehabilitation were offered the choice between psychotherapy or drug therapy.

The purpose of the study was to find patterns of social and psychological characteristics that predict which modes of treatment a given patient will accept, and what the outcome will be once he has accepted one or the other treatment programme.

At the start of treatment, all patients were given a social interview and a number of psychological tests. Patients who, for example, were married, had 12 or more years of education, had a professional, clerical, or skilled occupation, and had not been arrested for any crime, were classified as socially stable. The psychological tests measured, among other characteristics, intelligence and 'field dependence' (the terms field dependence and field independence are put in quotation marks when they denote low or high cognitive restructuring ability as measured by the Embedded Figures Test, EFT; cf. Section 21.3).

Follow-up was carried out approximately one year after intake. It is not clear what this means in terms of follow-up time after discharge for each programme. However, an average follow-up interval of six to ten months is a reasonable conjecture (see e.g. Smart 1978*b* on length of stay in treatment). The follow-up interview was possible in only about 50 per cent of the original patients. Patients who were lost to follow-up were classified as treatment failures.

Kissin and his co-workers found that a combination of social and psychological background characterstics appeared to influence both acceptance of a treatment and treatment outcome. More socially and psychologically intact alcoholics tended to prefer outpatient psychotherapy to inpatient rehabilitation, while the opposite held true for less socially and psychologically intact alcoholics. However, these patient characteristics had no influence on whether or not drug treatment was accepted.

The evaluation criterion included improvement of drinking behaviour and psychosocial adjustment during the six-month period prior to follow-up. The treatment was considered successful if alcohol consumption was reduced to no more than one-fourth of its original level while psychosocial adjustment was markedly improved.

The research group found a statistically significant interaction at the 0.001 level between patients' social stability, treatment setting, and outcome. The successes in both of the outpatient programmes were significantly more socially stable than the failures, while the successes in the inpatient programme were significantly *less* socially stable than the failures.

Effects of interaction involving psychological characteristics were also reported. For example, those who succeeded with drug therapy were significantly more 'field-dependent', those who succeeded in psychotherapy were significantly more 'field-independent', while there was no difference in 'field dependence/independence' between those who succeeded and those who failed in the inpatient rehabilitation programme.

According to the authors' summary, the study shows that:

(1) socially stable and psychologically more sophisticated (high intelligence, 'field independent') patients did best in psychotherapy;

(2) socially stable and psychologically less sophisticated (low intelligence, 'field dependent') patients did best in drug therapy; while

(3) socially unstable and psychologically more sophisticated (high intelligence, 'field independent') patients did best in the psychosocially oriented inpatient programme.

Kissin *et al.* (1970) suggest that social and psychological characteristics should be attended to in the selection of treatment. At the same time, however, the authors feel that some choice should be offered, since the patients' preferences led to a fairly good match between their needs and the kind of treatment entered.

Kissin's study has several methodological shortcomings that make it difficult to generalize the results. Among other things, patients in the psychotherapy group were significantly more stable and sophisticated than patients in the rehabilitation programme (Ogborne 1978). This could have occurred by chance, but Kissin and his co-workers also note that certain clinicians tended to circumvent the random assignment procedure. Moreover, the treatment programmes varied considerably in terms of attractiveness and availability for choice. Of those who were assigned to inpatient rehabilitation, only one-fourth began this treatment, while many more patients entered drug therapy than were originally assigned to this treatment modality.

Persons who dropped out of treatment within a month were not followed up on the grounds that they had not been adequately exposed to any specific treatment (Kissin 1977b). Most other evaluations of alcoholism treatment have about five days as the minimum length of stay. All of this, in combination with the dropout rate of about 50 per cent and the questionable (LaPorte et al. 1981) method of classifying those who were not followed up as treatment failures, renders it extremely difficult to distinguish differential effects of treatment from methodological artefacts.

There are, however, several studies (e.g. Ludwig et al. 1970; Pattison et al. 1968, 1969, 1973; Schmidt et al. 1968; Trice et al. 1969) that point in the same direction as those carried out by Kissin and his co-workers. They confirm that socioeconomic status largely determines which programme an alcoholic will enter and what his response will be. There are, however, significant psychological differences between alcoholics in similar social conditions. One must therefore, it is argued, take into account both social and psychological factors to be able to predict preferences and outcomes.

According to Pattison (1974), who has summarized these studies, there is some empirical support for the following conclusions:

1. Alcoholics who have high 'social competence' (here: socioeconomic status) and high psychological competence with 'field independence' (i.e. high restructuring ability) would be candidates for psychotherapy.

2. Alcoholics who have high 'social competence' and high psychological competence with 'field dependence' would be suitable for aversion conditioning methods and perhaps for AA.

3. Alcoholics with high 'social competence' and low psychological competence would benefit from medical regimes and supportive types of psychotherapy.

4. Alcoholics with low 'social competence' and high psychological competence would respond to AA and to programmes emphasizing social and vocational rehabilitation.

5. Alcoholics with low 'social competence' and low psychological competence will require continuing supportive services; they are not likely to affiliate with AA, and will not benefit from solely medical or psychological regimes.

Homeless alcoholics, for example, have low socioeconomic status. However, this population includes individuals with both markedly low and relatively normal psychological competence. Homeless alcoholics are not a homogeneous group. But their deviant lifestyle is so conspicuous that personal resources are not noticed until they are actively sought out (cf. the Skid Row Scale; Halikas 1980).

The research which Pattison has summarized is open to criticism in various respects. Nevertheless, it has had a certain influence, at least in the US, as a guideline for the planning of treatment.

There are at least three reasons why the studies by Kissin and his successors have had this impact, despite their methodological shortcomings. In the first place, they take into account recent research, showing that alcohol dependence is a multivariant syndrome and suggesting that treatment services should be diverse. Secondly, the combination of social and psychological factors makes the research clinically relevant. Controlled studies of single client attributes often lead to results that are difficult to translate into clinical practice, since treatment must be based on an overall assessment of clients' resources.

Thirdly, the results obtained are congruent with 'clinical experience', or the implicit matching hypotheses that many practitioners embrace. Like Kissin, Pattison, and others, administrators and therapists tend to think of interventions in terms of 'packages', for example medically, psychologically, or socially oriented, rather than in terms of narrowly defined treatment methods.

The line of research described above takes account of the pluralism that characterizes alcoholism treatment today. Since the findings are based on experience from relatively conventional types of treatment, there is a risk that the recommendations will entrench the status quo. However, refraining from investigating what types of clients available programmes are likely to help will not reduce this risk.

20.2   Gibbs

Leonard Gibbs (1980, 1981; Gibbs and Flanagan 1977) has tried to compensate for some of the methodological shortcomings inherent in the research tradition represented by Kissin, while preserving its broad approach. Gibbs' goal was to develop a clinically useful procedure for classifying alcoholics. He pointed out that no existing classification met basic standards that are set in logic texts and in discussions of taxonomy.

According to Gibbs (1980), a classification must fulfil four requirements to be acceptable. It is *reliable* if individuals to be classified are consistently assigned to the proper category. This requires

(1) that the categories be mutually exclusive so that an individual cannot fall into several categories at the same time;

(2) that they be comprehensive so that every individual fits into some type; and

(3) that they be clearly defined so that different persons make the same classification decisions.

The classification is *valid* if the chosen characteristics are relevant to the purpose of the classification. With regard to treatment research in the field of alcoholism, this requires

(4) that the classification be based on those characteristics of alcoholics that have proved to be statistically associated with the prognosis, either in general or with treatment of a certain kind.

This last requirement reveals the Achilles' heel of alcoholism research. Gibbs and Flanagan (1977) found, from 1937 and onward, 45 methodologically acceptable studies of prognostic indicators. The studies, which followed up 55 treatment groups, investigated no fewer than 208 different indicators for their predictive efficiency. The diversity of indicators selected by investigators is assumed to reflect widely differing theoretical approaches to the problem of alcoholism, or perhaps a helter-skelter approach based on no theory at all.

The authors were not able to find any highly stable prognostic indicators, i.e. indicators which had been investigated in six or more treatment groups and which had predictive power in all of them. This result is hardly surprising, given the variety of therapists, treatments, definitions of alcoholism, treatment populations, sample sizes, follow-up intervals, and outcome criteria investigated or employed. However, Gibbs and Flanagan did identify a set of indicators that were associated with treatment response in at least half of six or more studies. These personal characteristics were assumed to have some general predictive value.

In a second research phase, Gibbs (1980) listed the 50 prognostic indicators that were most frequently evaluated and most powerful. These indicators were assigned to four hypothetical groups or clusters: social stability, intellectual functioning, general severity of the problem, and outliers/non-outliers. The hypothetical groups were compared with the groups of indicators obtained from a hierarchical cluster analysis based on interviews measuring all 50 of the prognostic indicators and administered to 80 male subjects at five treatment facilities. Two of the hypothetical groups passed the empirical test, so that Gibbs obtained one cluster called *social stability* (16 prognostic indicators) and another called *intellectual functioning* (eight prognostic indicators).

In a third phase, Gibbs (1980) devised standardized scales for both of the dimensions expected to have predictive value. These scales were used to assign each interviewed alcoholic to one of four categories: (Type I:) higher social stability and lower intellectual functioning; (Type II:) higher social stability and higher intellectual functioning; (Type III:) lower social stability and lower intellectual functioning; and (Type IV:) lower social stability and higher intellectual functioning. With one exception, all alcoholic types were represented at each of the five treatment facilities from which the subject group had been drawn. From this, Gibbs inferred that alcoholics at each facility were not matched to treatments according to personal characteristics that may be relevant to the prognosis within specific treatment modalities.

In a fourth research phase, Gibbs (1981) reviewed the empirical literature suggesting patient–treatment interactions. He found it 'as fascinating as it is meagre'. Besides Kissin's work and some of the other studies examined in the present book, he identified an undated research report published by the US Public Health Service (Treffert, n.d.). These studies indicated that intellectual functioning and social stability are differentially associated with outcome in different treatments.

By means of a matching model based on the review, Gibbs exemplified how treatment programmes can be tailored to meet the needs of each of the four alcoholic types described above. His hypotheses on how type of treatment and client characteristics should be matched for the interventions to be as effective as possible agree for the most part with the assumptions formulated by Pattison (p. 200 above). The only essential difference is that Gibbs's carefully derived social resource dimension places the emphasis on clients' social stability (length of period worked at last job, length of longest employment with same employer, marital status, length of time lived with present woman, etc.), while Pattison concentrated on socioeconomic status.

Gibbs's research project is interesting as an attempt to formulate clinically useful prognostic indicators on the basis of previous studies. The inadequate reliability and uncertain validity of client variables is a great obstacle to a consistent and relevant individualization of alcoholism treatment. Gibbs's studies also show that matching models of the type outlined by Kissin and Pattison in the early 1970s have not become obsolete. Models of this multivariant type meet the need for typologies that can be immediately translated into clinical practice. One such model is presented in Section 24.5 below.

McLellan and his co-workers (1980c, 1981a, 1981c, 1983a, 1983c) also took into account a combination of social and psychological resources. They especially drew attention to the fact that the psychiatric severity of patients determines whether their social resources will have any differential effect on the outcome of different kinds of alcoholism treatment. However, the main purpose of these authors was not to define generalized indications for the selection of treatment. Their intention was rather to arrive at a generally applicable *method* for determining indications for various programmes. This is the reason why their research and development project is presented in Part III (Chapter 16), where interest is focused on the systems approach.

21 Cognitive styles

21.1 McLachlan

John McLachlan's study of the relationship between cognitive style, degree of structure of the treatment, and outcome (McLachlan 1972, 1974) provides perhaps the most illustrative example of the potential value of the matching concept for alcoholism treatment. Ogborne felt in 1978 that McLachlan's small-scale study provided the only truly convincing evidence to date to support the hypothesis that an interaction of patient and treatment variables influences outcome. He found it remarkable that this study was the only methodologically acceptable study to consider psychological variables in interaction with treatment variables.

McLachlan applied Kurt Lewin's (1935, 1936) classic formula, $B = f(P,E)$, which considered behaviour (B) to be a joint function of the person (P) and the environment (E). Patient improvement (B) was thus regarded as an interactive function of patient characteristics (P) and characteristics of the therapeutic environment (E) created by the therapist. Lewin's formula may appear to be a pedantic repetition of the obvious. Translated into therapeutic terms, however, it entails a challenge to ask questions different from the usual ones and to formulate treatment theories that take individual differences seriously, rather than regarding them as error variance or the source of exceptions to the general rule.

Harvey, Hunt, and Schroder (1961) were inspired by Lewin's model to formulate a cognitive personality theory, *conceptual systems theory* (see research review by Miller 1978), which describes human development along a dimension called *conceptual level*. Since the end of the 1960s, methods have been developed to assess conceptual level (CL) and to measure environmental factors in comparable terms (Hunt 1971; Schroder, Driver, and Streufert 1967). A person's conceptual level is assessed by a sentence-completion test (The Paragraph Completion Method, PCM; Hunt *et al.* 1978) that describes the examinee's attitudes towards absence of structure ('When I am not sure . . .'), towards externally imposed standards ('What I think about rules . . .', 'When I'm told what to do . . .') and towards interpersonal conflicts ('When I'm criticized . . .', 'When someone disagrees with me . . .'). The subject is requested to respond with three or four sentences indicating his personal reactions. The responses are scored according to a standardized procedure.

CL is a measure of both *conceptual complexity* (differentiation, discrimination, integration) and *interpersonal maturity* (self-responsibility). The conceptual systems theory assumes that a person at a higher CL is better able to pursue an independent, complex line of reasoning, to act under his own responsibility, and to adapt to a changing environment than a person at a lower CL.

Studies of the validity of the concept have been summarized by Hunt (1971, pp. 38–42) and Schroder (1971; Schroder *et al.* 1967). In a sample of about a thousand students, no clear-cut relationship was found between CL and social class. The most notable finding was the greater variability among lower-class students. Proportionately more lower-class students were found at the lowest of Hunt's three conceptual levels, but they also contained a slightly greater proportion (almost all female) at high CL.

By contrast, positive relationships have been found between CL and other measures of personality and developmental maturity, such as Kohlberg's Moral Maturity Scale (Hunt 1971). The body of evidence suggests that CL is a significant and relatively stable aspect of an individual's *cognitive style* (Witkin and Oltman 1967), i.e. his or her characteristic way of interpreting and responding to the environment.

David Hunt, a psychologist at the Ontario Institute for Studies in Education in Toronto, applied the CL concept to education and investigated its predictive validity (see reviews by Hunt 1971, 1975, 1978, 1979; Miller 1981). In an influential study of teacher effectiveness, Brophy and Good (1974) noted: 'Of the variables studied, Conceptual Level seems the most promising as a basis for optimizing matching teachers and students' (p. 269). Thus, conceptual level has proven to be a useful concept in both educational and treatment research. Since McLachlan used Hunt's theories and findings as the starting point for his work on alcoholism treatment, an elaboration of Hunt's matching models is warranted.

Hunt (1975) asked the standard question of how education can 'meet the needs of the student'. If this question is to be given an adequate answer, it is not enough to ask 'Which instructional approach is better?' It is necessary to add 'For whom?' and 'For what purpose?' The student and the educational environment must be described in theoretically relevant and objective terms that also have a bearing on educational practice. The term matching was used to describe person–environment combinations that are likely to promote the attainment of educational objectives. Hunt differentiated between contemporaneous and developmental matching.

Figure 21.1 describes personal and environmental dimensions in Hunt's *contemporaneous matching* model. The theoretically relevant environmental variable is *degree of structure*, or the degree of organization provided by the learning environment. A high degree of structure means that the environment is organized primarily by the teacher and that the student has little responsibility. With a low degree of structure, the student is much more responsible for organizing the environment.

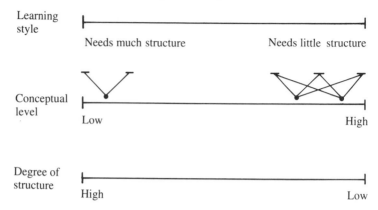

Fig. 21.1   Contemporaneous matching model.

David Hunt (1971) summarized his basic matching hypothesis as follows:

Thus, the heart of the CL matching model is a generally inverse relation between
CL and degree of structure: Low CL learners profiting more from high structure
and high CL learners profiting more from low structure, or in some cases, being less
affected by variations in structure. (p. 44)

In other words, it is predicted that learners who are unable to generate their
own concepts, who are categorical in their thinking, and who are dependent
on external standards (low conceptual level) will profit more from a highly
structured instructional approach. Students who are capable of generating
new concepts, are guided to a greater extent by internal standards, and are
able to adopt different perspectives (high conceptual level), are predicted to
profit more from a loosely structured approach or to be unaffected by the
degree of structure.

In discussing educational practice, Hunt (1975) uses the term *learning style*
to describe the student's CL. The term is defined in terms of how much
structure the student needs to learn efficiently (see Fig. 21.1). As every
experienced teacher knows, some students learn by listening to the teacher,
others benefit from group discussions, and yet others do well in working on
their own.

Hunt's contemporaneous matching hypothesis is supported by several
experimental studies. These show how learning in environments with a varying
degree of structure is moderated by the conceptual level of the student. In
almost all studies, students of differing CL, but on the same level of ability,
were compared. Controlling for ability is important because of the weak but
positive correlation (around 0.20 in heterogeneous groups) between
conceptual level/learning style and *intelligence* (Hunt 1971).

McLachlan and Hunt (1973) found, in an experiment involving discovery
learning, that this approach was differentially effective as predicted by the

matching hypothesis. Low CL students learned significantly better with a lecture (high structure) than with a discovery approach (low structure), whereas high CL students performed well in both conditions.

Tomlinson and Hunt (1971) drew similar conclusions from an experiment that varied the order between rule and example. Low CL students learned better with the rule presented before the example (high structure), whereas high CL students performed fairly well in both conditions (although their performance was poorer in the high-structure environment).

Studies have shown that the individual's CL is related to outcome when the task requires higher-order skills, for example the ability to draw conclusions concerning cause and effect. Performance on simple memory tests, on the other hand, does not seem to be affected by CL (Hunt 1978). The effect of psychosocial treatment aimed at changing an individual's perception of his problems should therefore be influenced by the client's CL.

CL variation is considered to be a significant dimension in a long-term view of the influence of educational environments as well. Figure 21.2 describes personal and environmental dimensions in Hunt's *developmental matching* model.

From a developmental perspective, conceptual level can be considered in terms of increasing conceptual complexity, increasing interpersonal maturity, and increasing understanding of oneself and others (Hunt 1975). The sequence of stages in Figure 21.2 can be summarized as proceeding from an immature, unsocialized stage (A) to a dependent, conforming stage (B) to an independent, self-reliant stage (C). Hunt (1975) referred to a three-year longitudinal study of approximately 125 students, which showed that the proportion of Stage C students increased from 27 per cent in the eighth grade to 56 per cent in the tenth grade.

The developmentally matched environments in Figure 21.2 were derived by asking the question: 'Given the conceptual work required to progress from

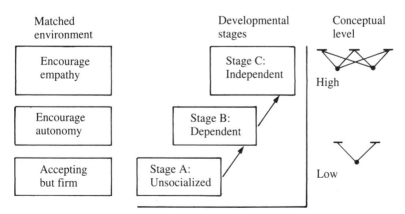

Fig. 21.2 Developmental matching model.

one stage to the next, what is the environment most likely to facilitate such stage-specific work?' Hunt (1975) replied: For the Stage A person to progress to Stage B, he must understand and incorporate the cultural rules. Since rules are learned best when they are clearly defined, the matched environment to foster development to Stage B is a clear, consistent, highly structured one. Following similar logic, the matched environment for progressing from Stage B to stage C is moderately structured with encouragement for self-expression and autonomy.

There are few studies that shed light on the validity of the developmental matching hypothesis. There is above all a lack of longitudinal studies of how persons pass from one stage to another, whether the stages always occur in the same sequence, whether every individual passes through each and every one of the stages, etc. The most interesting clue from the viewpoint of treatment research is provided by a study by Brill (1977, 1978). Brill applied Hunt's matching model to study the differential effects of treatment at reform schools. The schools accepted delinquent boys who were generally at a fairly low CL, although variations occurred even within this lower range of the scale. The boys were registered for at least one year in one of two treatment programmes that differed in degree of structure. A follow-up after termination of treatment showed that very low CL boys were better adjusted, with a lower incidence of problem behaviour, if they had received treatment in the highly structured programme, while low CL boys did better if they had been registered in the somewhat less structured programme.

Hunt and his co-workers have put the question of 'the needs of the student' into a new perspective. In conclusion, I would like to discuss one other aspect of this question, since it is clearly relevant to treatment research guided by the matching hypothesis. Hunt (1975) gave an account of the research by Robertson (1973) on student reactions to traditional class instruction (the lecture approach) versus a less structured approach (either group discussion or discovery learning). As predicted, low CL students judged the lecture more valuable for learning than did high CL students. However, when asked for preference for instructional modes, there was no difference between the two CL groups.

This finding epitomizes the necessity of distinguishing between the educational environment a student *requires* and the one he or she *prefers*. A high CL student can choose on the basis of his preference, since he is presumably capable of learning in environments of varying degrees of structure. However, a low CL student requires a structured educational environment, but may not prefer this alternative if allowed a free choice. Hence the 'cafeteria approach' does not guarantee optimal conditions for learning and development. This latter conclusion, which applies not only to the need for structure but to the educational environment in its entirety (Cronbach and Snow 1977, p. 476ff.), is probably applicable to other fields than educational research as well.

As mentioned above, McLachlan (1972, 1974) wanted to determine whether the concept of 'conceptual level' (CL) is fruitful for psychotherapy research. He chose to study alcoholism treatment, since he assumed that alcoholics as a group exhibited wide variation from the 'psychopathological' viewpoint. Subjects in this study were 100 patients (78 men and 22 women) admitted to the Donwood Institute, a conventional alcohol clinic in Toronto. All subjects were given the sentence completion test used to measure conceptual level.

The degree of structure of the treatment environment is the key dimension against which patients' CL was matched. The environment was judged to be *unilateral* or *interdependent*. A unilateral environment consists of ready-made rules which clearly set forth the required normative behaviour, while an interdependent environment gives feedback as a result of questions and explorative behaviour. Midway are those environmental conditions which encourage autonomy and independence.

Educational research (Hunt and Joyce 1967) had reported a direct relationship between the personality of the teachers and the kind of learning environment they provided. Low CL teachers provided unilateral conditions while high CL teachers created interdependent conditions. McLachlan (1972) showed that an equivalent relationship exists in group therapy between therapist CL and therapist style. High CL therapists were more non-directive than low CL therapists.

According to McLachlan's matching hypothesis (Table 21.1), low CL persons tend to benefit most from a consistent and well-organized treatment environment that compensates for their lack of resources to structure experience. These persons require guidelines from others to function adequately. A loosely structured environment creates uncertainty and confusion. The therapy should, however, especially in the later phases, encourage independence within the psychologically safe conditions provided by a normative structure.

Table 21.1 McLachlan's model for matching of treatment and conceptual level (CL)

Cognitive style	Patient characteristic	Matched therapy conditions
Low CL	Dependent on authority Concerned with rules Compliant	Moderate structure: Encouraging independence within normative structure (Therapist of moderate CL)
High CL	Independent Questioning Self-assertive	Low structure: Allowing high autonomy with numerous alternatives and low normative structure (Therapist of high CL)

High CL persons, however, who endeavour to generate their own guidelines, are assumed to benefit most from non-directive therapy. These persons require a minimum of normative pressure together with a maximum opportunity for independence and self-delineation. If the environment is too highly structured, it interferes with their efforts to explore their own potential and limitations. The result is assumed to be the same in an environment that is excessively complex and prematurely makes high demands on empathy and interdependent functioning.

After detoxification, patients in McLachlan's study participated in 26 hours of group therapy during three weeks of inpatient treatment. The therapy method is described as reconstructive, essentially client-centred, and with frequent use of psychodrama techniques. Therapy groups were heterogeneous in patient CL. The structure of the treatment was defined in terms of the therapist CL and the kind of aftercare provided. The 'low CL' therapists were low only in comparison with other therapists and were a stage above the low CL patients.

The aftercare that was available varied depending on where the patients lived. Those who lived in Toronto were encouraged to participate for one year in a highly structured programme, with both visits to the clinic and telephone contact or a personal interview once a week. Out-of-town patients were contacted by the clinical secretary and encouraged to communicate with another patient belonging to the same therapy group. In other words, the aftercare environment for out-of-town patients can be described as loosely structured. Low CL patients were designated as matched if provided the highly structured aftercare programme, while high CL patients were described as matched if provided the loosely structured programme. Other combinations (high CL–high structure; low CL–less structure) were classified as mismatching. In summary, McLachlan's study permits the examination of outcome for clients who have been matched to therapy, to aftercare, and to both.

Information on drinking behaviour was obtained for 94 of the original 100 patients 12 to 16 months after discharge from inpatient treatment. Sixty-one per cent of the patients were classified as 'recovered'. They were no longer drinking, they had been abstinent for at least the past three months, and they had not had more than three slips of short duration since treatment. Taken in isolation, neither patient CL, therapist CL, nor type of aftercare was related to outcome. However, when patient CL was analysed in conjunction with therapist CL (i.e. degree of structure of therapy) and the degree of structure of aftercare, statistically significant differences in recovery rates emerged (Table 21.2).

Patients who were matched to therapy or aftercare did significantly better than those who were not. Patients who were matched to both therapy and aftercare environments had a somewhat higher recovery rate than those who were matched to only one of these conditions. The gap between the

Table 21.2 Outcome of therapy and after-care by degree of match to patients' conceptual level

Matching model	Per cent recovered of patients	
	Matched	Mismatched
To structure of therapy	70*	50*
To structure of after-care	71*	49*
To both[a]	77	38

*$p<0.05$; [a]Probability level was not reported.

consistently matched patients and those who were mismatched to both conditions was considerably greater.

The results support McLachlan's hypothesis that treatment will be more successful if the client's cognitive style and need for structure are taken into account. Low CL patients appear to function best when rules and expectations are clearly expressed. Thus, a consistent and directive, highly structured therapy is to be recommended. A therapy that is non-directive and encourages self-expression and autonomy should be preferred only for the high CL patient. It is presumably no coincidence that Carl Rogers' non-directive therapy was developed with students as subjects, while his method generally fails when applied to case-work with the heavily drinking clientele of social welfare agencies.

Lewin's (1935) formula for predicting behaviour and Harvey, Hunt, and Schroder's (1961) concept of 'conceptual level' appear to be fruitful in treatment research. This impression is reinforced by an early doctoral thesis by Brook (1962), which studied the cognitive style of alcoholics who were more versus less successful with AA. Subjects who functioned on a concrete level and accepted external authority proved to benefit more from AA than subjects who questioned authority and tested limits.

No attempt to replicate McLachlan's findings has been reported. However, there are very few studies of interaction of any kind in alcoholism treatment research. And as mentioned above, a number of educational studies by Hunt and his co-workers contribute indirectly to making McLachlan's conclusions plausible.

Nor has anyone reported a prospective study that matches clients of varying CL to treatments of varying degree of structure. Such a study would clarify the issue of whether the cognitive style of the client interacts directly with the structure of the treatment or whether the interaction is moderated by the social context. It is, for example, not certain that therapists and clients will communicate in the same way in homogeneous therapy groups created by matching as they did in heterogeneous groups created by random assignment. Different group level effects (see Cronbach and Webb 1975;

Finney and Moos 1986) should be considered when discussing matching models.

Finally, the question immediately suggests itself as to whether other aspects of an individual's cognitive style, in addition to conceptual level, should be taken into account in the selection of treatment. McLachlan's (1972, 1974) studies are rather unique in alcoholism treatment, but there are studies in related fields that illustrate the need for a closer study of how cognitive factors influence outcome of psychosocial treatment. *Cognitive matching* is a topical concept in both psychotherapy (e.g. Weiner and Crowder 1986) and education (e.g. Brooks, Fusco, and Grennon 1983; Dunn 1984; Shipman and Shipman 1985).

21.2 Conceptual differentiation

John Carr and Allan Posthuma (1975; Posthuma and Carr 1975; Carr 1980) summarized a series of studies designed to investigate the hypothesis that the success of social interaction is determined by the extent to which the participants are matched in the complexity, or level of *differentiation*, of their cognitive structure. Differentiation in the social context is defined as: 'the tendency to make fine distinctions among people and thus to perceive them as different from one another' (Shrauger and Altrocci 1964, p. 292).

Conceptual differentiation has usually been measured by a shortened and less complex alternative to G. A. Kelly's Role Construct Repertory Test, Rep Test (Kelly 1955), called the Interpersonal Discrimination Task, IDT (Carr 1965). Differentiation was suggested as a useful mediating construct in accounting for many interactions between the environment and the individual. A fundamental thesis in Kelly's personality theory, from which the original Rep Test was derived, is that the conceptual structure that the individual uses to interpret the world exerts an important influence on his behaviour.

Carr and Posthuma (1975) maintain that successful communication is dependent upon the degree to which a common language exists or can be developed between the participants. This does not just mean sharing a number of conceptual dimensions. Common constructs also have to be differentiated to a similar degree. To choose an example from alcoholism treatment, the patient and the therapist must agree on what should be considered an 'improvement'. If the patient only has a 'cure' in view, while the therapist is referring to a whole spectrum of changes, there is a great chance that they will misunderstand each other. In this case, the therapist has a more differentiated idea than the client about what 'improvement' implies, even though both use the same construct.

Carr (1970) was interested in whether conceptual compatibility versus discrepancy between patient and therapist influences the outcome of psychosocial treatment. The subject group consisted of 24 adult patients with mainly neurotic problems. During the first week of treatment, the patients were asked to complete a test (Carr's IDT) intended to rate the level of cognitive differentiation and a standardized questionnaire (The Cornell Index) that was used to assess their psychiatric symptom level. The therapists, who were similar with regard to age, educational level, socioeconomic class, experience, and theoretical orientation, took only the cognitive test.

After 12 weeks of outpatient therapy, assessment of the patients' psychiatric symptom level was repeated, and they were also asked to estimate the size of the change on a seven-point scale from 'significantly improved' to 'significantly worse'. The results showed that compatible (matched) patients—i.e. patients who were on 'the same wavelength' as the therapist in terms of conceptual differentiation—improved significantly more than discrepant (mismatched) patients, in terms of both symptom reduction and perceived improvement. While the symptom level in the discrepant group either remained unchanged or increased slightly, patients in the compatible group evidenced a statistically significant ($p < 0.025$) reduction in the number of psychiatric symptoms reported (Fig. 21.3).

In a similar study, Landfield (1971) found that the rate of premature termination of therapy (his criterion for treatment failure) varied with the degree of divergence between patient and therapist in conceptual differentiation. Carr's (1970) and Landfield's (1971) results rest on a shaky empirical foundation, however. Moreover, since neither author evaluated the symptom level some time after termination of treatment, the studies do not permit any conclusions about rehabilitation.

Hunt, Carr, *et al.* (1985) further tested the relationship between patient–therapist matching on conceptual differentiation and the outcome of

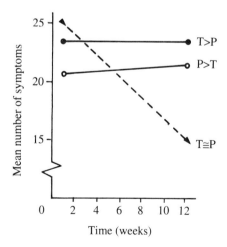

Fig. 21.3 Patient syndrome change in three groups differing in initial patient–therapist compatibility. P = patient's differentiation level, T = therapists's differentiation level.

psychotherapy. Sixty-three psychiatric outpatients were randomly assigned to therapists, who were more experienced than in the study by Carr (1970). Twenty-two therapist–patient pairs satisfied the criteria for a match, while 41 were mismatched on cognitive structure.

Premature termination, or irregular discharge during the first eight weeks of treatment, occured for 63 per cent of the unmatched pairs and 37 per cent of the matched pairs. Assessments of the symptom level indicated a significantly faster rate of improvement for the remaining matched pairs during the first 12 weeks of follow-up. The unmatched pairs eventually reached similar endpoints, with outcome measures at 24 weeks being unable to distinguish between the two groups. In summary, patient–therapist cognitive match seemed to effect a more rapid response to therapy.

According to Carr (1980), research on conceptual differentiation, as well as several other studies dealing with some form of similarity between patient and therapist (reviewed by Luborsky et al. 1971), indicate that the key to the matching effect is to be found in the area of cognitive process rather than personality. In other words, degree of communicability seems to be a more powerful predictor of psychotherapy outcome than therapist traits.

21.3   Field dependence and restructuring

There is a large body of research on individual differences in the tendency to function autonomously of external referents and in the ability to restructure and go beyond the information given. The foundation was laid by Herman Witkin and his co-workers in a series of studies on perception of the upright (see Witkin et al. 1954). The group of researchers originally tried to determine how people locate the upright as quickly and accurately as they ordinarily do. Quite unexpectedly, this study revealed marked and consistent differences between subjects in their performance on orientation tasks.

In some of the studies, the subject was seated in a dark room and viewed a luminous rod, surrounded by a luminous square frame, which was tilted at an angle of 28 degrees in relation to the upright. The subject's task was to adjust the rod to the upright, while the frame remained in its initial position of tilt. Most subjects positioned the rod slightly tilted in relation to the upright. According to Witkin and his co-workers, this was because people in general make use of information both from the external visual field and from the body with its organ of balance (the vestibular apparatus in the inner ear).

Some subjects tilted the rod far towards the tilted frame, which indicated that they oriented themselves with the prevailing visual field as the primary referent. Other subjects adjusted the rod more or less close to the upright, regardless of the position of the frame. This suggested that they relied primarily on sensations from the body. These two characteristic modes of orienting oneself in space were called *field dependent* and *field independent*, respectively. Nowadays they are usually measured by Oltman's Portable Rod and Frame Test, PRFT (Oltman 1968).

In a study of other perceptual tasks, Witkin and his co-workers (1954) found a close relationship between performance on the rod-and-frame test and scores on a conventional spatial test called the Embedded-Figures Test, EFT (Witkin 1950; Witkin *et al.* 1971). Subjects who take the EFT are shown a simple figure and then asked to find it in a complex design that is so patterned that each component of the simple figure is made part of a clear-cut subwhole of the pattern, so that the figure is effectively hidden (see Fig. 21.4).

These and other findings suggested that the field dependence–independence dimension was a more general cognitive dimension than it had first appeared. Perhaps, assumed Witkin *et al.* (1954), both the rod-and-frame test and the EFT measure an underlying ability to separate the relevant aspects of a perceptual field (the rod and the simple figure) and disregard other aspects (the frame and the complex design). Put in everyday terminology, field dependence–independence was redefined as an ability to perceive a wide range of situations analytically. The EFT, which is relatively simple to administer, often came to be used instead of, or together with, the rod-and-frame test to measure 'field dependence–independence' in this broader sense (with the terms put in quotation marks).

More recent research has found a connection between field dependence–independence and the intellectual ability of people to impose structure on a field lacking it (Witkin *et al.* 1962) and with their mode of cognitive functioning within a variety of areas (Witkin 1954, 1962, 1979). Many of these are ordinarily subsumed under 'personality', for example nature of defences (undifferentiated versus specialized), possible psychopathological symptoms, body concept, and self-image. On the basis of these results, Witkin and his co-workers (1962, 1979) drew the conclusion that field

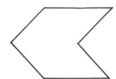

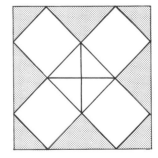

Fig. 21.4 Example of simple figure and complex design similar to those used in the Embedded-Figures Test.

dependence–independence constitutes one of the manifestations of the individual's level of psychological *differentiation*.

In the 1970s, field dependence–independence was also linked to specialization of function at the neurophysiological level (Witkin, Goodenough, and Oltman 1979) and to social behaviour. Field-dependent persons were described as more attentive to social cues, more interested in people, and less in need of autonomy in interpersonal situations than is the case with field-independent persons, resulting from a weaker differentiation between self and others (Witkin and Goodenough 1977).

These findings, however, also led to a re-evaluation of the interpretation of the rod-and-frame and the EFT tests as measures of a generalized ability to perceive a part of a field as separate from the field as a whole. Witkin and Goodenough (1981) introduced a distinction between two cognitive dimensions, one referring to a *style* (manner of moving towards a goal) and the other to an *ability* (competence in goal attainment).

The cognitive-style dimension is represented by *field dependence–independence* as originally defined. According to this definition, field-dependent persons are influenced more by external frames of reference, particularly in conflict situations that lack a clear structure, than field-independent persons, who rely more on their own internal frames of reference in processing information. To earlier characterizations of this dimension, the authors added that it is neutral with regard to value. That is, each pole has qualities that are adaptive in particular circumstances. The rod-and-frame test is considered to measure field dependence–independence in this narrower sense (with no quotation marks around the terms).

The EFT, in contrast, is said to measure functioning on a related spatial and verbal dimension, which Witkin and Goodenough (1981) call cognitive *restructuring ability*. This dimension involves the ability to break up an organized field so that its parts are experienced as being discrete from the background, to give a structure to a field that lacks it, and to impose a different organization on a field from the one suggested by its inherent organization.

On purely logical grounds, restructuring ability should be relevant in psychosocial treatment, which often persuades clients to view their problems in a new perspective. There is also empirical evidence indicating that both restructuring ability and field dependence–independence influence outcome of treatment in ways predicted by the theory.

Witkin (1965) assumes that the person who is 'field dependent' tends to differ from 'field independent' persons in the way he relates to the therapist. With his less developed sense of separate identity, the field-dependent patient is more likely to experience 'fusion' with the therapist. This is a possible explanation for why field-dependent patients often say they 'feel better' at an early stage in treatment, before any real problems have been worked through.

It is not unusual for the field-dependent patient to solicit support from the therapist by asking questions such as 'Is it normal to feel like this?' or 'Do you think I'm mentally ill, Doctor, from the way I'm talking?' The field-dependent patient also seems to accept the therapist's suggestions and interpretations more readily, which may make him feel better. He typically agrees to such suggestions with a 'You're right, Doctor' or by repeating a part of the therapist's statement. Relatively field-independent patients, on the other hand, are apt to be more cautious in the establishment of their relationship with the therapist. They are also, according to Witkin, more inclined to sift the suggestions of the therapist through a value hierarchy of their own.

Witkin's (1965) early speculations have received some support from more recent investigations. Witkin, Lewis, and Weil (1968), Russakoff *et al.* (1976), Dowds *et al.* (1977), and Austrian and Goldbergèr (1982) have shown, in studies with the rod-and-frame test (RFT) alone or in combination with the EFT, that field-dependent persons require a great deal of structure and guidance, and the assurance that they are responding as expected of them. Furthermore, there are results indicating that field-independent persons might become bored or 'turned off' in a highly structured therapy situation (Austrian and Goldbergèr 1982). According to Austrian and Goldbergèr, the correlations were higher with the EFT (restructuring ability) than with the RFT.

Therapists may be able to perceive this difference in need for structure at an early point during therapy. This is suggested by an analysis carried out by Witkin and his co-workers (1977) of therapy transcripts from Witkin, Lewis, and Weil's (1968) study. Therapists in this latter study put significantly more open questions to patients who were field independent on the RFT and who did well on the EFT. Conversely, they put more questions with yes-or-no answers to patients who were on the opposite end of these tests. In general, therapists were more active with field-dependent than with field-independent patients.

Yet another analysis of transcripts from therapy sessions from Witkin, Lewis, and Weil's (1968) study was performed by Sousa-Poza and Rohrberg (1976). These authors found that field-independent patients were task-oriented in their relation to the therapist, while field-dependent patients established a person-oriented relationship. The latter expressed more frequently how it felt to converse with the therapist. The highly personal communicative style of these patients may have reinforced their sense of self, which is more dependent on external referents.

Pardes, Papernik, and Winston's (1974) study of 60 patients and their therapists at a psychiatric hospital in New York is particularly interesting, since the authors tested both patients and therapists with the RFT to measure their field dependence–independence. It was found that the field-independent therapists achieved the best results regardless of patient category (three levels of field dependence–independence) and evaluation criterion (length of hospital stay, improvement in the hospital, and rate of readmission within three years after discharge).

The working style of the field-independent therapists can be summarized by the words 'get the job done', while the field-dependent therapists had a more nurturing style that may be characterized by the phrase 'come in and let me help you' (cf. Pollack and Kiev 1963; Shows and Carson 1965). The nurturing style led to good results with field-dependent patients. However, the duration of the patients' stay at the hospital was prolonged by an average of 80 per cent, which the authors explained by suggesting that this kind of support may be difficult to surrender.

Pardes and his co-workers argue, on the basis of these results, that psychotherapy with hospitalized patients should be conducted by field-independent therapists. However, it should be borne in mind that long-term accommodation in a supportive environment may be a desirable goal for certain client populations, such as the homeless and psychiatrically disabled alcohol abusers described by Leach and Wing (1980).

Karp, Kissin, and Hustmyer (1970) found that alcoholics who had a low score on the Embedded-Figures Test (EFT) were selected less often for psychotherapy than alcoholics who did well on the EFT. The former alcoholics also tended to drop out of insight-oriented therapy more often once they had begun it. There was, however, no difference in the tendency to drop out of drug therapy. The authors recommended that the EFT, which measures restructuring ability (Witkin and Goodenough 1981), be tried as a means for screening psychotherapy candidates.

Kissin, Platz, and Su (1970; Kissin 1977b) drew a similar conclusion in another study, reviewed in Section 20.1. It should be added that if the psychotherapy offered focuses on underlying dynamic structures, as in the case of Karp, Kissin, and Hustmyer (1970), then a measure of the severity of alcohol dependence should also be used to select patients (see Chapter 8).

Finally, Erwin and Hunter (1984) studied the dropout rate among 80 patients in an aftercare rehabilitation programme for middle-class alcoholics. The patients took the EFT and were asked to solve two problems devised by Jean Piaget and his associates: the pendulum problem and the plant problem. The Piagetian tasks are measures of *formal operations*, typically manifested in thinking that considers the real as one among other hypothetical possibilities. The high correlations among test scores indicated, according to the authors, that the EFT, the pendulum problem, and the plant problem measure different facets of the same cognitive ability.

Thirty-one patients remained in treatment throughout the ten weeks of aftercare. There was a highly significant correlation between cognitive ability and dropout rate. Patients who had a low score on the EFT or who (in Piagetian terminology) performed on a *preoperational* to *concrete operational* level in solving the pendulum problem and the plant problem, dropped out of treatment two and a half times as often as patients who did well on the EFT or who performed on a formal operational (hypothetico-deductive) level. The best predictor, the plant problem, accounted for 36 per cent of the variance in attendance. Furthermore, the cognitive tests accounted for about three times as much variance in attendance as did education or occupational level.

Erwin and Hunter (1984) assumed that these results were partially a consequence of the orientation of the programme. They exemplified this by describing a group exercise in which each participant was asked first to describe a future situation in which he or she would be tempted to drink and then to devise a constructive counter-response to it. The exercise, in effect, called on patients to think conditionally or hypothetically, i.e. a type of abstract thought which Piaget characterized as formal operational. A typical preoperational patient responded:

I really don't know what it will be like. You don't know something that hasn't happened yet. I will know after it happens. . . . This assignment isn't helpful because I can't say what I will do before it happens.

The authors drew two major conclusions. The first is that cognitive factors probably play a more important role for how well alcoholics respond to treatment than had previously been assumed. The other is that since most alcoholics do less well on the EFT and, judging from this study, are cognitively concrete rather than abstract, rehabilitation programmes should include as much concrete skills training and as little verbal-symbolic material as possible (cf. Intagliata 1978).

The latter conclusion is essential. The observation that alcoholics deficient in abstract reasoning ability have a high rate of dropout from psychosocial treatment does not relieve health and social services agencies of the responsibility to further develop the services provided, so that *all* alcoholics can receive appropriate treatment. Witkin (1965) maintained that:

it is hard to accept the idea that the one kind of patient is amenable to psychotherapy and the other not. Even if there is some difference between them in this respect, it may very well be that each will benefit from quite different treatment procedures. Perhaps the core issue is not suitability for psychotherapy, but which form of psychotherapy for which kind of patient. Focusing on the kinds of therapy that may help persons who show the characteristics associated with field dependence may aid us in finding ways of treating at least some of the field-dependent patients who now seem to be rejected en masse. (p. 329)

There seems to be a need, not least in alcoholism treatment, for a psychosocial approach that provides a high degree of structure and directiveness. There is ample evidence showing that active alcoholics are in general more field-dependent than other people (see reviews by Sugerman and Schneider 1976; Barnes 1983). Many of them are also more or less disabled by cognitive deficiencies.

The relationship between alcoholism and brain damage has been verified in numerous studies (see reviews by Wilkinson and Carlen 1981; Parsons and Leber 1982; Porjesz and Begleiter 1983; Ryan and Butters 1983). Mild symptoms of brain damage have even been discovered among heavy drinkers with early symptoms of dependence (see e.g. Bergman 1985, 1987). Research results obtained in recent years indicate that neuropsychological dysfunction is a very common alcohol-related disability. In less severe cases, however, the brain largely recovers its normal function after an extended period of abstinence (see Muuronen *et al.* 1989; reviews by Goldman 1983; Porjesz and Begleiter 1983).

One often finds already among young alcohol abusers an impaired capacity for abstract thought, problem solving, analogical reasoning, and learning, while memory deficits and generalized intellectual impairment appear only in the higher age groups. As assessed by conventional tests, the intelligence of alcoholics is most often normal. Cognitive differences between alcohol abusers without severe brain damage and the rest of the population can generally only be detected by using more demanding spatial or verbal tests (e.g. Bergman 1987; cf. Section 8.2 above).

Erwin and Hunter's (1984) study indicates that ordinary forms of psychotherapy are not suited for alcoholics with cognitive deficits. These treatment modalities require an ability for cognitive restructuring (EFT) or formal operational thinking (the pendulum problem, the plant problem), i.e. an ability for problem solving at a relatively advanced level. Research findings on the prevalence and character of neuropsychological dysfunctions among alcoholics underscore the importance of tailoring treatment to the needs of the client (see also Guthrie and Elliott 1980; Wilkinson and Sanchez-Craig 1981; Goldman 1986; McCrady and Smith 1986; McCrady 1987; Hulbert and Lens 1988).

However, treatment variables have to be chosen with great care. Donovan, Walker, and Kivlahan (1987) summarized a few studies investigating the interactive effects of neuropsychological impairment and length of inpatient hospitalization on treatment outcome among alcoholics. It was hypothesized that alcoholics with a high degree of impairment would be more affected by the length of stay than alcoholics with no or minimal impairment.

Subjects were randomly assigned to either a two-week or a seven-week programme. The findings from follow-up at nine months after discharge indicated that, overall, length of stay had no bearing on subsequent outcome (cf. Section 3.1). Furthermore, there was only marginal evidence for an effect of interaction between neuropsychological status, length of stay, and outcome. Donovan and his co-workers (1987) assumed that cognitive deficits represent only one of a number of possible factors contributing to treatment outcome. The above review indicates that such deficits may be particularly relevant when treatment content is taken into account.

21.4   Locus of control

The cognitive factor which—along with conceptual level and Piaget's cognitive operations—offers the most promise for matching is *locus of control*. This concept, developed out of Julian Rotter's (1954) social learning theory, refers to the degree to which an individual sees himself in control of his life and the events that influence it. *Internal control* is defined as a generalized expectancy that events are contingent upon one's own behaviour and therefore under personal control. *External control*, on the other hand, refers to the perception that events are unrelated to one's behaviour and are primarily the result of fate, chance, powerful others, or unpredictable external forces (Rotter 1966, 1975).

The concept of locus of control is akin to Seeman's concept of alienation and its *powerlessness* component (Seeman and Evans 1962; Tolor and LeBlanc 1971) and to Maier and Seligman's (1976) *learned helplessness* construct. All of these concepts describe the extent to which a person feels he is able to control events by means of his own actions.

Locus of control is usually measured by Rotter's Internal–External Locus of Control Scale, I–E (Rotter 1966). There is a large body of research on the concept and its relation to a variety of personality attributes and behaviours, for example susceptibility to influence, cognitive activity, tolerance of frustration, achievement behaviour, and response to success and failure (see reviews by Lefcourt 1966, 1972; Joe 1971; Throop and MacDonald 1971).

The research suggests that an indivual's background and current life situation play a major role in determining his perception of control. But there is also evidence that psychosocial treatment is able to modify an individual's locus of control, at least temporarily. Lesyk (1969), Dua (1970), Gillis and Jessor (1970), and Smith (1970) found that patients who were judged as being improved exhibited a significant shift in the direction of internal control expectancy. Pierce, Schanble, and Farkas (1970) were able to train externally oriented individuals to adopt a more internal-controlled orientation during psychotherapy.

In an evaluation of alcoholism treatment, Abbott (1984) used two measures of locus of control, a generalized measure (I–E, see above) and a drinking-related one (The Drinking-Related Locus of Control Scale, DRIE; Donovan and O'Leary 1978). Abbott found a statistically significant shift in the direction of internal control from admission to follow-up three months after completion of treatment. The change was greatest on the drinking-related scale. It was also greater in patients whose perception of control was rated as more external. The drinking-related measure (DRIE) appeared, in contrast to the generalized one (I–E), to be of value in predicting drinking outcomes.

A couple of attempts at treatment using what Hunt (1975) calls contemporaneous—in contrast to developmental—matching provide the most encouraging results, however. One example is a study presented by Bernard

Liberman (1978*b*; see also Frank 1974*b*), a member of Jerome Frank's research group at the Johns Hopkins University School of Medicine in Baltimore.

Liberman and his co-workers designed an ingenious experiment to explore how the experience of mastery influences the outcome of psychotherapy. The research sample consisted of 32 psychiatric outpatients who had been referred for psychotherapy. All patients were aware that they were taking part in a trial programme and that more traditional therapy was available for those who wished it. None of the patients took advantage of this offer, however.

The experimental tasks were designed in such a way that they would be psychotherapeutically 'neutral', i.e. that no current specific theory of psychotherapy could account for the treatment outcome solely on the basis of performance of the particular tasks. This design was intended to reduce the probability of alternative explanations of the experimental results. At the same time, however, the tasks had to be of such a nature that patients perceived the treatment as being credible.

Three tasks were devised:

(1) a psychophysical task where the patients' reaction time and ability to discriminate between light stimuli of different colours were measured;

(2) a perception task in which patients viewed tachistoscopically presented pictures and were required to answer content and mood questions about what they saw;

(3) a 'biofeedback' task in which patients observed and attempted to modify perceived physiological feedback on an oscilloscope screen in response to stressful and non-stressful visual and auditory stimuli.

The tasks were carried out during eight sessions at weekly intervals. During an introductory session, the patient was provided with an individualized rationale and explanation of the treatment programme. At the beginning of each task session, the patient was given the opportunity to speak into a tape recorder about his problems for half an hour. A staff member whom the patient never met listened to the tape and wrote a brief, supportive note which the patient received at the following session. This procedure was aimed at preventing the patient from forming an affective relationship to the task trainer, who was able to concentrate on the tasks that had been prepared.

At the end of each session, the patient was shown graphs that were said to indicate how he had improved on each task. In fact, the graphs had nothing to do with the patient's actual performance. They were drawn so that the patient would experience a steady progress over the course of treatment.

'Progress' was given different explanations in experimental and control conditions. In the former condition 'improved' performance was attributed solely to the patients' own efforts, while in the latter condition it was attributed to external factors in the form of a placebo, which only this group received. The placebo medication was discontinued at the final treatment session with the explanation that the treatment programme was completed and that the gains it produced would be expected to continue.

Patients were evaluated three months and one year after termination of the treatment programme. Their symptom level on the follow-up evaluations was compared with their symptom level at discharge using a standardized questionnaire (The Hopkins Symptom Checklist, HSCL). Three months after the conclusion of treatment, patients in the experimental group showed significantly better results than those in the control group, as expected. One year after the close of therapy, the difference between the groups was still in the expected direction, but was not statistically significant. Moreover, the results from the second follow-up must be taken with a pinch of salt, since only half of the original sample returned for this evaluation.

Liberman and his co-workers also investigated how the outcome was influenced by the attribution orientation of patients. They devised an instrument, based in part on Seeman's Powerlessness Scale (Seeman and Evans 1962). Those who scored in the top third (self-attribution) on admission to treatment were compared with those who scored in the bottom third (external attribution) with respect to their responsiveness to the experimental (mastery) and control (placebo) conditions. The results three months after conclusion of treatment are shown in Figure 21.5.

The effect of interaction was notable. Patients who were oriented towards self-reliance showed a more favourable three-month and one-year response to therapy when exposed to a mastery-oriented treatment approach, i.e. when told that their 'progress' was due to their own efforts. Patients whose initial orientation indicated greater reliance on external forces and agents, on the other hand, showed more improvement when given treatment where 'progress' was attributed to the external agent of medication.

The study suggests that attribution orientation (i.e. internal vs. external locus of control) is a suitable criterion for selection of patients to treatments based on either internal or external rationales. This conclusion has been corroborated by other studies of locus of control and treatment outcome under different treatment conditions in non-alcoholic populations (Abramowitz *et al.* 1974; Friedman and Dies 1974; Johnson and Meyer 1974; Kilmann and Howell 1974; Balch and Ross 1975; Kilmann, Albert, and Sotile 1975; Best 1975; Best and Steffy 1975; see also review by Foon 1987). So far, however, Liberman (1978*b*) and Best (1975; Best and Steffy 1975) are rather alone in having worked with clinical samples.

Bandura (1977) pointed out that a careful distinction should be made between expectations concerning the causal relationship between action and outcome (locus of control) and expectations concerning self-efficacy. A person can be convinced that a given course of action will lead to a desired result

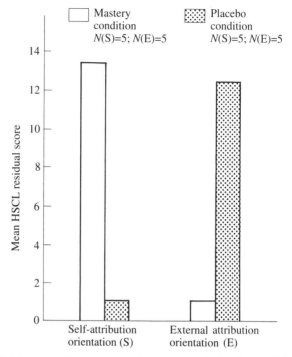

Fig. 21.5   Maintenance of improvement in mastery and placebo conditions, classified by patients' attribution orientation (high scores reflect greater maintenance of improvement from discharge to follow-up). N.B. Data on patients in the middle range as regards attribution orientation ($N = 12$) are lacking.

(internal locus of control) but still feel incapable of acting in the manner required (low self-efficacy). Such a person can be helped by someone who persuades him that he is actually capable of doing something about his problems. Frank (1968) emphasizes here the 'role of hope' as an effective, non-specific factor in psychosocial treatment.

    People with an external locus of control do not necessarily doubt their own competence, but they find efforts futile. They do not believe they are in a position to control events that affect them. The observation that persons who improve in psychotherapy often exhibit a shift from external to internal locus of control does not necessarily mean that any real change has taken place. As Rohsenow and O'Leary (1978a) pointed out, it can just as well be interpreted as a social desirability effect (the patient has been told repeatedly during treatment that everything is up to him, and he responds accordingly) or a statistical regression artefact (the patient answers the questionnaire initially in a situation when he feels unusually helpless; after a while, his strength and confidence begin to return).

Liberman (1978*b*) and his co-workers' success with placebo medication of patients with external locus of control is interesting, but such medication cannot be continued indefinitely. The question therefore arises how long improvement can be maintained after the reliance on an external agent has been discontinued. Best and Steffy (1975) found that smokers with external locus of control did well with a behaviour analysis of how situational factors influenced their smoking. Other researchers to whom reference is made above have shown that persons with external locus of control prefer or do best with directive therapies.

There is a substantial body of literature dealing with the relationship of locus of control to alcoholism and its treatment (see reviews by Hinrichsen 1976; Rohsenow and O'Leary 1978*a*, 1978*b*; Donovan and O'Leary 1979). Only a few studies, however, have investigated whether there is an interaction between locus of control, treatment modality and outcome.

Spoth (1983) applied relaxation training to an alcoholic population. Thirty-seven male volunteers were randomly assigned to either externally or internally oriented therapy groups. The former groups were characterized by high structure, including daily practice, and a treatment rationale which emphasized factors beyond the direct control of the patient, such as neuropsychological processes. The latter groups were provided with less structure; relaxation was presented as an active coping skill and was to be applied only in stressful situations. At a follow-up eight weeks after completion of treatment, there was no significant difference in general anxiety between internally and externally oriented therapy groups.

However, a significant interaction between treatment orientation, locus of control, and outcome was found. Alcoholics with an internal locus of control benefited more from internally oriented treatment, while those with an external locus of control benefited more from externally oriented treatment. Although this study suggests the utility of a differential approach to relaxation training, several methodological limitations, such as the short follow-up interval and a response rate of only 57 per cent, should be kept in mind.

Hartman, Krywonis, and Morrison (1988) designed a clinical trial in which 45 outpatients with a primary alcohol problem were randomly assigned to an unstructured, minimal intervention or a more intensive, structured intervention. Data on change in general anxiety, number of days abstinent, and number of drinks per drinking occasion were collected 30 days after the last treatment session. Overall, on each dependent variable, both intervention approaches were found to be equally effective. The intensity or structure of treatment seemed to be of no importance, regardless of whether the patient had a high or a low degree of alcohol dependence.

However, patients with an external locus of control achieved better outcome, across measures, after the more intensive, structured intervention than after brief, non-directive counselling. Patients with an internal locus of control responded equally well to both intervention approaches. Hartman and his co-workers concluded that people who believe that they exert independent control over their lives can get started on the road to recovery with only a minimum of encouragement, guidance, and support. By contrast, people who view themselves as somewhat helpless and victims of their environment may require more structure, direction, and support in order to initiate and maintain significant changes.

These assumptions are, of course, highly speculative. It is open to question whether any conclusions at all can be drawn from a study with a follow-up interval of only one month. On the other hand, if no short-term effects have been observed, there is no reason to look for effects over a longer range. Spoth's (1983) and Hartman and his co-workers' (1988) studies may thus—like findings from non-alcoholic populations—have a heuristic value, that is, they may help us to identify patient characteristics and treatment dimensions that are worth testing in further alcoholism treatment research. Skinner's hypothesis, to be described in next section, has been included on similar grounds.

21.5   Skinner's hypothesis

Harvey Skinner (1980a) at the Addiction Research Foundation in Toronto has presented a paper on anti-alcohol drugs in which he illustrated how research and development work in alcoholism treatment could benefit from the results of cognitively oriented research. Skinner noted that two anti-alcohol drugs are available today: disulfiram (Antabuse) and calcium carbimide (Temposil). These two drugs have somewhat different actions. Antabuse has a slower onset (usually 12 hours after ingestion) and longer duration of reactivity to alcohol (7–12 days). Temposil acts much faster but during a shorter period of time (1–24 hours), and has less adverse potential side effects.

The pharmacological difference between Antabuse and Temposil suggests a rationale for their differential use. Antabuse administered daily would provide a better protection for persons who need a relatively continuous, external support for abstinence. Temposil, in contrast, would be a more favourable option for individuals who are capable of taking the drug themselves on an 'as required' basis, for example before a party.

Skinner proposed that two intervention strategies be tried. The first, which represents, in Hunt's (1975) terminology, a *contemporaneous* matching model, entails referring patients to different programmes on the basis of an assessment of their locus-of-control orientation (e.g. Rotter 1966). Skinner referred to a research review by Beutler (1979) as support for the hypothesis that clients with an external locus of control (low reactance) fare better with a well-structured behaviour therapy combined with Antabuse ingested daily.

Clients with an internal locus of control (high reactance), in contrast, are assumed to benefit more from a form of cognitive therapy, supported by Temposil which the client takes at his discretion. Within this experimental design, the author also wished to investigate the effectiveness of the therapies and the anti-alcohol drugs, each by themselves.

In addition to the evidence referred to by Skinner (1980a), there are a few other studies that indirectly support the contemporaneous matching hypothesis. In an outpatient study from Boston, for example, Mayer and Myerson (1971) found that Antabuse was associated with greater therapeutic success for socially unstable alcoholics. For socially stable alcoholics, in contrast, Antabuse was less successful. Rose, Powell, and Penick (1978) found a tendency towards external locus of control among socially unstable alcoholics and internal locus of control among socially stable alcoholics. Perhaps the external locus of control of the socially unstable alcoholics may explain their relative success with Antabuse in Mayer and Myerson's study. The lower rate of success of the socially stable alcoholics in Antabuse treatment could, analogously, possibly be explained by the more internal orientation of this group.

In support of this contention, Obitz (1978) found that male alcoholics who elected to take Antabuse were significantly ($p < 0.001$) more externally oriented than were those who did not. There was no significant difference between the Antabuse and non-Antabuse groups in age, years of education, or employment. Although treatment preference is not to be equated with treatment effectiveness, Obitz's study, as well as the rationale provided by Skinner and previous research, suggests that patients' control orientation should be included in future evaluations of Antabuse treatment.

Skinner's (1980a) second intervention strategy, illustrated in Figure 21.6, exemplifies a *developmental* matching model (Hunt 1975). All clients are offered supportive therapy (including help with practical problems), with individualized drug therapy as a supplement.

Clients who enter at the lowest treatment level are given Antabuse daily. This phase is limited in time (e.g. six weeks), and progress to the next phase is contingent on achieving specified goals (e.g. finding a job). In the second phase of the model, the client receives Temposil daily and is expected to take successively more responsibility for the use of this anti-alcohol drug. On the third level, Temposil use is entirely at the discretion of the client, who takes it on an 'as required' basis. Finally, the fourth step involves the absence of any anti-alcohol drugs, pending the termination of therapy.

Clients can enter at any stage in this hierarchical sequence, and are naturally allowed to step down to a lower level. The most appropriate stage to enter is determined after an assessment of the client's locus-of-control orientation. The goal is that clients should gain more control over both the treatment and their life.

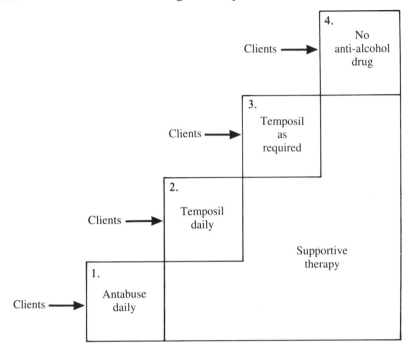

Fig. 21.6   Skinner's developmental model for supportive therapy with differential use of anti-alcohol drugs.

As noted above (p. 224), it is questionable whether psychosocial treatment is truly able to bring about a lasting shift from external to internal locus of control. Skinner's hypothesis about a sequence of interactions between locus of control (reactance), treatment modality, and outcome is nevertheless worth testing. At least, like Liberman's (1978*b*) trials (Section 21.4), the proposed model meets with Frank's (1961) requirements for successful psychotherapy, that is, a therapeutic alliance, a reasonably optimistic rationale, and a task that actively involves both the client and the therapist.

21.6   Therapist–milieu interaction

The studies presented above have all focused on the interaction between patient characteristics and treatment conditions. Arlene Frank and John Gunderson at Harvard Medical School and McLean Hospital in Belmont, Massachusetts, made a study that brings another dimension to the research on interaction effects. Frank and Gunderson (1984) examined how the interaction between *therapist* and *treatment milieu* affects the patient's engagement and continuance in treatment. Therapists and treatment milieus were classified as being either insight-oriented or control- and reality-oriented. This way of categorizing treatment conditions is not unlike that applied by McLachlan (1972, 1974) in alcoholism treatment (Section 21.1).

The subject group consisted of 60 young, well-to-do schizophrenic men and women who had consented to participate in the study and had not previously received extensive psychotherapy. Frank and Gunderson believed, with some justification, that the results obtained can be generalized to other diagnostic groups that are given psychosocial treatment. Since the study, furthermore, has significant clinical implications that require neither extra resources nor complicated administrative arrangements, it is worthy of closer examination.

The study can be divided into three phases. Frank and Gunderson started by having 12 experienced psychiatrists at McLean Hospital classify the treatment milieus as either *control-oriented* or *insight-oriented*. Both kinds of milieus had active treatment philosophies and were considered to be representative of the milieus that are commonly available in psychiatry today.

Four milieus were classified as control-oriented. Milieus of this kind place a premium on control of disturbed behaviour, suppression of symptoms, and rapid transition out of the hospital. They are hierarchically organized and place a heavy emphasis on a medical model of illness. The treatment activities are structured and task-centred. Regressions are discouraged and strict limits are employed. Such milieus are common in general hospitals with many acutely ill patients.

Five milieus were classified as insight-oriented. Milieus of this type place a premium on personal growth, self-understanding and improved ego function. Staff attempt to provide a corrective experience by supervising the treatment and giving close attention to personal problems. Less structured groups and informal talks with nursing staff are the rule. Open expression of feelings is encouraged and regressions can be coped with. Lengthy stays are not unusual. Such milieus are common in private psychiatric hospitals in the US.

The second phase of the study involved classifying therapists both according to their treatment orientation and their style of interacting with the milieu. On the basis of self-reports and information from other sources, 21 therapists were judged as being *reality-oriented, adaptive* and *supportive (RAS)*, while 17 were classified as *expressive* and *insight-oriented (EIO)*.

According to Frank and Gunderson's (1984) definition, RAS therapists view schizophrenia as an illness with a strong biological/hereditary component and with ego deficits that are likely to persist even after treatment. They try to prevent regressions within therapy and avoid uncovering activities. Their primary aim is to restore the patient to his premorbid level of functioning and to help him maintain it. They focus on the present situation, not the past. These therapists are open, supportive, and advising.

EIO therapists, on the contrary, consider environmental and developmental factors as more important in the aetiology of schizophrenia than biological/hereditary factors. They also believe that the schizophrenic's ego deficits are reversible with treatment. Their primary aim is to increase the patient's understanding of himself and why he became psychotic. Hence, they focus on the past. They believe that regressions within therapy sessions need not be harmful. These therapists tend to be non-directive and to refrain from giving advice or revealing personal information. They place less emphasis than the RAS therapists on drug therapy.

The therapists were further classified as either *administratively involved* or *uninvolved*, depending on their style of interacting with the treatment milieu. Administratively involved therapists participate in making decisions regarding the patient, while administratively uninvolved therapists are only willing to serve as consultants or advisers to the milieu staff. The therapists were fairly evenly divided into these two categories.

In the third and last phase of the study, Frank and Gunderson assessed how a match or mismatch between therapists and milieus affected patient engagement and continuance in psychotherapy. Table 21.3 shows that patients were significantly more deeply engaged in therapy after three months and were more likely to still be in therapy at six months and at two years, if their therapist's treatment orientation was congruent with that of the milieu staff than if it was not. When therapists and milieus were matched, 55 per cent of the patients remained in psychotherapy throughout the two-year period of the study, as compared to only 23 per cent if they were mismatched. This interaction effect was found no matter how brief the hospitalization was or what particular orientation therapists and milieus adhered to.

Table 21.3 Effects of milieu orientation (insight vs. control) and therapist orientation (EIO vs. RAS) on patient engagement and continuance in psychotherapy

Milieu and therapist	Three-month ratings of engagement		Still in therapy at 6 months		Still in therapy at 24 months		Total months in therapy in 2 years	Months of hospitalization
	N	X^a	N	%	N	%	X	X
Insight								
EIO	24	2.45	16	67	11	46	14.80	5.75
RAS	12	2.86	6	50	2	17	8.83	7.37
Control								
EIO	10	2.74	4	40	3	30	10.25	2.61
RAS	14	2.03	12	86	10	71	17.83	2.52
Good match	38	2.27	28	74	21	55	15.75	4.46
Poor match	22	2.80	10	45	5	23	9.54	5.10
	$p<0.05$		$p<0.05$		$p<0.05$		$p<0.05$	—

[a]The higher the score, the less engaged.

These results are notable, since long-term treatment (18 months or more) is required for meaningful and significant change to occur with schizophrenic patients. Moreover, previous studies have shown that even under optimal conditions, no more than two of five patients can be expected to remain in psychotherapy for the time required. The presented study indicates that a match between the therapist's and the milieu staff's orientation is more important for patient engagement and continuance in psychotherapy than is the particular treatment orientation.

Frank and Gunderson believed that the outcome of psychotherapy with inpatients depends as much on the match between therapists and milieus as on the match between therapists and patients (Gunderson 1978) or between patients and milieus (Almond 1983). The study illustrates the importance of taking into account the context in which psychotherapy is conducted. Taken alone, neither milieu orientation nor therapist orientation had any discernible effect on patient engagement or continuance.

By itself, it also did not seem to make any difference whether the therapist was administratively involved or not. However, Table 21.4 shows that the therapist's style of interacting with the treatment milieu did, in fact, affect patients' attitude towards psychotherapy. But this influence is only noticeable when the therapist's style is considered in conjunction with both the therapist's and the milieu staff's treatment orientation.

Therapists who not only had a philosophy that differed from the predominant orientation in the treatment milieu, but who also interfered in

Table 21.4   Effects of milieu orientation, therapist orientation, and therapist style on patient engagement and continuance in psychotherapy

Milieu–therapist–style–	Three-month ratings of engagement		Still in therapy at 6 months		Still in therapy at 24 months		Total months in therapy in 2 years	Months of hospitalization
	N	X^a	N	%	N	%	X	X
Insight–RAS–involved or Control–EIO–involved	11	3.08	4	36	1	9	6.77	4.22
Insight–RAS–uninvolved or Control–EIO–uninvolved	6	2.15	5	83	3	50	16.40	3.94
Insight–EIO–uninvolved or Control–RAS–involved	19	2.27	16	84	12	63	18.43	3.62
	$p = 0.08$		$p < 0.05$		$p < 0.05$		$p < 0.01$	—

[a]The higher the score, the less engaged.

the work of the staff had the most trouble engaging and maintaining patients in therapy. Only 36 per cent of their patients were still in therapy at six months, and only one person (9 per cent) remained for a full two years. By contrast, therapists who not only shared the orientation of the milieu staff, but who also had a style of interaction that conformed to the expectations of the staff (involved therapist in control-oriented environment, uninvolved therapist in insight-oriented environment) had the greatest success in engaging and maintaining patients in therapy. Fully 84 per cent of their patients remained in therapy for at least six months, and almost two-thirds (63 per cent) were still in therapy at two years. Finally, Table 21.4 (the line in the middle) shows that if the therapist did not become involved in the work of the staff, the fact that his or her treatment orientation conflicted with that of the milieu mattered little.

Frank and Gunderson drew the conclusion that if a psychotherapist is forced to work in a milieu whose theoretical orientation he does not share, he should keep his differing opinions to himself. This approach conflicts with the widely accepted idea, promulgated by Stanton and Schwartz (1954), that covert disagreements are harmful and should be openly acknowledged and dealt with. Frank and Gunderson's empirical data, however, indicate that covert disagreements between therapists and milieus scarcely affect patient engagement or continuance in psychotherapy.

It is not a foregone conclusion that patient engagement and continuance affects treatment outcome. The authors' assumption that these factors are correlated is, however, not unreasonable. It is also open to question whether Frank and Gunderson are correct in assuming that the results obtained are generalizable to other diagnostic groups. One may, for example, ask: How long a period of hospitalization is required for therapy-milieu interactions to have effects? Is sensitivity to open conflicts particularly great among schizophrenic patients compared with other clinical populations?

Despite its limitations, however, Frank and Gunderson's (1984) study is very fruitful. It illustrates the multidimensional nature of interaction effects, and it underscores how important it is for evaluators to take into account values and attitudes in the client's social environment. The study shows that psychotherapy is facilitated by a common theoretical orientation on the part of the therapist and the hospital staff. However, attitudes towards deviant behaviour and how people can be improved vary outside the hospital walls as well. It would therefore be of interest to examine how the interaction between the therapist's orientation and expectations in the client's natural environment affect the outcome of psychotherapy. Frank and Gunderson's study may provide fresh impetus for a deeper investigation of psychosocial treatment as a culturally mediated phenomenon.

22 Degree of alcohol dependence

22.1 Edwards and Orford

Griffith Edwards, Jim Orford, and their co-workers' study of 100 married male alcoholics at a Maudsley Hospital outpatient clinic in England (Edwards, Orford, *et al.* 1977*a*; Orford and Edwards 1977) gained a worldwide reputation within a few years as the study that definitely confirmed what everyone already 'knew': that it is useless to treat alcoholism.

How can a study that seems to show that treatment does not make any difference be interpreted as a support for the matching hypothesis? And how can a result that only confirmed what everyone felt they already knew be regarded as 'a milestone in clinical research in alcoholism' (Kissin 1977*a*, p. 1804)? An answer to these questions requires closer scrutiny not only of the study itself but also of the discussion about fundamental assumptions in alcoholism care to which the study gave rise. For the fact is that the renown of the study can ultimately be attributed to the fact that the right problem was formulated at the right time and—one is tempted to add—by the right persons.

Behind the treatment study of 100 marriages in which the husband was an alcoholic stood a well-established and internationally acknowledged team of researchers under the leadership of Edwards and Orford at the University of London's Institute of Psychiatry, Addiction Research Unit. The design of the study is illustrated by Figure 22.1.

The study included only physically and mentally intact patients with a diagnosed drinking problem. In the 100 couples, both man and wife were willing to participate in one initial counselling session. The drinking problem and various social and psychological background factors were assessed during a three-hour examination at the outpatient clinic. The information was gathered independently from the man by a psychiatrist and a psychologist and from the wife by a social worker. When the assessment had been completed, the families were assigned randomly to a treatment group and an advice group.

The husband and the wife then jointly attended a counselling session with the treatment team for half an hour. The psychiatrist clearly stated during the conversation that the man was an alcoholic, that the preferred goal was abstinence, that the man should continue working or return to work, and that the husband and wife should attempt to make their marriage viable. A free discussion then followed with a more individual and personal interpretation given to the situation.

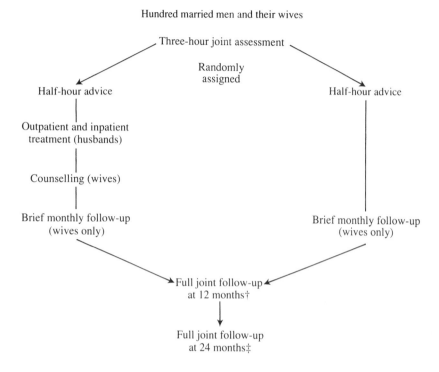

Fig. 22.1   The research design applied by Edwards and Orford.
†Edwards *et al.* (1977); ‡Orford *et al.* (1976).

The couples in the *advice group* were told, in sympathetic and constructive terms, that responsibility for attainment of the stated goals lay in their own hands. It could not be taken over by anyone else. It was explained that the patient would not be offered a further appointment at the clinic, but that someone would call the wife each month and inquire about the progress. The patient was advised to contact his general practitioner if he should be suffering from withdrawal symptoms. No medication was to be given by the clinic.

In the *treatment group*, all patients were offered an introduction to AA, a prescription of an anti-alcohol drug, and drugs to cover withdrawal if indicated. Further appointments were made with the psychiatrist for discussions of appropriate ways to prevent relapse, of personal difficulties, interpersonal and marital problems, etc. If the patient failed to respond to outpatient care, he was offered admission to a specialized six-week inpatient alcoholism unit for detoxification, group therapy, occupational therapy, and milieu therapy. The social worker was available for counselling. She also saw the wife for work on marital and other problems. The psychiatrist and social worker met regularly and sometimes proposed conjoint sessions with husband and wife.

The treatment programme was described as an 'average package of help', i.e. the kind of regimen that a well-supported treatment centre anywhere in the western world would have offered. The much less intensive advice programme would, in contrast, usually have been dismissed as inadequate.

During a period of twelve months from initial assessment, brief monthly follow-up information was obtained from the wives alone, in both advice and treatment groups. At the end of the twelve-month period, a complete follow-up session was held with the husband and wife. During the second year, no attempt was made to maintain any distinction between the treatment experience of the two groups. The men were followed up at twenty-four months with special reference to variations in drinking pattern and evidence of 'controlled drinking'.

The results of the study were conclusive. At twelve months there were no statistically significant differences between the advice group and the treatment group (Edwards, Orford, et al. 1977a). The evaluation criteria included measures both of social adjustment in the family and at work and of the scope and character of the drinking problem, with independent accounts obtained from both the patient and his wife and with information collected both by an independent psychologist and by the treatment staff. Information was also obtained from AA and other helping agencies for the twelve-month period, and it was concluded that the advice group did not have more contacts with agencies outside the clinic than did the treatment group.

The negative results obtained by Edwards, Orford, and their co-workers are noteworthy, but should not come as any surprise. Levinson and Sereny's (1969) comparison between intensive psychiatrically-oriented treatment and a programme that simply offered a period of rest and diversion, for example, gave at least as gloomy a picture of the effectiveness of widespread techniques of alcoholism treatment. A review of more recent research that arrived at similar results is given in Section 3.1.

However, the Maudsley Hospital study was exceptionally rigorous. It also came at an opportune moment. At the end of the 1970s, alcoholism treatment research was sufficiently well established to stand up to a constructive self-examination. The majority of commentators accepted the main results of the study. The discussion instead came to focus on how the findings should be interpreted. Edwards, Orford, and their co-workers (1977a) themselves did not at all give up on alcoholism treatment. In their eyes, the results indicated rather 'a need for development of new treatment techniques and their rigorous testing' (p. 1028). They emphasized:

The implications of this study must not be seen as nihilistic. In an area of health care so much in need of development it would be sad indeed if a research report were misread as evidence that treatment of alcoholism must forever be a worthless enterprise. The practical implication from which one should not turn away, however, is that the received wisdom as to what constitutes effective and economic treatment of alcoholism may be in need of revision. (p. 1027)

Edwards, Orford, *et al.* (1977*a*, p. 1004) noted that the current treatment philosophy was based on the classical disease model of alcoholism. In a commentary, Glaser (1977) claimed that what mainly needs to be reconsidered is this unitary disease concept and the fruitless search for an 'average package' of help. If alcoholics are a heterogeneous group, then any particular therapy may only be appropriate for a minority. The matching hypothesis was proposed as an alternative to the package policy. According to Glaser, the most reasonable conclusion of the study is not the one that seems to have been the most common, namely that treatment is no more effective than advice. The study shows rather that if the same treatment is indiscriminately applied to all patients, the overall result will be no better than what can be achieved in a counselling session. Interpreted in this manner, the study provided impetus for a novel approach to treatment at the Addiction Research Foundation in Toronto, according to Glaser *et al.* (1985; see Chapter 15 above).

Glaser's (1977) indirect argumentation on behalf of the matching hypothesis may have logical appeal, but it carries little weight as empirical evidence. However, the *two-year* follow-up of the 100 alcoholic men and their wives (Orford *et al.* 1976) provided direct evidence of interaction between patient, treatment, and outcome.

This study was based on the 65 couples for whom it was possible to obtain complete two-year follow-up data from both marital partners. For 19 alcoholics, two-year follow-up data were obtained from only one spouse, and for the remaining 16 men, no data at all were obtained. The latter subjects were left out of the analysis instead of being classified as failures or mainly failures according to common practice. This source of bias, in combination with the high dropout rate and the small number of subjects, means that the results, even though they may be interesting, must be interpreted very cautiously.

The drinking pattern during the second year of follow-up was classified as 'good' (26 men), 'bad' (19 men), or 'equivocal' (20 men). The latter category included ten men whose drinking pattern was considered neither good nor bad and ten cases where the husbands and wives differed in their estimates of how often excessive drinking occurred.

Based on the initial assessment, subjects were divided into 'Gamma alcoholics' (20 men) and 'non-Gamma alcoholics' (45 men). The term Gamma alcoholism was introduced by Jellinek (1960) to designate a drinking pattern distinguished by increased tolerance, withdrawal symptoms, morning drinking, 'loss of control', and other signs of 'physical dependence'. In current terminology, these symptoms would indicate a well-established *alcohol dependence.*

Orford, Oppenheimer, and Edwards (1976) wanted to know whether Gamma alcoholics responded differently than non-Gammas to more intensive treatment compared with brief counselling. The data presented in Section 12.4 above suggest that such an interaction did exist at the two-year follow-up. Gamma alcoholics tended to do well and non-Gammas poorly in intensive outpatient treatment, while the reverse was true with brief counselling alone. However, since no such interaction was observed at the 12-month follow-up, these findings are problematic. The lack of consistency may be an effect of bias due to dropout at the two-year follow-up rather than of differential response to treatment and advice.

A closer examination of patients who did well during the second year (26 out of 65) indicated that there was an interaction between patient characteristics and the nature of the improvement. Those with a good outcome were almost equally divided into abstainers (11 men) and 'controlled drinkers' (10 men). 'Controlled drinking' defined by Orford *et al.* (op. cit.) was not more than 200 grams of alcohol (16 *drinks* defined as 1.5 oz. of liquor 40 per cent) on any single day and no drinking that was unacceptable to the wife. In the remaining five cases, a clear categorization as abstainer or controlled drinker was prevented by disagreement between husband and wife on the details of drinking.

Age and problem chronicity were not predictive of abstinence versus 'controlled drinking'. Table 22.1, however, shows that Gamma alcoholism versus non-Gamma alcoholism, or the severity of alcohol dependence, did predict the nature of improvement. Dependent or Gamma alcoholics did well through total abstinence (significant), while non-Gamma alcoholics tended to do well through 'controlled drinking'.

The results confirm findings by, for example, Davies (1962) and Armor *et al.* (1978), which showed that periods of controlled or attenuated drinking among alcohol abusers are not an unusual phenomenon, but rather an important outcome of treatment. But they also support Edward's (1977) and others' assumption that alcohol dependence can reach such a degree of severity that a return to controlled drinking is highly unlikely.

Edwards (1977) pointed out that a treatment goal has certain prospects of being achieved if the patient himself regards it as realistic and as a logical

Table 22.1 Nature of improvement by severity of alcohol dependence

Severity of alcohol dependence	Nature of improvement	
	Abstinence	'Controlled drinking'
Non-dependent	5	10
Dependent (Gamma)	6*	0*

*$p < 0.025$

consequence of an accurate diagnosis rather than a form of punishment and control. The vague and all-encompassing use of the term 'alcoholism', which does not distinguish the medical and social complications of drinking from the actual dependence symptoms and their severity, has made it difficult to make an individual prognosis and arrive at a rational plan of treatment. The Maudsley Hospital study suggests that the graduated dependence concept (Edwards and Gross 1976) can facilitate the choice of realistic treatment goals. This conclusion is supported by Rand Report II (Section 22.2), which, however, indicates that the interaction between patient characteristics and an outcome of abstinence versus 'controlled drinking' is complex and includes more factors than the degree of alcohol dependence.

Another conclusion drawn by Edwards and Orford (Edwards *et al.* 1977*a*; Orford and Edwards 1977) is that we should perhaps not look so much for more intensive versions of conventional treatment, but rather develop and test less intensive treatments than have previously been thought adequate. It is important to realize that the advice offered in the study was partially individualized and presented as a credible option. It was quite different from control conditions such as 'no treatment' or 'waiting list'. It has been argued that the advice, rather than being a pale shadow of alcoholism treatment, actually constituted an appropriate and qualified crisis intervention (Orford 1980).

Trice and Beyer (1981) pointed out that the advice offered is similar to a *constructive confrontation* strategy that has been found effective in American job-based alcoholism programmes. Here employees are confronted with evidence of their impaired job performance and simultaneously offered non-judgemental rehabilitative help. There are also similarities to a promising French intervention strategy, which uses education and feedback of health consequences as a means to persuade the non-dependent problem drinker to reduce his consumption (Babor *et al.* 1983; Chick 1984).

In Sweden, Hans Kristenson (1987; Kristenson *et al.* 1983) has developed a method of counselling and repeated feedback of values on the Gamma-GT test for early liver disorder (popularly known as the 'nagging method'). Kristenson's method is a successful attempt to treat heavy drinkers identified by a general health screening project. All these programmes, i.e. advice offered to alcoholics with intact families, constructive confrontation of employed alcohol abusers, feedback of health consequences to non-dependent problem drinkers, and a regular check-up for drinkers with elevated Gamma-GT values, exemplify carefully planned low-cost interventions that show considerable promise for alcohol abusers with a relatively favourable prognosis.

22.2   Rand Report II

The second Rand report, written by Michael Polich, David Armor, and Harriet Braiker (1981), is a very sophisticated attempt to describe the course of alcoholism among patients after treatment. The first Rand report (Armor *et al.* 1978) sparked widespread public interest and debate in the United States that mainly centred around its inclusion of 'normal drinking' as a form of remission. 'Normal drinking' defined by the Rand report was not more than an average of three ounces of absolute alcohol (five to six drinks of 1.5 oz. liquor 40 per cent) a day *and* no 'serious symptoms'. 'Serious symptoms' were frequent episodes of blackouts, missing work, morning drinking; missing meals, and being drunk. This broad definition of 'normal drinking', including also what most people would regard as alcohol abuse, was taken by some as evidence to suggest that alcoholics may safely resume drinking.

In the preface to the second edition of the original Rand report, Armor, Polich, and Stambul (1978) emphasized that they had chosen the term 'remission', and not 'recovery', since the study spanned only 18 months after initial treatment. Whether the outcome would prove stable over a longer period of time remained an unanswered question. Added to this uncertainty were the methodological limitations, which, the authors admitted, reduced the validity of the findings.

In the second Rand report (Polich *et al.* 1981) non-problem drinkers were distinguished not by the controversial 'normal drinking' criterion, but rather by the absence of any symptoms of alcohol dependence (blackouts, tremors, missing meals, morning drinking, or drinking continuously over 12 hours) and the absence of any serious consequences of drinking, such as medical complications, arrests, or job problems.

Rand Report II traces patterns of change in a large, nationally representative cohort of alcoholics from admission to treatment via follow-up at 18 months to a follow-up four years after initial contact. An extensive body of data was collected, covering drinking behaviour and adverse effects of drinking, psychosocial functioning, physical health, and previous treatment experiences. The validity of self-reports was checked both by measurements of blood alcohol concentration and by interviews with a collateral (a person who knew the subject well).

Hodgson (1980*b*) said about this second Rand report that it is not as controversial as the original, but it provides more solid evidence and deserves more attention. Among other things, the size of the study cohort permitted a detailed examination of multifactorial relationships that determine the probability of remission and relapse. This analysis is of particular interest from the viewpoint of the matching hypothesis.

The cohort in this analysis of relapse (Polich *et al.* 1980, 1981, Ch. 7; Armor 1980) was a random sample of male individuals who had been admitted to treatment at any of eight NIAAA-funded alcoholism treatment centres during a given period of time and who could also be interviewed at a follow-up 18 months later. Of those subjects who had been interviewed on two occasions (admission, 18 months), approximately 15 per cent had died four years after the initial contact. Ninety per cent of the survivors, or 474 persons, were available for follow-up at four years. Of these subjects, 29 per cent had been abstinent for six months or more; 18 per cent were non-problem drinkers during the six-month period before follow-up; while 53 per cent were experiencing problems defined as either symptoms of alcohol dependence or serious adverse consequences of drinking.

The analysis of factors that might explain the differences in relapse rate was focused on those clients who were improved at follow-up after 18 months but who, at follow-up after four years, had lost control over their drinking. Subjects in 'remission' at 18 months included (a) 115 persons who had been abstinent for six months or longer, and (b) 85 persons who drank in the past month but with no symptoms of dependence (blackouts, tremors, missing meals, morning drinking, or drinking continuously over 12 hours).

The relapse analysis is thus based on the select one-third (200 persons) of the original study cohort that remained after subtracting persons who either died between 18 months and four years or were problem drinkers at the 18 month follow-up. Compared with all men who had been admitted to treatment, the clients studied appear to have been younger, less mobile, somewhat more socially stable and well-off, drinking less, and to have had less serious symptoms and fewer treatments for alcoholism.

On the basis of a smaller sample and a shorter observation period, the first Rand Report had suggested that some alcoholics can resume 'normal' drinking without relapsing into problem drinking. This position was highly controversial. In the second Rand Report, the authors therefore wanted to extend the analysis by comparing the relapse rate of abstinent and 'normal' drinkers over the longer four-year follow-up period.

The evaluation at four years showed that those who had been long-term abstainers at 18 months had a slightly lower relapse rate than those who had been drinking without any symptoms of dependence. The difference was not statistically significant, however. This result brought up the question of whether there are any intervening variables that influence the probability of relapse with non-problem drinking versus abstinence. Such multifactorial relationships, if they exist, would facilitate an understanding of the processes that cause relapse. Perhaps, it was assumed, there are some alcoholics who have a better prognosis if they abstain, while others have a better prognosis if they engage in non-problem drinking.

Polich, Armor, and Braiker examined a number of individual background characteristics by means of multiple regression analysis to determine whether they had any impact on the risk of relapse. The definition of 'relapse' was drinking with symptoms of dependence in the month prior to the four-year follow-up. The analysis included factors that previous research had shown to be generally related to remission, such as severity of alcohol dependence, socioeconomic status, marital and employment status, age, race, and previous treatment experience.

Table 22.2 Expected relapse rates at 4-year follow-up for abstainers versus non-problem drinkers at 18 months by age, severity of alchol dependence, and marital status

	Age under 40		Age 40 or over	
Background characteristics at admission	Abstaining 6 months or more at 18 months %	Non-problem drinking at 18 months %	Abstaining 6 months or more at 18 months %	Non-problem drinking at 18 months %
High severity of dependence[a]				
Married	7	17	4	50
Unmarried	16	7	10	28
Low severity of dependence				
Married	16	7	11	28
Unmarried	32	3	22	13

[a]High severity of dependence represents 11 or more symptom events (blackouts, tremors, missing meals, morning drinking, drinking continuously for 12 hours) during the 30 days preceding admission to treatment. Low severity of dependence represents 1 to 10 such events. Subjects with no dependence symptoms at admission are excluded from the table.

The research group found statistically significant interaction effects showing that age, severity of dependence, and marital status influenced the probability of relapse following abstention and non-problem drinking. These background characteristics were considered to be the most interesting ones from a theoretical point of view as well. Table 22.2 shows expected relapse rates for the sub-groups formed by the intervening variables. The proportion of variation in the data explained by the model is 7 per cent for abstainers and 14 per cent for non-problem drinkers. With so little predictive ability, the model must—despite the significant interaction effects—be regarded as highly preliminary (see Smith and Jackson 1982).

The table tells us that older men with high severity of alcohol dependence at admission for treatment had a much lower risk of relapse if they abstained rather than engaged in non-problem drinking at 18 months, regardless of marital status. The reverse was true for younger men with low severity of dependence: abstainers had higher expected relapse rates than non-problem drinkers, regardless of marital status. For the other two groups—older men with low severity of dependence and younger men with high severity of dependence—the interaction was more complex. Marital status appeared to play an important role: those who were married had lower expected relapse rates if they abstained, whereas the unmarrieds had lower expected relapse rates if they were non-problem drinkers.

The analysis of expected relapse rates indicates that the process leading to relapse involves a number of predisposing factors. No individual factor was of decisive importance in predicting the course of alcoholism after treatment. Persons with severe alcohol dependence, for example, generally had a better prognosis if they abstained—with the exception of the younger unmarrieds, for whom predicted relapse was lower if they were non-problem drinkers. Furthermore, those under 40 generally had lower relapse rates if they were non-problem drinkers—with the exception of severely dependent married persons, for whom abstention yielded the better prognosis. These results, if replicated, suggest a far more complex picture of remission and relapse in alcoholism than has been previously acknowledged.

Existing theories of alcoholism provide no complete explanation for the specific variables that, according to Polich, Armor, and Braiker, intervene in the relapse process. The authors did, however, offer some hypotheses that include both *biological* and *psychosocial* factors.

From a psychobiological point of view, the results are consistent with the assumption that when alcohol dependence has reached a certain degree of severity, the likelihood of being able to resume moderate drinking is very small. Persons who are not severely dependent may, however, be able to resume non-problem drinking without relapse. Advancing age may complicate the picture by bringing about psychobiological changes that intensify the effects of the dependence.

The role of dependence is underscored by the observation (Polich *et al.* 1981, Ch. 3; Polich 1980) that the *quantity* of alcohol consumed did not influence the expected relapse rate for alcoholics who engaged in non-problem drinking at 18 months. The presence of *symptoms*, in contrast, increased the risk of relapse, regardless of the quantity of alcohol consumed. The study thus confirms the usefulness of the graduated concept of dependence and its potential value for matching clients to treatments (cf. Chapters 7, 11).

The importance of age and marital status indicates that psychosocial factors influence the relapse process. Sometimes, the impact of the environment seems to be strong enough to reverse the probability of remission versus relapse. Of the severely alcohol-dependent men, the younger and unmarried ones tended to do *worse* after abstention than after engaging in non-problem drinking. Polich, Armor, and Braiker guessed that many of these men found themselves in a subculture where frequent drinking is the norm. Younger or unmarried men who try to maintain abstention in such a non-supportive environment may find it so stressful that the probability of relapse is increased.

Of men who were not severely dependent on alcohol, the older and married ones departed from the general pattern by doing worse after engaging in non-problem drinking than after abstention. The authors of Rand Report II make the assumption here that married male alcoholics who abstain receive considerable support from their wives, while they may not receive support when they attempt moderate drinking. Because of the widely held belief that alcoholics cannot return to moderate drinking, attempts to do so may be regarded as failures. This attitude may be so stressful for the alcoholic that attempts at attenuated drinking will lead to relapse. Probably, one may add, attempts at moderate drinking can be so frustrating for the wife as well that she is simply unable to provide the support her husband may need to recover.

The analysis in the second Rand report raises provocative questions and inspires hope that findings from different fields of alcohol research may be integrated in a biopsychosocial perspective. It should be born in mind, however, that the analysis is based on observations made under non-experimental conditions. The study does not tell what would happen if alcoholics were advised to engage in non-problem drinking. Moreover, it offers a description of how people actually behave, not a recommendation as to how they should behave. Polich, Armor, and Braiker (1981) explicitly warn against immediate and sweeping changes in the current treatment policy with its emphasis on abstinence:

Although there is a definite trend toward controlled-drinking methods in the treatment of alcoholism (Sobell and Sobell, 1978), it appears that most alcoholics in treatment, being older and highly dependent on alcohol, would have a poor prognosis with nonproblem drinking. In addition, attempts at nonproblem drinking are inappropriate for those alcoholics who have physical conditions exacerbated by drinking (e.g., liver disease) and for those who have repeatedly attempted but failed at controlled drinking. Nonetheless, an expansion of treatment approaches, including goals other than the traditional demand for abstinence, might offer advantages for some alcoholics. We recommend that well-controlled experimental studies be undertaken to investigate the efficacy of varying treatment goals. (p. 220)

This cautious interpretation of the research results is justified, considering that:

(1) only a small percentage of variation in the data has been explained;

(2) the analysis concerns a select sample of alcoholic clients;

(3) the definition of non-problem drinking at 18 month follow-up is based on symptom events in the past month only; and

(4) a 30-day window only was used to assess outcome at four-year follow-up, which permits some bout drinkers to be classified as being in remission.

The results regarding expected relapse rates for abstainers versus non-problem drinkers are, nevertheless, consistent and plausible. The authors' recommendation for more rigorous research on whether a matching of clients and interventions might lead to improved outcomes therefore seems well-founded.

22.3 Welte

In a review in 1983, William Miller cited the results of the second Rand report as major evidence that moderation-oriented approaches hold promise in treating the less dependent problem drinker. At the same time, however, John Welte, Joseph Lyons, and Lloyd Sokolow (1983) at the Research Institute on Alcoholism in Buffalo, New York, published findings that were at variance with those of the Rand Study.

The research group followed up 1340 clients of both sexes from 17 inpatient alcoholism rehabilitation units three and eight months after discharge from treatment (see Section 19.3). At three months, 72 per cent of the clients were interviewed. At eight months, interviews were obtained with 67 per cent of the clients, including 79 per cent of those who had been interviewed at three months.

The analysis was done in two stages. First the overall relationship between drinking pattern at the three-month follow-up and the relapse rate at eight months was examined. The criteria for relapse versus non-problem drinking were borrowed from the authors of Rand Report II (Polich et al. 1981; see Section 22.2). Welte and his co-workers found that only 12 per cent of those clients who were abstaining at the three-month follow-up had relapsed at eight months. By contrast, 32 per cent of those who were drinking with no symptoms of dependence at the three-month follow-up had relapsed five months later. The difference eight months after treatment between the abstaining group and the group that was drinking without symptoms at three months was significant at the 0.001 level.

In the next stage, researchers looked for interaction effects that indicated that the relationship between drinking pattern and relapse rate varied with different groups of clients. Thirteen demographic and clinical variables were examined, including age and severity of alcohol dependence. However, the authors were unable to identify any sub-population of clients who were more successful at avoiding relapse with non-problem drinking than with abstinence.

This result is different from that described by the second Rand report (Polich et al. 1981). Welte, Lyons, and Sokolow (1983) advocated, as did the Rand authors, caution with controlled drinking. But they were not opposed to the development of programmes with alternative drinking goals. Welte and his co-workers pointed out that the validity of their findings was limited by the fact that all subjects had received treatment aimed at total abstinence.

Nor did these authors—in contrast to the Rand researchers—examine the existence of theoretically meaningful multivariate interactions. Welte and his co-workers also included women in the subject group, which means that a direct comparison with the second Rand report would require a study of interaction effects involving sex in addition to degree of alcohol dependence, age, and marital status.

22.4   Foy, Sanchez-Craig

In all of the studies discussed above, treatment programmes have aimed at total abstinence. The cited research thereby has only indirect relevance to the debate about controlled drinking as a treatment goal. In recent years, however, a few evaluations have been presented of treatment specifically designed to achieve controlled drinking.

The best of these studies was carried out in conventional alcoholism treatment by David Foy, Bruce Nunn, and Robert Rychtarik (1984). Foy and his co-workers at the Veterans Administration Medical Center in Jackson, Mississippi, had reported over a number of years on experiments with social skills training and training in controlled drinking skills. The research group was therefore well qualified for the task of comparing traditional treatment of alcoholics with treatment aimed at controlled drinking.

Foy, Nunn, and Rychtarik (1984) tried to control for major sources of confounding present in earlier treatment experiments, which, according to these authors, were hampered by such methodological flaws that it was impossible to draw any conclusions about the effects of training controlled drinking skills.

Sixty-two male alcoholics without severe physical or psychiatric complications or cognitive deficits were assigned randomly to either of two broad-spectrum four-week inpatient treatment programmes. The goal in the one programme was abstinence. In the other, subjects were administered 15 hours of controlled drinking skills training. The staff had long experience of alcoholism treatment, were behavioural in their theoretical orientation, and were cautiously optimistic about the clients' chances of learning to drink in a controlled manner. Posttraining tests showed that clients actually had learnt the purported controlled drinking skills.

The outcomes of the two programmes were compared six and 12 months after discharge. The six-month follow-up revealed that subjects in the drinking skills condition had significantly fewer abstinent days ($p < 0.05$) and more abusive days ($p < 0.05$) than subjects in treatment aimed at total abstinence. The proportion of abstinent days in the former group was 60 per cent as compared with 75 per cent in the latter group. The proportion of abusive days was 24 per cent among those in the drinking skills condition as compared with 12 per cent among those who had been recommended to abstain. Although the trends continued, differences between the groups were no longer statistically significant at the twelve-month follow-up. At the five to six-year follow-up (Rychtarik *et al.* 1987), the two groups were virtually indistinguishable in outcome.

Foy and his co-workers (1984) did not, however, find any differences between different programmes as regards number of days with reduced or controlled drinking. Nor was there any difference with regard to social adjustment. Reduced drinking here was three to eight ounces of 80-proof distilled spirits (5–11 drinks of 1.5 oz. liquor), while controlled drinking was less than three ounces (five drinks) each day.

The research group also investigated the relationship between pretreatment alcohol dependence and drinking behaviour at follow-up. It was found that the severity of alcohol dependence (measured by the symptoms of the second Rand report: blackouts, tremors, missing meals, morning drinking, and drinking continuously over 12 hours) affected the type of drinking that occurred after treatment. For men with high severity of dependence (three or more symptoms), 75 per cent of the drinking was abusive. The corresponding figure for men with low severity of dependence (no more than one symptom) was 47 per cent. The percentage of abstinent days was, however, not significantly affected by the severity of alcohol dependence.

The study suggests that alcoholics who have been trained in controlled drinking skills generally run a greater risk of relapse than alcoholics who have been recommended to abstain. However, this negative effect—like positive effects of treatment—seems to be of a transient nature. Since the percentage of days with moderate (reduced and controlled) drinking was the same regardless of treatment received, the study does not lend any support to the assumption that lack of specific skills contributes to the impaired ability of alcoholics to control their drinking. Foy's and his co-workers' study is, however, consistent with the hypothesis that the severity of alcohol dependence influences the probability of a controlled drinking outcome.

These conclusions are also consistent with the results obtained by Sanchez-Craig, Annis, Bornet, and MacDonald (1984) in a study of secondary preventive measures, i.e. early intervention strategies offered to the less serious type of problem drinker. Seventy such subjects were randomly assigned to two treatment programmes that were identical, except that the goal in one was abstinence while the goal in the other was controlled drinking. The clients in the latter condition were trained for six 90-minutes sessions in controlled drinking skills.

Sanchez-Craig et al. (1984) found no statistically significant differences between the two programmes, in terms of either dropout rate or outcome six months and two years after discharge. The majority of clients reduced their alcohol consumption to a 'moderate' level (here: less than 21 drinks of 1.5 oz. liquor per week) without becoming abstinent, no matter which treatment programme they entered. In the controlled drinking condition, three per cent of the clients were abstinent while 69 per cent drank 'moderately' at six months. In the abstinence condition, the corresponding figures were seven and 67 per cent respectively.

Sanchez-Craig and Lei (1986) argued that some drinkers may have gained more than others from entering the controlled-drinking programme instead of treatment aimed at abstinence. However, the difference in outcome was not statistically significant, no adjustment was made for dropouts, and the subjects available for the relevant comparisons were so few that reclassification of two clients would have made the '21 per cent difference' disappear. Nevertheless, controlled drinking was found to be a more acceptable goal than abstinence. Sanchez-Craig and colleagues (1984) therefore recommended this drinking goal for programmes recruiting early-stage problem drinkers.

The controversy of whether there are clients even in conventional alcoholism treatment that may benefit from a controlled drinking goal has, however, not been settled yet. Notwithstanding the results obtained by Foy and his co-workers (1984), there may be a minority for whom controlled drinking is an appropriate goal.

22.5   Long-term outcome

The controlled drinking debate culminated in the mid 1980s. The *British Journal of Addiction* published 17 sets of comments by leading clinicians and researchers on a paper by Stockwell (1986) raising the question: 'Is controlled drinking possible for the person who has been severely alcohol dependent?' Stockwell (1988) interpreted the replies as showing an emerging consensus that 'the eventuality is so unlikely as to be unimportant' (p. 149).

During the same period, four critical reviews were published. Taylor, Helzer, and Robins (1986) and Chick (1987) recommended total abstinence as a provisional guideline for those who suffer from severe dependence on alcohol. Peele (1987) and Sobell and Sobell (1987), on the other hand, warned against premature closure on this issue and emphasized the importance of expectations, beliefs, and cultural differences.

Two kinds of empirical studies have been much quoted in the debate. First, a set of long-term follow-up studies shed light on the question of whether severely alcohol dependent persons are able to sustain controlled drinking over time. Secondly, a few short-term follow-ups were reported, which studied severity of dependence as a predictor of abstinence versus moderation outcome (see Section 22.6).

Among the first set of studies is the one by Vaillant and Milofsky (1982*a*) following 110 Core-City alcohol abusers until 47 years of age. Among those 71 men who had ever met the DSM-III criteria for alcohol dependence, six (8 per cent) resumed non-problem drinking for two years or more (average, ten years). In contrast, 15 men (21 per cent) became abstinent for three years or more (average, ten years). The severity of alcohol dependence was a strong predictor of the ability to engage in non-problem drinking over time. In Vaillant's (1983*b*) clinical sample, drawn from a hospital detoxification unit, only five out of 106 patients (5 per cent) had returned to non-problem drinking after eight years.

Edwards *et al.* (1983) found eight cases of sustained controlled drinking in their ten to 12-year follow-up of 100 married male alcoholics (cf. Section. 22.1). Only one of these drinkers had ever met the Severity of Alcohol

Dependence Questionnaire criteria for severe dependence. This man reduced his consumption due to extreme loss of tolerance to alcohol.

Helzer *et al.* (1985) studied the five to seven-year outcome for 1289 patients who had been treated for alcoholism. In the three years before interview, 41 subjects (6 per cent) were moderate drinkers, as defined by criteria allowing up to six drinks a day, or were mostly abstinent but did drink occasionally. Eighty-four subjects (15 per cent) had been totally abstinent during all 36 months before the follow-up interview. Predictors of moderate and occasional drinking were female sex and a history of less severe drinking problems.

Other studies following severely dependent drinkers have similarly reported that no more than ten per cent will resume a stable pattern of controlled drinking (e.g. Smart 1978*a*; Finney and Moos 1981; Pettinati *et al.* 1982*a*). However, according to Peele (1987) and the Sobells (1987), recent long-term studies by McCabe (1986), Nordström and Berglund (1987*b*), and Rychtarik *et al.* (1987) question the *severity of dependence hypothesis*, i.e. the assumption that there is a reverse relationship between severity of dependence and the likelihood of controlled drinking outcomes.

McCabe (1986) reported a 16-year follow-up of 57 married individuals who at treatment entry were classified as alcohol dependent. Forty-six per cent of the sample were Gamma and Epsilon alcoholics. These diagnoses require repeated withdrawal symptoms and thus indicate at least moderate dependence on alcohol. In the year prior to follow-up, eight individuals (15 per cent) were abstinent, while 11 (20 per cent) were drinking in a controlled manner, i.e. without dependence or alcohol-related problems. This large proportion of controlled drinking is intriguing. However, small sample size, follow-up interval of one year only, and lack of analysis of outcomes related to initial severity of alcohol dependence, make any far-reaching implications hazardous.

Nordström (1987; Nordström and Berglund 1987*b*) reported on a 21-year follow-up of 324 male alcoholics admitted to inpatient treatment. Of these, 70 men (15 per cent if deceased patients are included) fulfilled the study criteria of good social adjustment. Among those 55 men, of 60 interviewed, who had ever met the DSM-III criteria for alcohol dependence, 21 had resumed non-problem drinking at follow-up (approx. 8 per cent of all alcohol dependent men). Eleven patients in the good adjustment group were abstainers (approx. 4 per cent of all dependent men). During the first seven years after treatment admission, in contrast, abstinence was the dominating type of successful adjustment.

This study indicates that alcohol dependence does not preclude a return to social drinking. The findings do not, however, challenge abstinence as the primary drinking goal of inpatient alcoholism treatment. Half of those who eventually practised controlled drinking did achieve this after a sustained period of abstinence (average, three years). The other half attained social drinking by gradually reducing their drinking, often as a consequence of decreased tolerance for alcohol. The latter course seems no more safe than Russian roulette, however, since 30 per cent of all patients in the original sample were deceased at follow-up.

Rychtarik *et al.* (1987) examined stability of drinking patterns and predictors of outcome in a five to six-year follow-up of those subjects studied by Foy *et al.* (1984; see Section 22.4). They found that abstinent days at one year was positively related to abstinent days at five to six years, while a moderation outcome at one year was not predictive of a stable moderation pattern over the long term. Of the seven subjects drinking moderately at the end of the first year, six were in a predominantly abusive drinking category over the long term, while one subject died (non-alcohol related). At the end of the follow-up, however, two of these subjects had been drinking moderately for the last six months.

There was an inverse relationship between the presence of social supports at treatment entry and quantity of alcohol consumed at long-term follow-up. However, no significant relationship was found between number of pretreatment withdrawal symptoms and alcohol consumption at follow-up. Whatever implication this fact may have for the dependence hypothesis, Foy and Rychtarik (1987) are perfectly right in concluding that their study is 'not encouraging for an immediate goal of moderation for severely dependent individuals' (p. 72).

22.6   Persuasion versus dependence

Orford and Keddie (1986*a*) introduced the *persuasion hypothesis* as 'the major alternative' to the dependence hypothesis. The former hypothesis states that the more a person is persuaded that one goal is possible for him, the greater is the likelihood of attaining this goal.

In a test of this hypothesis, Orford and Keddie (1986*b*) assigned subjects who strongly preferred a goal of abstinence or controlled drinking to treatment aiming at their preferred goal. Subjects who did not express a strong goal preference were randomly assigned to abstinence and controlled drinking-oriented treatments. In a third step, patients were assigned either to intensive or brief treatment. The sample consisted of 46 clients representing a broad range of severity of dependence on alcohol.

At follow-up one year after treatment admission, the success rate did not differ between those in abstinence treatment and those in controlled drinking treatment. Nor were there any differential effects of intensive versus brief treatment. The criteria for success allowed for a few slips during the past six months and drinking at 'harm-free levels' throughout the period. Drinking success did not depend upon whether the treatment received was matched or mismatched according to the dependence hypothesis. Severely dependent alcoholics did as well in controlled drinking treatment as in abstinence treatment. In contrast, personal persuasion at treatment entry, and the treatment orientation, were predictive of type of outcome. Clients who strongly preferred a controlled drinking goal, and those who received controlled drinking treatment, were significantly more likely than others to attain this goal.

Orford and Keddie (1986b) concluded that the type of treatment outcome seem to 'depend upon the personal persuasion of a client, the persuasion of treatment personnel, and the compatibility of these two' (p. 502). They cautioned, however, that clients' personal beliefs and preferences were typically in line with the orientation of the treatment received. This contamination was caused by the experimental design, which did not enable a full random assignment to treatment groups. They noted, furthermore, that neither abstinence nor controlled drinking was very often well established by the end of the follow-up year. Six clients were, in fact, still in treatment at one year, and the posttreatment follow-up period varied widely for the rest of the sample. It may be added that the tests of the dependence and the persuasion hypotheses were based on data from 22 clients only and that the criteria for 'harm-free' or 'controlled' drinking were somewhat loose.

In the study by Elal-Lawrence, Slade, and Dewey (1986) subjects were free to select either abstinence or controlled drinking-oriented treatment. At one-year follow-up 50 successful controlled drinkers, 45 abstainers, and 44 relapsers were compared on 32 pretreatment variables. Subjects who dropped out from outpatient treatment or could not be unequivocally classified at follow-up were excluded from the analysis.

Number of alcohol-related symptoms and other indicators of a severe drinking problem did not predict type of outcome. The most powerful predictors, besides the presence of liver damage, were instead AA attendance and previous abstinence. Most controlled drinkers had not been exposed to a strong abstinence ideology through AA or medical agencies; and they had not attempted abstinence, or else they had been unsuccessful at it. Results were interpreted as suggesting that drinking goals should be matched to clients' beliefs and experiences.

In contrast to Orford and Keddie (1986b), however, Elal-Lawrence and his co-workers found no relationship between clients' goal choice and type of outcome. Thus, the study does not offer any consistent support for the former authors' persuasion hypothesis. It rather demonstrates—in the words of Elal-Lawrence et al. (1986)—that 'factors influencing outcome are likely to be complex and interactive' (p. 46). Finally, the validity of the study as a test of the dependence hypothesis may be questioned on the grounds that alcohol dependence—as distinct from alcohol-related disabilities etc.—was not actually measured.

The third study relevant to the severity of dependence hypothesis was conducted by Heather, Whitton, and Robertson (1986). These authors studied problem drinkers who responded to a newspaper advertisement offering free help to cut down drinking. About half of the respondents agreed to initial assessment. Although the intervention (a self-help manual) was intended for early-stage problem drinkers, one third of the subjects interviewed showed evidence of 'late dependence' (restlessness, tremor, relief drinking). What is more, the reduction in consumption shown by the late-dependence group ($N = 10$) was not significantly different from that shown by subjects exhibiting early or no dependence ($N = 22$). If anything, subjects showing late dependence seemed to benefit more from the moderation instructions than did other problem drinkers.

Again, the sample size was very small, outcome was assessed by a seven-day window only, and the effects of dropout are difficult to assess. Like the other two studies examined above, this study does not provide sufficient evidence for a rejection of the severity of dependence hypothesis (cf. Heather 1989a). Indeed, Heather (1987) himself was explicit on this issue, saying that:

severely dependent problem drinkers should normally be advised to abstain entirely from alcohol. The main reason for this is simply that, at the present stage of our knowledge, the evidence shows abstinence to be the less risky option. (p. 254; italics in original)

The latter conclusion is confirmed by this review, with the addition that some alcoholics may be able to resume drinking after an extended period of abstinence, if their social support system and other conditions are favourable (Nordström 1987; Rychtarik et al. 1987). Heather et al.'s (1986) and Orford and Keddie's (1986b) studies highlight, however, the needs of those alcoholics who refuse to consider abstinence. Such individuals should not be turned away, but might instead benefit from treatment aimed at reduction of their consumption to a less problematic level. In this sense, the persuasion of the client should be considered in *addition* to the severity of his dependence in selecting an appropriate drinking goal.

Part V

Selection of treatment

Part V draws general conclusions and examines the scientific and clinical implications of the facts and analyses presented in this book. The first chapter attempts to answer the question of whether the matching hypothesis is a fruitful perspective on treatment. The two following chapters formulate assumptions as to how and why the outcome of alcoholism treatment can be improved by deliberately and consistently pairing clients and interventions.

23 Treatment in perspective

The matching hypothesis, or the assumption that improved treatment outcomes can be achieved by means of a differential approach that deliberately and consistently matches clients and interventions, may appear intuitively plausible. And yet it has still not been established whether the choice of treatment for alcohol problems has any effect whatsoever on outcome. There is only one evaluation (McLellan *et al.* 1983c) of an organization in which selection of treatment for each patient was based on empirically derived indications. According to this evaluation, matching achieved a number of positive effects during and after treatment, but did not affect patients' alcohol consumption.

As far as patients' drinking behaviour is concerned, support for the matching hypothesis is of an indirect nature. In the problem section of this book, it was stated that three conditions have to be satisfied in order for the matching hypothesis to be regarded as a fruitful perspective for research and development work:

1. No single treatment has been found superior for all alcoholics.

2. No valid evidence exists for the assumption that alcoholics are essentially alike.

3. Interaction takes place between type of client, form of intervention, and outcome in the treatment of alcoholism.

The arguments for and against these statements will be summarized and evaluated below.

23.1 Is there a superior method?

Research on the outcome of alcoholism treatment has a short history. It still suffers from methodological defects, although significant improvements have taken place in the last decade. Claims regarding the presence or absence of differences between treatment methods must therefore be interpreted with caution. It has been noted that the more rigorously the evaluation is designed, the less favourable are its results. Experimental studies with control or comparison groups have found only weak and short-term effects of alcoholism treatment. Moreover, in unselected groups of alcoholics very little or no outcome differences have been demonstrated between different treatment settings and orientations or between programmes of varying length and intensity. No single treatment has been found superior for all alcoholics.

However, programmes that have been subjected to scientific evaluation have generally been geared towards immediate change rather than to a process of long-term rehabilitation. Hence their focus has been on the individual alcoholic rather than on healing processes in his or her natural environment. Medical and psychological aspects have dominated over social and cultural aspects of treatment. Approaches emphasizing environmental resources and long-term support deserve more attention in development work and research (see Chapter 10). The same is true of preventive measures for early-stage problem drinkers, which have yielded results that are far more promising than those of conventional alcoholism treatment.

Furthermore, most early studies of alcoholism treatment focused on abstinence as the criterion of successful outcome. Today, more precise and differentiated measures of drinking behaviour and of social adjustment and physical and psychiatric health are being introduced. However, those aspects of rehabilitation that do not correlate exactly with drinking behaviour need still more emphasis in treatment outcome research.

23.2   Are all alcoholics alike?

The lack of reliable research results has contributed to a proliferation of philosophies and rationales within alcoholism treatment. Like the speculative medical schools at the time of Hippocrates (Section 2.1), many treatment rationales of today are based on a set of postulates taken at face value. Alcoholism is still often perceived as a unitary and well-defined phenomenon and defined either as a disease with a predictable course, or as a symptom of underlying social or psychological problems.

The symptomatic concept once had a great influence on alcoholism treatment. However, its impact is currently declining even among former adherents (Section 8.2). Prospective, longitudinal studies of samples randomly selected from the general population suggest that the conception of alcoholism as merely symptomatic of underlying problems is based on a retrospective illusion. There is support for the assumption that youths with antisocial personality traits run a greater risk of developing alcoholism than their peers. Otherwise, future alcoholics do not seem to differ psychologically or socially from the rest of the population. An over-representation of social and psychological problems probably does not arise until after alcohol dependence has developed.

The classical disease model, as it was presented by Mortimer Jellinek in 'Phases of Alcohol Addiction' (1952), has been the target, too, of growing, empirically-based criticism. According to most researchers, the concept of natural history does not take enough account of how the career of the alcoholic is influenced by aberrant learning. It has also been shown that 'loss of control' is relative. Moreover, outside AA the disease model has often been associated with a sick role emphasizing biological processes and professional help. This concept of alcoholism tends to discourage preventive policies aimed at the control of alcohol and to absolve society from long-term responsibility for those alcoholics who do not satisfy the expectations associated with the sick role.

Behavioural psychologists have maintained that the contingencies that reinforce a person's alcohol use are so varied that every alcoholic's drinking pattern, problems, and prospects for change are unique and must be analysed as such. The behavioural theories that have been presented so far do not, however, provide any exhaustive explanation of alcohol problems. In some respects, they can be regarded as antitheses to the assumptions that are usually associated with the disease model.

Initiatives do, however, exist for a scientific synthesis that integrates elements from both the biological disease model and the behavioural model. In 1977, Griffith Edwards and his colleagues introduced the concept alcohol-dependence syndrome, which, in contrast to previous diagnostic classifications, distinguishes the state of dependence (characterized by an empirically definable drinking pattern) from physical, psychological, and social complications of drinking (alcohol-related disabilities). The authors did not take any position on whether alcohol dependence should be regarded as a disease or as a behavioural disorder.

Edwards and his WHO group (1977b) provided a biopsychosocial description of alcoholism which, besides physiological factors, also takes into account aberrant learning, cognitive factors, socio-cultural influences, etc. By taking into consideration the varying degree of alcohol dependence, this model permits an analysis of how the interaction of physiological, psychological, and socio-cultural variables changes from one phase to another in the addictive cycle. In an early phase, a complex interaction of genetic, psychological, and socio-cultural variables has a decisive influence on how much and how often a person drinks. Later, when drinking has been cued to relief and avoidance of the discomfort associated with withdrawal, the addiction probably enters a new phase. At this point, psychobiological processes begin to play a dominant role for the drinking pattern.

The WHO group of investigators assumed that there are different types of alcoholism that can best be interpreted as culturally, environmentally, or personally patterned manifestations of the fundamental dependence syndrome. In summary, the graded dependence concept and the multivariate analysis of the addictive cycle rest on the assumption that alcoholics are different from one another. In a biopsychosocial perspective, neither the classical disease model, the behavioural model, nor the methods of treatment based on these theoretical perspectives seem to be valid for all alcoholics.

This appears to be true also of ideas and treatments based on the emerging social model of alcoholism.

23.3   Are there effects of interaction?

The question of whether an interaction exists between client characteristics, treatment dimensions, and outcome in alcoholism treatment was long debated. Several major studies that tried to identify effects of interaction arrived at negative results (Chapter 18; Section 22.3). The authors of the first Rand report (Armor *et al.* 1978) stated, without qualifications, that 'the specific type of treatment is largely irrelevant to the client's prospect for remission' (p. 151). Other researchers have drawn more cautious conclusions from their negative results. They did not rule out the possibility that the design of the study may have been flawed or that the combinations of patient and treatment variables may have been irrelevant.

Small sample sizes, non-random assignment of clients to treatment conditions, and unreliable procedures for measuring prognostic indicators and treatment outcomes may help to explain the difficulties of detecting interactions between client, treatment, and outcome.

It is hardly a coincidence that of five major studies that did not support the thesis of interaction effects, all except one (Stinson *et al.* 1979) were observational. Most studies that did find effects of interaction have had an experimental design (Wallerstein 1957; Kissin *et al.* 1970; McLachlan 1974; Orford *et al.* 1976; Azrin *et al.* 1982; Spoth 1983; Hartman *et al.* 1988; Annis and Davis 1989*a*; Kadden *et al.* 1989). Controlled studies with each client type randomly assigned to interventions offer the best conditions for the observation of interaction effects.

The poor reliability and validity of prognostic indicators can be illustrated by the definition of alcoholism (Chapter 7). Until fairly recently, when the international classification of diseases was revised, the customary definition focused on complications of excessive drinking. However, criteria of this kind are greatly influenced by the individual's general physical, psychological, and social resources as well as by the norms, values, and sanctions of society. Studies that have found interactions between client characteristics and type of successful treatment outcome (abstinence vs. controlled drinking) did, in contrast, assess degree of alcohol dependence (Orford *et al.* 1976; Polich *et al.* 1981; Foy *et al.* 1984). Other common criteria of alcoholism, such as chronicity of the drinking problem and quantity of alcohol consumption, have not been shown to interact with the nature of improvement. However, no fully adequate instrument exists for measuring components of the alcohol-dependence syndrome (Stockwell 1988). The more reliable the instruments for assessing degree of dependence and other client characteristics become, the fewer subjects will be required to identify interaction effects.

Furthermore, treatment conditions must be clearly differentiated and well defined to enable interactions between client, treatment, and outcome to be observed. This has not very often been the case in studies looking for interaction effects. Firstly, programmes that have been evaluated are mainly of a short-term nature, with intensive intervention followed by more or less sporadic contacts. Moos and Finney (1983) assumed that observed interaction effects (e.g. McLachlan 1974) can be reinforced if the behaviour of clients in their 'natural' environment is examined and is influenced through supportive networks.

Secondly, it is questionable whether the treatments that have been examined differed very much (see Section 12.5). Studies of interaction effects have often focused on the treatment setting, e.g. outpatient versus inpatient care (Armor *et al.* 1978), or have compared group therapy with individual therapy (Smart 1978*b*). Only in a few studies, such as those by Wallerstein (1957), Azrin *et al.* (1982), Annis and Davis (1989*a*), and Kadden *et al.* (1989), has the theoretical orientation or the specific content of treatment been varied.

Studies of interaction effects in alcoholism treatment can also be criticized for having used too narrow outcome criteria, often only a set of measures of the client's drinking pattern (see Section 12.1). But even if no effects of interaction on the drinking career are found, treatments might have differential effects on the physical, psychological, and social concomitants of drinking. McLellan and his co-workers (1983*c*) observed with the aid of a multidimensional evaluative instrument, the Addiction Severity Index (ASI), a number of positive effects of matching that would have been neglected if the follow-up had focused on drinking behaviour alone. In fact, the research group did not find any effect of client–treatment matching on the drinking problem itself.

One criticism that deserves particular attention is that interaction research has often studied irrelevant combinations of client and treatment variables. Studies that found no evidence of interaction typically observed a heterogeneous set of demographic and clinical characteristics. Data on gender, age, and social class or quantity of consumption and chronicity of the drinking problem are readily accessible and easy to quantify, which is undoubtedly one of the reasons they are still so prevalent in studies of interaction. However, the literature indicates that these background factors have, at best, only an indirect relation to the personal characteristics that are relevant in selecting treatment setting, treatment modality, and therapist.

The evidence to support client–treatment matching comes from studies that examined psychological variables (including degree of alcohol dependence), sometimes in combination with demographic characteristics. The most promising of the research efforts focused on personality traits (Chapter 19), a combination of social and psychological resources (Chapters 16, 20), cognitive styles (Chapter 21), and degree of alcohol dependence (Chapter 22). The theoretical implications of the observed interaction between psychological characterstics, treatment dimensions, and outcome of alcoholism treatment will be discussed in Chapter 25.

Certain results suggest that it is necessary to explore client–treatment interactions of a more complex nature than most of those examined in the past (see Chapter 16; Section 22.2). The research by McLellan and his co-workers (1983a) is particularly illustrative here. The authors found no statistically significant interaction between patient characteristics, programme type, and outcome until they divided the clinical sample on purely statistical grounds into a low group, a middle group, and a high group with respect to psychiatric severity. This classification revealed significant interactions in the middle group which, owing to the dominant role of psychiatric severity, had been masked in the initial analysis of the outcome for the subject group as a whole. Thus, powerful prognostic indicators, such as psychiatric severity and perhaps degree of alcohol dependence, must sometimes be controlled in order for interaction effects to be detected.

Nevertheless, a number of alcohol studies have demonstrated the existence of interactions between client characterstics, treatment dimensions, and outcome (Wallerstein 1957; Kissin et al. 1970; Mayer and Myerson 1971; McLachlan 1974; Glaser's 1980 reanalysis of Reynolds et al. 1977; Sokolow et al. 1980; Azrin et al. 1982; Lyons et al. 1982; McLellan et al. 1983a, 1983c; Spoth 1983; Hartman et al. 1988; Annis and Davis 1989a; Dahlgren and Willander 1989; Kadden et al. 1989; Longabaugh et al., in press) or have found a relationship between client type and nature of improvement (Orford et al. 1976; Polich et al. 1981; Vaillant and Milofsky 1982a; Edwards et al. 1983; Foy et al. 1984; Helzer et al. 1985; Elal-Lawrence et al. 1986; Orford and Keddie 1986b). Similar interactions have been observed in related disciplines, such as psychotherapy research, educational studies, and correctional research.

Together, empirical evidence and plausible explanations of conflicting findings support the assumption that client–treatment interactions do affect the outcome of alcoholism treatment. The recognized difficulty of demonstrating interactions can be partially explained by methodological flaws and irrelevant client or treatment variables. In summary, the literature suggests that the prospects of identifying interaction effects are most favourable under the following conditions:

1. A large sample.

2. A controlled study with each client type randomly assigned to treatment conditions.

3. Reliable and valid instruments for measuring prognostic indicators and outcome criteria.

4. Clearly differentiated and well-defined treatment conditions.

5. A multidimensional evaluative instrument (such as the Addiction Severity Index).

6. Inclusion of both psychological variables (including degree of alcohol dependence) and demographic characteristics.

7. Analysis of complex interactions, with controls for powerful prognostic indicators.

23.4   Conclusion on matching

Since the requirements set forth in Section 1.2 are met, i.e. there is no superior treatment, alcoholics constitute a heterogeneous group, and client-treatment interactions affect outcome, the matching hypothesis can be regarded as a fruitful perspective for research and development work in the treatment of alcoholism.

A few retrospective studies (Wallerstein 1957; Kissin *et al.* 1970; McLachlan 1974; Longabaugh *et al.*, in press), have demonstrated effects of interaction between client characteristics and type of treatment one year or more after discharge from inpatient treatment or admission to outpatient treatment. These findings are particularly promising in view of the short-term impact of alcoholism treatment that has generally been observed. We do not know, however, whether the effects would be as pronounced in a prospective study that matches clients and treatments in accordance with a preconceived and explicit plan.

In the only prospective study of matching, McLellan and his co-workers (1983c) followed some 250 alcoholics for an average of four months after termination of treatment (Section 16.4). In this study, matching did not affect the drinking problem. It did, however, make patients more motivated for treatment and contributed to significant improvements with respect to medical condition, employment, drug use, legal status, and family/social relations. Considering the generally weak effects of alcoholism treatment, this result is encouraging.

Studies of interaction and other literature reviewed suggest that the specific type of treatment is in fact of importance for alcoholics' prospects for remission. This conclusion may appear obvious. However, outcome studies that have not taken account of interaction effects have repeatedly reported that different kinds of treatment produce basically the same outcome. They have therefore tended to favour the least expensive programme. Now we see that this programme is not necessarily the most cost-effective alternative for all types of alcoholics.

The interaction between type of client, form of intervention, and outcome is, however, multidimensional. Lee Cronbach (1957), in a famous essay entitled 'The two disciplines of scientific psychology', introduced the concept of interaction as a link between experimental psychology and the study of individual differences. The possibility of generalizing *main effects* within both disciplines is limited by interaction effects, he argued. Two decades later, Cronbach (1975) lamented that he had been shortsighted not to apply the same argument to interaction effects themselves, since the possibility of generalizing effects of first-order interaction (patient characteristic $P_1 \times$ treatment dimension T_1) is always limited by *effects of higher-order interaction* (e.g. patient variable $P_1 \times$ patient variable $P_2 \times$ treatment dimension T_1). Cronbach (1975) pointed out: 'Once we attend to interactions, we enter a hall of mirrors that extends to infinity. However far we carry our analysis—to third order or fifth order or any other—untested interactions of a still higher order can be envisioned' (p. 119).

Kissin, Platz, and Su's (1970) study of social and psychological characteristics that predict the outcome of different kinds of treatment in inpatient and outpatient settings provided an early example of the effects of second-order interaction.

The authors of the second Rand report (Polich *et al.* 1981) had to investigate effects of third-order interaction (degree of alcohol dependence × age × marital status) in order to describe which clients did well following abstinence versus non-problem drinking. The general rule that men with high severity of alcohol dependence did better with abstinence while men with low severity of dependence did better with non-problem drinking had two exceptions. Younger unmarried men with a high degree of dependence had a lower relapse rate if they engaged in non-problem drinking after treatment. Older married men with a low degree of dependence, on the other hand, had a lower relapse rate if they abstained from alcohol.

McLellan and his co-workers' (1983a) retrospective study of 460 alcoholics in outpatient and inpatient treatment found effects of interaction of an even higher order. Single or unemployed patients had a better prognosis in inpatient care only if they belonged to the group characterized by middle-severity psychiatric problems. For patients in the low and high psychiatric severity groups, the type of treatment setting did not seem to make any difference. Patients in the middle psychiatric severity group who, besides employment or family problems, also had a criminal record, had to be assigned to a highly structured programme (the combined clinic) in order to benefit from inpatient care. In other words, the research team had to take into account effects of fourth-order interaction (psychiatric status × employment status × family/social status × legal status) in predicting treatment response and matching patients to treatment.

If results are to be generalized to other treatment settings, however, even more factors must be considered. The three studies just mentioned, for example, only included male alcoholics. Moreover, they confined themselves to selected groups of clients. Kissin *et al.* (1970) excluded all subjects who stayed in treatment for less than a month; the comparison in the second Rand report (Polich *et al.* 1981) between abstinent and non-problem drinking subjects is based on the one-third of the original study sample that had neither relapsed at the first follow-up nor died at the second; McLellan *et al.* (1983*a*) disregarded the approximately 17 per cent of alcoholics admitted to treatment who dropped out within five days.

Similar limitations afflict many other studies that have demonstrated the presence of interaction effects in alcoholism treatment. Wallerstein's (1957) subject group consisted of men at the clinic of a famous school of psychiatry, who volunteered for an experimental programme lasting for two months or more; McLachlan (1974) selected his subjects at a hospital in Toronto whose patients were mainly recruited from the middle and upper class; Orford, Oppenheimer, and Edwards' (1976) studied married male patients at the outpatient department of a well-known university hospital in England.

Furthermore, most studies of interaction have assumed, without explicitly stating so, that individual patients are exposed and respond to treatment independently of each other. In Sections 19.3 and 21.1, it has been argued that group effects can make it more difficult to generalize results and to say which treatment is the most appropriate for each individual (see also Cronbach and Webb 1975; Finney and Moos 1986).

In evaluating McLachlan's (1974) findings concerning group therapy, for example, one must take into account the possibility that therapists and patients communicate differently in homogeneous therapy groups created by matching than in heterogeneous groups created by random assignment. Lyons' (1982) observation that women did better in medically oriented programmes while men gained more from peer group oriented programmes should be evaluated in the context of the sexual distribution in alcoholism treatment. Sokolow *et al.* (1980) found that more women were abstinent when treated in a programme with a lower proportion of women, while men had a more successful outcome when treated in a programme with a higher percentage of women. However, in both conditions most clients were men. A study by Dahlgren and Willander (1989) suggests that the benefit for women of self-help groups would be greater if the groups were composed solely of women.

Finally, in studying human affairs one must pay attention to social, political, and cultural differences and changes (cf. Gergen 1973). Cronbach (1975) speaks here about *time* as an important source of interactions in social and behavioural science: 'Generalizations decay. At one time a conclusion describes the existing situation well, at a later time it accounts for rather little variance, and ultimately it is valid only as history' (pp. 122–3).

Culture-based interactions are well known within alcoholism treatment research (see Section 4.2). Fifty years ago, Voegtlin and Lemere (1942), using the prescription of strychnine in the 1920s as an example, warned against an excessive faith in new, promising treatment methods that have not been subjected to the test of time. More recently, Vaillant (1983*b*) commented on some treatments that showed superior outcomes at first, but were unable to replicate these outcomes later on. According to Vaillant, the initial success of the treatments can be explained by the fact that, in addition to a helping relationship, they offered a rationale compatible with the prevailing cultural world view, coupled with a ritual that required the active participation of patients and therapists.

Interactions of the kinds illustrated above complicate the picture for every researcher who synthesizes observations from different treatment settings. In principle, human events are not unpredictable. Like everything else in nature, they conform to certain laws. But the possibility of generalizing findings is always limited by interactions which—like the reflections in a 'hall of mirrors' (Cronbach 1975)—enter into systems of a higher order. These systems are so complex that no one will be able to predict the behaviour of individual people with a high level of confidence.

Considering the complexity of the task, no dramatic breakthrough should be expected as a consequence of the matching of clients to treatment. Research on alcoholism treatment has thus far, with few exceptions (Kissin *et al.* 1970; Sokolow *et al.* 1980; Polich *et al.* 1981; McLellan *et al.* 1983*a*; Longabaugh *et al.*, in press), only identified effects of first-order interaction. However, by incorporating our knowledge of interactions into more comprehensive matching models, we may gradually develop more effective approaches to the treatment of alcohol problems.

24 Matching clients to treatments

An assessment of the implications of matching for alcoholism treatment must take into account both present limitations and future potential. The limitations are in part a result of the complex nature of client–treatment interactions and our inadequate state of knowledge. Since the validity of empirical generalizations is always threatened by higher-order interactions, a sound policy has to recognize the limits of the plannable (cf. Glass 1979). Cronbach (1975; Cronbach and Snow 1977), aware of the complexity of the task, recommended that matching be regarded as a process of adjustment encompassing multiple stages, rather than a single event based on prior experience with other people or in other settings. Luborsky and his co-workers (1988; Luborsky and McLellan 1981) in the Penn Psychotherapy Project put forth similar views.

The Penn researchers found that a rating of the therapeutic relationship at an early stage of psychotherapy gave a good indication of the final outcome. Since crucial prognostic indicators often only emerge after client and therapist have met, Luborsky and his co-workers tried out an assignment model in which the client is given an opportunity for 're-pairing'. Clients admitted at a psychiatric outpatient clinic were allowed to have two sessions with two different therapists before making a decision about which therapist to continue therapy with. Although the data have not been completely analysed, two findings were evident to Luborsky *et al.* (1988): Patients like having a choice, and they often have a clear preference for one or the other therapist.

Finney and Moos (1986) pointed out that the benefits achieved by differential treatment may be so modest at the beginning that they do not outweigh the increased costs of implementing new assessment procedures, providing alternative forms of treatment, and operating a system of outcome determination. Assuming constant resources, the rising expenses may lead to fewer clients receiving treatment. The absolute number of clients who experience improvement may thereby be unchanged at the beginning, or may even decrease. Nevertheless, Finney and Moos (1986) consider the matching hypothesis to be 'the best hope for improving treatment services for alcohol-dependent patients, as well as for persons suffering from other types of psychological-behavioral disorders' (p. 132).

Incremental efficiency is, however, not the only, or perhaps not even the strongest, argument for a deliberate and consistent pairing of clients and interventions. At least as important is the possibility that certain kinds of treatment can make certain clients worse than they would have been with no or minimal treatment (see reviews by Lambert, Bergin, and Collins 1977; Bergin and Lambert 1978). Examples of treatments where negative effects have been observed are highly confrontational group therapy for alcoholics with a negative self-image (Annis and Chan 1983), therapy focusing on underlying dynamic structures for alcohol-dependent patients (Olson *et al.* 1981), and relationally focused treatment for persons who are highly sensitive to their social environment but experience little support for abstinence (Longabaugh *et al.*, in press). According to the Hippocratic oath, the first duty of a physician is to do no harm to anyone (*primum non nocere*). The same guiding principle should apply to alcoholism treatment. This requires a systematic study of the interaction between client characteristics, treatment modalities, and outcome.

The literature on interaction suggests that in a number of areas, clinical decisions can be guided by research-supported methods of matching. The most important areas will be summarized here under the following headings: abstinence versus controlled drinking; inpatient versus outpatient treatment; degree of structure and directiveness; and kind of treatment task.

24.1   Abstinence versus controlled drinking

The question of whether alcoholics can be taught controlled drinking is a controversial one. The divergence of opinions can be partially explained by the use of different definitions and criteria. The term controlled drinking sometimes designates the drinking pattern of alcoholics who have reduced their alcohol consumption, prolonged abstinent periods, and become less intoxicated during relapses. Such *attenuated drinking* (Pattison 1976) may be an acceptable goal in conjunction with improvement in other areas of life. But it is still an alcohol-dependent drinking pattern. No one today would deny the fact that alcoholics sometimes attenuate their drinking in the described manner. But there are different opinions about whether it is possible—by means of behaviour therapy, for example—to teach alcoholics true control over when, where, and how to drink.

Everyone agrees that liver damage and other medical complications may be sufficient reasons for recommending an alcoholic not to opt for a goal of controlled drinking. But that is about as far as the consensus goes. The research on interaction effects arrives at seemingly contradictory conclusions.

Welte, Lyons, and Sokolow (1983), in a large follow-up of alcoholics after discharge from treatment, were unable to identify any sub-population which was more successful at avoiding relapse with non-problem drinking than with abstinence. The background characteristics that were examined included age and degree of alcohol dependence. Welte and his co-workers did, however, make the qualification that all clients had received treatment aimed at total abstinence.

Foy, Nunn, and Rychtarik (1984) studied the outcomes of two broad-spectrum treatment programmes that differed only with regard to the drinking goal. The one programme trained clients in controlled drinking skills, while the other recommended abstinence. Clients were randomly assigned to the two programmes. A follow-up six months after discharge showed that those clients who had trained controlled drinking skills had a higher relapse rate than those who had been advised to abstain. The former clients had fewer abstinent days, but just as many days with reduced or controlled drinking. In this study, the degree of alcohol dependence, rather than the type of treatment, determined whether clients would be able to engage in non-problem drinking. Only male alcoholics were included in the trial.

Studies by Orford, Oppenheimer, and Edwards (1976), and Polich, Armor, and Braiker (1981), however, indicate that certain clients, after discharge from conventional treatment for alcohol problems aimed at abstinence, have at least temporarily resumed controlled drinking without having an increased risk of relapse. In examining which clients had been successful during the second year of follow-up, Orford et al. (1976) found that persons with a high degree of alcohol dependence (Gamma alcoholics) did well through abstinence, while persons with a low degree of dependence tended to do well through controlled drinking. Age and chronicity of the drinking problem showed no correlation with type of successful outcome. The study included only married men.

Polich et al. (1981) found that the probability of achieving long-term remission following abstention and non-problem drinking was a function of the degree of alcohol dependence, age, and marital status. The quantity of alcohol consumed, however, was not a reliable predictor. All subjects were men in a positively selected sample.

In a screening and intervention study, Kristenson et al. (1983; Kristenson 1987) advised heavy drinkers to reduce their overall consumption and to abstain for at least two days a week. This drinking goal was supported by Gamma-GT tests administered by a nurse at regular intervals. Subjects were informed of the condition of their liver and were encouraged to develop interests in hobbies, exercise, and other alternatives to drinking. Kristenson's study was one of the first randomized controlled trials of a secondary prevention programme for problem drinkers, and it has attracted great attention due to its promising results in terms of sick absenteeism, hospitalization, and mortality.

Sanchez-Craig et al. (1984) reported on an experiment in which early-stage problem drinkers were randomly assigned to identical treatment programmes with a goal of either abstinence or controlled drinking. No statistically significant differences were demonstrated between the groups as regards dropout rate or outcome two years after discharge. A goal of controlled drinking was found to be more acceptable for the majority of the clients, however. Most of the clients who were assigned to abstinence also developed moderate drinking on their own.

The studies cited above indicate that it is necessary to consider the *degree of alcohol dependence* in deciding what drinking goal to prefer. They confirm the importance of current efforts to devise and test standardized instruments for the assessment of alcohol dependence (Chapter 7). Frequently used criteria of addiction severity, such as the quantity of alcohol consumed and chronicity of the drinking problem, do not appear to be reliable prognostic indicators.

Studies by Orford *et al.* (1976), Kristenson *et al.* (1983), and Sanchez-Craig *et al.* (1984) have shown that, for heavy drinkers with early symptoms of dependence, controlled drinking can be an effective goal that is *more acceptable* than abstinence. This finding is particularly important for *secondary prevention programmes* in primary health care, occupational, and other settings.

In *conventional alcoholism treatment* with its more alcohol-dependent clientele, controlled drinking is usually not a realistic treatment goal. Polich *et al.* (1981), Welte *et al.* (1983), and Foy *et al.* (1984) have arrived at results that indicate that controlled drinking cannot be recommended without qualifications even for clients with a low degree of dependence. This conclusion appears to be inconsistent with the results presented by Orford *et al.* (1976), Kristenson *et al.* (1983), and Sanchez-Craig *et al.* (1984).

One reason for the discrepancy may be that different definitions of alcohol dependence have been used. Problem drinkers in Kristenson *et al.*'s and Sanchez-Craig *et al.*'s early-intervention programmes, and non-Gamma alcoholics at Orford *et al.*'s outpatient family clinic, probably had a more favourable prognosis than those clients who were considered to have a low degree of dependence in the studies carried out by Polich *et al.*, Welte *et al.*, and Foy *et al.* Subjects in the last-cited studies were selected from programmes in conventional alcoholism treatment.

Furthermore, there is a difference of opinion as to what is 'controlled' or 'normal' drinking. The first Rand report (Armor *et al.* 1978), for example, applied a very broad definition. The same can be said about the study by Orford *et al.* (1976). Some of the clients that were judged to drink in a 'controlled' manner in these studies would presumably have been classified as relapsed by other investigators.

Another reason for the conflicting results may be that only Polich *et al.* (1981) looked for higher-order interactions. Welte *et al.* (1983) examined more than a dozen client variables, including degree of alcohol dependence and age. But they studied each variable individually, hoping to find effects of first-order interaction. The results of the second Rand report, however, indicate that persons with a low degree of dependence have a favourable prognosis following non-problem drinking only under certain conditions related to age and marital status.

Orford and Keddie's (1986*b*) and Elal-Lawrence, Slade, and Dewey's (1986) studies suggest that among those additional factors that should be considered in selecting drinking goals are also expectations, beliefs, and cultural differences. Moreover, some alcohol-dependent clients refuse to consider total abstinence. As suggested by Heather, Whitton, and Robertson (1986), Elal-Lawrence *et al.* (1986), and Orford and Keddie (1986*b*), these clients may nonetheless benefit from treatment aimed at reduction of their consumption to a less problematic level.

Thus, the choice between controlled-drinking and abstinence goals seems to require more than clear definitions and more reliable measures of alcohol dependence. It is just as important to develop good theories and a comprehensive understanding of alcohol dependence as a biopsychosocial phenomenon, and to respect the client's wishes for change.

24.2   Inpatient versus outpatient treatment

Alcoholism treatment has traditionally begun with hospital or other residential care for one or two months. This setting was considered to promote a 'massive confrontation' of the alcoholic's denial of his disease (Moore and Buchanan 1966). In the last decades, however, the utility of extended hospital care for purposes other than the treatment of severe medical or psychiatric complications has been questioned. Nevertheless, a recent four-year longitudinal study of US federal employees (Holder and Blose 1986) found that although the average length of stay was no more than three weeks, inpatient care accounted for 95 per cent of all alcoholism treatment costs.

The vast increase in health expenditure and the fiscal crisis of the state are important reasons why policy makers and administrators have begun to look around for less expensive alternatives. In the US, for example, the number of specialist treatment programmes for alcohol problems has increased from less than 400 in 1967 to over 5000 today (IOM 1990). At the same time, the treatment population has changed from a relatively homogenous group of persons in hospital care to a large number of different people who are provided treatment in a variety of settings.

Behaviour therapists (e.g. McCrady *et al.* 1983) have emphasized the advantages of the outpatient and day care setting. They have argued that hospital care provides an artificial environment in which the patient easily forgets that abstention from alcohol is a difficult task that requires new skills and a change in lifestyle. Outpatient and partial-hospital care permit a more accurate assessment of drinking patterns and high-risk situations, and provide increased opportunity for rehearsal of new skills and coping strategies in the natural environment.

In the first randomized controlled trial of inpatient and outpatient care, Edwards and Guthrie (1967) found that the outpatients did, in fact, slightly better in terms of drinking behaviour and social adjustment than the inpatients. The difference was not statistically significant, however. Several reviews of subsequent research have concluded that outpatient and partial-hospital care are at least as effective as inpatient care for alcoholics (Baekeland 1977; Emrick 1979; Miller and Hester 1980, 1986*b*; Cole *et al.* 1981; Annis 1986, 1987).

As early as 1938, Seliger proposed that the choice between outpatient and inpatient alcoholism treatment should be made on the basis of explicit criteria, and he suggested that outpatient care was indicated for patients who have 'good intelligence and some maturity' and whose 'life habits and contacts are not too bad' (p. 704). Nevertheless, the issue of whether there is a subgroup of alcoholics who are more likely to improve their drinking behaviour and social adjustment in inpatient than in outpatient care has not been finally settled.

Armor, Polich, and Stambul (1978) in the US and Smart (1978*b*) in Canada followed up large randomly selected samples of alcoholics treated in both outpatient and inpatient settings. Both studies investigated the presence of client–treatment interactions. Armor and his co-workers studied differential effects of a variation of the client's social stability, socioeconomic status, and severity of alcoholism, while Smart similarly examined 31 client characteristics: 12 demographic variables, 11 scale scores, and eight assessments of drinking habits. None of the two follow-ups found any effect of interaction to indicate that some clients did better with one treatment setting than with another.

However, the results of these studies are difficult to interpret. For example, clients who chose to enter outpatient treatment may have differed in some respects from those who entered inpatient treatment, and these differences may have had a bearing on the follow-up status. Furthermore, both studies used clients' drinking behaviour as the only evaluation criterion. Finally, neither study looked for effects of higher-order interaction taking into account, for example, a combination of social and psychological resources.

Kissin, Platz, and Su (1970) carried out a controlled trial with the purpose of randomly assigning alcoholics to outpatient and inpatient treatment. Clients' rehabilitation potential was assessed by a social interview and a number of psychological tests. Persons who were married, had 12 or more years of education, had a professional, clerical, or skilled occupation, and had not been arrested for any crime were classified as socially stable. The psychological tests measured, among other things, 'field dependence' (cognitive restructuring ability).

As evaluation criterion, Kissin and his co-workers used an undifferentiated measure of changes in drinking behaviour and psychosocial adjustment. They found a highly significant interaction between patients' social stability, treatment setting, and outcome. Those who did well in outpatient treatment were significantly more socially stable than those who failed, while those who did well in hospital care were significantly *less* socially stable than those who failed.

Psychological characteristics seemed to affect treatment outcome in a more complex manner. Those who did well with outpatient drug therapy were significantly more 'field dependent', those who did well with outpatient psychotherapy were significantly more 'field independent', while those who did well in the hospital programme did not differ with regard to 'field dependence–independence' from those who failed.

Unfortunately, Kissin and his co-workers' study suffers from serious methodological shortcomings that limit the generalizability of results. However, the conclusion that socially unstable alcoholics may benefit from a stay in a protective environment receives indirect support from Edwards' (1970a) observation that the stability of clients with regard to family, employment, and housing influenced outcome more in outpatient than in inpatient treatment.

Also of interest here is the finding by Welte and his co-workers (1981) that length of stay in inpatient treatment did not affect outcome, in terms of average alcohol consumption, for patients with high social stability. Patients with low social stability, in contrast, reduced their posttreatment alcohol consumption as length of stay increased. The research group studied a variation of eight other patient characteristics relating primarily to severity of the drinking problem, but none of them had any differential effect on treatment outcome.

The Penn-VA Project, presented by McLellan and his co-workers (1983a, 1983c), reinforces the impression that social stability is of importance in comparing the efficacy of outpatient and inpatient treatment. McLellan et al. (1983a) identified statistically significant interaction effects only after dividing the sample into a low, a middle, and a high group in terms of psychiatric severity. Clients in the high- and low-severity groups did equally poorly or well regardless of which treatment they entered.

Clients in the middle-severity group with great work-related problems (e.g. unemployment, casual work), or great family-related problems (e.g. divorce, family involvement in abuse), did less well in the outpatient programme than in other programmes. These results agreed with the experience of the authors that severe alcohol abuse, as well as medical and legal problems, can often be dealt with in outpatient treatment. Clients with fairly severe psychiatric problems, in combination with employment or family problems, seemed to do better in inpatient treatment, however.

In a prospective study of matching effects, McLellan and his co-workers (1983c) confirmed that clients with little or no psychiatric problems can 'almost always' (except if they have severe employment/support problems) be treated in outpatient programmes. The Penn-VA researchers also found that clients with moderate psychiatric severity, in combination with severe work- or family-related problems, gained more from treatment in an inpatient setting. Inpatient treatment had a favourable effect on the physical health and social adjustment of these clients. The treatment setting seemed to have no effect, however, on alcohol use or psychiatric status.

In summary, comparative studies show that with heterogeneous groups of alcoholics, inpatient treatment is no more effective than treatment in outpatient or day care settings. The research provides no support for the view that treatment of alcoholics should routinely begin in a residential setting. Several weeks in a hospital for other than medical or psychiatric reasons are usually unnecessary, and may sometimes even be harmful. Inpatient care should rather be regarded as a last resort and should be preceded by careful individual assessment.

Studies of interaction between client, treatment, and outcome suggest that *social stability* should be a key criterion in selecting treatment setting. This client characteristic should not be confused with socioeconomic status which, judging from Welte *et al.* (1981), does not predict how length of inpatient stay affects outcome. Social stability provides a measure of the quality of the client's social network, i.e. the extent to which he or she can count on support from the natural environment in changing behaviour.

The results obtained by the Penn-VA group (McLellan *et al.* 1983*a*, 1983*c*) indicate that rehabilitation of, at least, alcoholics with psychiatric problems is facilitated in an environment that provides some protection and structure. If a supportive network with such qualities exists in the natural environment, outpatient treatment appear to be the better alternative, particularly if the therapy is behaviourally oriented. It is probably no coincidence that in Edwards and Guthrie's (1967) controlled study, where outcome tended to be in favour of outpatient treatment, 70 per cent of the clients were married and an equal number were of the middle class. In a similar study by Stein, Newton, and Bowman (1975), which found no difference between the outcomes of outpatient and inpatient treatment, only 36 per cent of the clients were married and 14 per cent were of the middle class.

The treatment setting describes the environment in which treatment takes place, but it says virtually nothing about the content of treatment. Kissin, Platz, and Su's (1970) study indicates that different approaches in outpatient treatment (drug therapy versus psychotherapy) have different effects on different types of alcoholics ('field dependent–independent'). McLellan and his co-workers (1983*a*) found that a less structured approach in a hospital setting was inappropriate for certain patients ('sociopaths'). The advantages that are usually associated with a given treatment setting can thus be cancelled out by the treatment content that is offered. This observation underscores the importance of taking into account effects of higher-order interaction in the selection of treatment setting as well.

Owing to the small differences in outcome and the high costs of inpatient programmes, which are on average ten times more expensive than comparable outpatient programmes, it is justified to conclude that inpatient treatment is cost-effective only for a small segment of the alcoholic population. Even detoxification can be safely managed in non-hospital settings for the great majority of alcoholics (see review by Annis 1986).

Severe psychiatric or medical complications necessitate hospitalization, however. Residential care is, moreover, legally mandated in many countries and states when an alcoholic becomes dangerous to himself or others, or is seriously deteriorating and cannot be cared for in a less restrictive community setting. Finally, there is a homeless and psychiatrically disabled subpopulation of alcoholics with a poor potential for rehabilitation. Instead of casual treatment, many of these individuals need accommodations that provide a good quality of life, where they can stay long enough to regard them as their home (see Leach and Wing 1980).

24.3   Degree of structure and directiveness

Conceptual level

Degree of structure draws attention to the treatment method and to the match between client and therapist. McLachlan (1972, 1974) was the first to demonstrate the relevance of this dimension for the selection of alcoholism treatment. This was done in an ingenious study based on the observation that there is a relationship between a therapist's personality and his or her therapeutic style. Group therapists at a high conceptual level (CL) were found to be more non-directive than others. By rating the CL of individual therapists, McLachlan obtained an idea of the structure provided by the inpatient treatment environment. By varying the degree of structure in aftercare as well, he was able to study whether there was any interaction between the cognitive style of patients, structure of treatment, and drinking outcome.

The study supported the author's hypothesis that clients at a low conceptual level benefit more from a consistent and directive, highly structured therapy with clearly expressed rules and expectations, whereas high CL clients benefit more from non-directive therapy that encourages self-expression and autonomy.

These findings were not just a fortunate coincidence. They were an offshoot of a body of educational research providing support for Hunt's (1971) hypothesis that there is an inverse relation between the conceptual level of students and their need for structure. According to Hunt, low CL learners profit more from high structure (e.g. didactive instruction), while high CL learners profit more from low structure (e.g. discovery learning) or are, in some cases, less affected by variations in structure.

Hunt's matching models are, in turn, founded on a cognitive personality theory, conceptual systems theory (Harvey, Hunt, and Schroder 1961), which, following Kurt Lewin (1935), assumes that behaviour is a function of the person and the environment. Advocates of this theory emphasize structural qualities of a person's conceptual system. They are mainly interested in *how* a person thinks, not *what* he is thinking about. They presume that although the cognitive content varies, the formal properties of the conceptual system (level of differentiation, discrimination, and integration) are relatively stable.

Most researchers assume that there is a relationship between a person's cognitive complexity and his 'interpersonal maturity'. Conceptually simple persons are described as conforming and dependent, while conceptually complex persons are described as self-responsible and interdependent. The instrument used by McLachlan and Hunt to assess conceptual level (The Paragraph Completion Method, PCM) emphasizes the structure of the conceptual system, however.

One of the merits of the conceptual systems theory is that it describes personality traits and environmental conditions in comparable terms. Approaches of this kind are very unusual in psychology (cf. Bem and Funder 1978). Degree of structure is the basic dimension of environmental variation. Since the description of conceptual level focuses on cognitive complexity, one would expect that the environmental description would also place an emphasis on the range and diversity of rules and expectations. However, Hunt's and his colleagues' classification of environmental conditions has still not reached the same standard as their assessment of psychological characteristics. This shortcoming reflects the general situation in psychology, which has only in recent years begun a systematic analysis of environments (see reviews by Frederiksen 1972; Moos 1973; Pervin 1978).

Examples have been given in Chapter 21 of a number of cognitive characteristics, all of which are likely to be relevant in matching clients to treatments that differ in degree of structure. McLachlan (1974) cited the study in social psychology carried out by Carr (1970). This study showed that cognitive compatibility between client and therapist can have a favourable effect on the outcome of psychotherapy. Similar findings have been reported by Landfield (1971) and Hunt, Carr, et al. (1985). Carr developed a test, the Interpersonal Discrimination Task (IDT), which measures the individual's conceptual differentiation, defined as a tendency to make fine distinctions among people and thus perceive them as different from one another. Carr's differentiation concept describes a dimension that is similar to what in conceptual systems theory is called a person's conceptual level.

Field independence and cognitive ability

The term psychological 'differentiation' is also central in the cognitive personality theory developed by Witkin and his co-workers (1962, 1979), but it is used here in a somewhat different sense than in Carr's socio-psychological research. An individual's differentiation has been measured by means of perceptual tests, usually Oltman's Portable Rod and Frame Test ([P]RFT) or the Embedded-Figures Test (EFT). Witkin and Goodenough (1981), however, arrived at the conclusion that these two tests measure different, although related, characteristics.

The RFT is described as a measure of the individual's cognitive style, as manifested in perceptual, intellectual, intra-personal, and interpersonal areas of function. The theoretically significant dimension here is whether the individual tends to rely on external or internal frames of reference in processing information. Persons rated as field-dependent on the RFT are assumed to orient themselves with the external field as the primary referent, while field-independent persons rely more on their own internal frames of reference.

Alcoholics are often more field-dependent than others (Sugerman and Schneider 1976; Barnes 1983). Psychosocial treatment research has shown that field-dependent persons prefer and need a great deal of structure, guidance, and reassurance (Witkin et al. 1968; Russakoff et al. 1976; Dowds et al. 1977; Austrian and Goldbergèr 1982). In this respect they are similar to persons who are at a low conceptual level according to conceptual systems theory. Pardes and his co-workers (1974) found, however, in a study of field dependence–independence of patients and therapists, that field-independent therapists achieved the best results regardless of how patients had been classified on the RFT. Thus, in contrast to what McLachlan (1972, 1974) and Carr (1970) had found regarding conceptual level, similarity between patient and therapist in cognitive style was not a reliable predictor of treatment outcome.

According to Witkin and Goodenough (1981), the EFT assesses the individual's cognitive restructuring ability. Studies by Kissin and his co-workers (1970; Karp et al. 1970) showed that this ability was of importance for the response of alcoholics to psychotherapy. Erwin and Hunter (1984) replicated this finding. In addition, they studied the fertility of Jean Piaget's stages of intellectual development for alcoholism treatment research.

Piaget's stages of development—the preoperational, the concrete operational, and the formal operational—were originally intended to describe differences in how children and young peole think at different ages. In recent years, however, studies have been performed showing that the same type of differences exist among adults. Renner et al. (1976) found that less than half of his adult subjects were able to solve problems of the type associated by Piaget with the formal operational stage, i.e. the stage of development where the individual becomes capable of abstract thought without having to experience through his senses the situation to which his cognitive operations apply. Moreover, neuropsychological research has shown that more alcohol abusers than previously realized have cognitive deficits, manifested primarily in a reduced capacity for abstraction and problem solving (see e.g. Bergman 1987).

Erwin and Hunter (1984) found that two indicators of the alcoholic's capacity for formal operational thought, the pendulum problem and the plant problem, were strongly correlated with his tendency to remain in a verbally oriented treatment programme. In summary, the available evidence indicates that verbal psychotherapy often requires an ability for 'cognitive restructuring' or 'formal operational thought', and it clearly suggests that clients' capability for abstract thought should be taken into account in deciding whether to choose an abstract-symbolic or a concrete-behavioural treatment approach.

Locus of control

Locus of control is a basic construct in Rotter's (1954) social learning theory and is measured by Rotter's Internal–External Locus of Control Scale (I–E) or similar instruments (e.g. Seeman's Powerlessness Scale). It refers to the degree to which individuals perceive the events that influence their lives as being a consequence of their own behaviour, and thereby controllable (internal control), or as being unrelated to their own behaviour and, thereby, beyond personal control (external control).

Experiments have demonstrated a relationship between locus of control and interpersonal behaviour (Lefcourt 1972). Individuals seem to be susceptible to influence under different conditions, depending on their locus of control. Those who view themselves as responsible for their own fates resist if they feel they are being manipulated. They are not captivated by statements presented by authorities. They respond to arguments that are in agreement with their own perceptions, and they can be induced to change their attitudes and behaviour when allowed more active participation, as in role-playing and group discussions. Persons who do not perceive themselves as being in active control of their fate appear to respond more to the prominence of the source of influence than to the merits of the arguments.

Psychotherapy researchers have shown, sometimes with clinical subject groups, that persons with external locus of control prefer and do best in directive therapy. Liberman (1978b) found, for example, that psychiatric outpatients who were oriented towards self-reliance did best when exposed to therapy emphasizing their own efforts, while persons whose orientation indicated greater reliance on external forces profited more from therapy that attributed progress to the external agent of medication. In a study by Best and Steffy (1975), smokers who perceived themselves as being internally controlled did best with an aversion therapy that emphasized subjective perceptions, while those who perceived themselves as being externally controlled did best with behavioural analysis, i.e. an analysis of how environmental events influenced their smoking.

Skinner (1980a) put forth the hypothesis that alcoholics with external locus of control do better with well-structured behaviour therapy combined with Antabuse ingested daily, while those with internal locus of control probably benefit more from some form of cognitive therapy, supported by Temposil (an anti-alcohol drug with a shorter duration of effect than Antabuse) taken 'as required'. Skinner's hypothesis, which was based on a literature review by Beutler (1979), receives some support from a study by Obitz (1978) showing that alcoholics who elected to take Antabuse were significantly more externally oriented than were those who did not.

Spoth (1983) reported that alcoholics with external locus of control benefited more from relaxation training emphasizing factors beyond the direct control of the client, such as neuropsychological processes. Alcoholics with internal locus of control, in contrast, did better in training where relaxation was presented as an active coping skill to be applied only in stressful situations. Hartman, Krywonis, and Morrison (1988), finally, found that externals improved more after discharge from intensive, structured treatment than from brief, non-directive counselling. Internals responded equally well to both approaches, which might indicate that they need little external encouragement, guidance, and support to improve.

One might expect a correlation to exist between locus of control and field dependence–independence. The constructs overlap, and both predict interpersonal behaviour: assertiveness, the experiencing of oneself as a distinct source of causation, and the tendency to be self-reliant rather than acquiescent and conforming (Lefcourt 1972). And yet neither Rotter (1966), Deever (1968), Lefcourt and Telegdi (1971), Roodin, Broughton, and Vaught (1974), or Tobacyk, Broughton, and Vaught (1975) were able to find any statistically significant relationship between an individual's locus of control and his dependence on or independence of external frames of reference.

It is reasonable to assume that these variables are complementary to each other, and that they must sometimes be used simultaneously to predict differential effects of treatment. This assumption receives indirect support from Lefcourt and Telegdi (1971), who, in an attempt to predict cognitive activity in responding to psychological tests, found effects of higher-order interaction. Neither field dependence–independence nor locus of control permitted any prediction, each taken by itself. Only in combination were significant results obtained. Subjects who were both field independent and had internal locus of control did best on the task. Field-dependent subjects with external locus of control did second best, surprisingly, while incongruent persons, i.e. those who functioned in one way but perceived the situation in another (field dependent with internal locus of control, field independent with external locus of control), had the poorest performance. Tobacyk *et al.* (1975) showed that this ranking was also valid for predictions of personality adjustment and performance on a perceptual task.

Since interactions always form part of higher-order systems, the many significant first-order interactions involving *cognitive styles*—such as conceptual level, conceptual differentiation, field dependence–independence, cognitive restructuring ability, capacity for formal operational thought, and locus of control—are both surprising and encouraging. They raise hopes that a combination of psychological indications will provide a solid basis for prognoses as to which degree of structure and directiveness offers the best conditions for treatment.

The constructs mentioned above are, however, multidimensional and partially overlapping. It should therefore be a research priority to define more precisely which cognitive and socio-psychological indications are the most useful in choosing between treatment methods that are highly structured, concrete, and directive, and approaches with a lower degree of structure, a more abstract-symbolic content, and greater opportunity for the client himself to control the course of events.

There is also reason to study other characteristics of alcoholics that might be of importance to the degree of treatment structure. Studies by Wilbur *et al.* (1966), Norman and Schulze (1970), McLellan *et al.* (1983*a*; p. 164), and Kadden *et al.* (1989) show that *sociopathic* alcoholics are likely to benefit from a highly structured treatment experience. Mayer and Myerson (1971) found that social stability had a bearing on outcome in Antabuse treatment, with unstable alcoholics improving more than others. Assessment of degree of alcohol dependence and the Drinking-Related Locus of Control Scale (DRIE) may prove to be useful predictors, too, as well Sjöberg and his co-workers' (Samsonowitz & Sjöberg 1981; Sjöberg, Samsonowitz and Olsson 1983) assessment of coping techniques that alcoholics use spontaneously in order to avoid relapse.

As was pointed out above, classification of treatment environments in general terms such as degree of structure, concrete versus abstract, directive versus non-directive, etc. is still undeveloped. Another problem concerns the integrity of treatment (see Yeaton and Sechrest 1981), i.e. the degree to which treatment is delivered as intended. Most classifications presume that there is a relationship between professed treatment orientation and what the therapist actually does. Beutler (1979) estimated the different types of psychological treatment at over 130. In a review of outcome research, he showed that a theoretical division of therapy approaches into directive and non-directive did, in fact, reveal client–treatment interactions similar to those described above. An optimal matching of client and treatment would, however, entail a systematic monitoring of critical treatment dimensions.

Conditions of relevance to the degree of structure, concretion, and directiveness of a treatment should be studied both individually and in combination. This is evidenced by a study in psychiatry by Frank and Gunderson (1984), which showed that therapists who had a philosophy that differed from the predominant orientation in the treatment milieu, had a more difficult time engaging and maintaining patients in therapy than therapists who shared the orientation of the milieu staff. Thus, reality-oriented, adaptive, and supportive therapists did best in a control-oriented milieu, while expressive and insight-oriented therapists were most successful in an insight-oriented milieu.

The degree of structure provided after discharge from intensive treatment should also be taken into consideration. McLachlan's (1974) study showed that well-organized aftercare was valuable for those clients who, judging from their conceptual level, had a greater need for structure. It is likely that these clients would also have benefited from attending AA (cf. Ogborne and Glaser 1981) or from becoming involved in a community-based treatment for alcoholics of the kind described by Hunt and Azrin (1973; Azrin 1976).

Azrin *et al.* (1982) showed that among single alcoholics, rearrangement of the social environment in such a way that other reinforcing activities competed with drinking behaviour, was essential for remission. Among married alcoholics, in contrast, supervised Antabuse was sufficient to produce abstinence. These clients usually obtained jobs and re-established satisfying marital and social relationships with no assistance from the counsellor. The study suggests that 'need for structure' is not solely an intra-personal characteristic, but depends on which environmental resources are available to the alcoholic as well (cf. Section 10.3).

In an early paper, Witkin (1965) drew attention to the fact that field-dependent persons were generally judged as unsuitable for psychotherapy. They often had to settle for drug therapy. The literature reviewed suggests that psychosocial treatments that provide a high degree of structure, active guidance, and concrete training may be helpful for persons who are at a low conceptual level, are field dependent, have a limited capacity for cognitive restructuring and abstract thought, or have an external locus of control. It should be a research priority to further test such approaches and to refine indications so that in the future all alcoholics can be offered qualified treatment tailored to their needs.

24.4   Kind of treatment task

The discussion in the two preceding sections has ultimately concerned what necessary conditions must be fulfilled in order for a therapeutic process to take place. An inpatient setting, for example, is therapeutic only through the protection and structure it affords certain patients, who, without this environment, would not be able to concentrate on any therapeutic procedures at all. Similarly, the degree of structure and directiveness creates the conditions required for any therapeutic message to be conveyed. Inadequate adaptation to the client's cognitive style and role expectations will impair or prevent communication.

Perhaps it is above all in these respects that treatment research can arrive at generalizable conclusions about how to match clients to treatments. The issue of what message should be conveyed, i.e. which content of treatment or *treatment task* should be selected, is much more complicated. A recent count (Karasu 1986) found more than 400 different types of psychotherapy offered to the public, and existing treatment philosophies give the impression that the number of critical client and treatment variables is virtually unlimited.

Yet the Hippocratic writings contain a general principle that might serve as a common denominator in efforts to match client with treatment task. According to the Hippocratics, *vis medicatrix naturae* or nature herself is the actual healer. The physician is merely nature's servant, who must carefully observe any 'pointings of nature' (indications) for a given remedy. In particular, he must avoid all arbitrary interventions that might interfere with the natural processes of healing.

Transferred to the treatment of alcoholism, this principle says that the therapist's primary responsibility is to facilitate the process of self-healing. The client is a human being with his own thoughts, feelings, and desires. He is not a passive organism that merely responds to external stimuli. Nor is there any way for the therapist to bypass the patient's knowledge, experience, and values in order to directly influence, say, the nervous system. Psychosocial treatment is a co-operative art. In order to bring about a therapeutic alliance, the therapist must apply techniques that agree with and support the 'natural' strategies of individual clients to cope with life and to change behaviour. Above all, the therapist should refrain from activities that might induce a deterioration.

Some studies discussed in previous chapters substantiate the validity of these guidelines. An early study by Wallerstein (1956, 1957) comparing Antabuse, aversion therapy, milieu therapy, and other therapeutic approaches, suggests the presence of interactions between the 'psychological meanings' of therapeutic procedures, the psychic 'needs' of individual patients, and the outcome of treatment.

Antabuse treatment, for example, entails that the alcoholic submits to a form of external control that inhibits relapses. Wallerstein found that patients with a compulsive character had a better prognosis than others in this therapy, since they managed to ritualize the intake of the drug. Improvement in individual patients was often accompanied by a gradual shift towards more compulsive personality traits. Many succeeded in maintaining their compulsive defences chiefly due to their close ties to the hospital and the therapist. Antabuse alone was an inappropriate treatment for 'latent schizophrenic' and severely depressive patients.

According to Wiens and Menustik (1983), aversion therapy is becoming increasingly popular in the United States. Most aversive alcoholism programmes give patients emetine, a nausea-inducing drug, in connection with five to six drinks. Wallerstein interpreted this treatment modality as representing a punishing agent, directed from the outside, which the individual is powerless to control, but must instead somehow internalize and assimilate. He found that aggressive patients were significantly less successful than others with this treatment. They construed the aversive threat as a provocation rather than a therapeutic tool. In this regime, however, depressive patients improved markedly.

In the milieu programme, patients had to assume the major responsibility for change. They could not rely on external agents, but were encouraged to discuss their own problems and feelings in therapy groups. Wallerstein found that the ability to form stable, predominantly positive attachments to other people significantly influenced outcome in this programme. This result has face validity and has been replicated by the findings of similar studies on both alcoholism treatment (Wilbur *et al.* 1966) and education (Chan 1980). However, the 'psychological meaning' of group therapy may vary with the composition of the groups. Wallerstein's study included only male alcoholics. Lyons, Sokolow, and their co-workers (1982) showed that female alcoholics benefited less than male alcoholics from peer-group oriented programmes. On closer examination, Sokolow *et al.* (1980) found that outcome was dependent on the male/female ratio, with women doing better in programmes with few other women. By contrast, Dahlgren and Willander (1989) found that early-stage female problem drinkers were most successful in a programme with all women. Although there is no obvious explanation for these findings, they do suggest that women have specific needs that should be taken into account in designing and selecting programmes for alcoholics and early-stage problem drinkers.

Longabaugh and Beattie (1985) introduced the construct *social investment* to describe the amount and quality of an individual's interactions with significant others. Longabaugh *et al.* (in press) found that alcoholics with high social investment treated in relationally focused treatment had good drinking outcomes when they received high posttreatment support for abstinence, but they had extremely poor outcomes when support was low. It could be that a patient slip after treatment caused a withdrawal of support, rather than that lack of support preceded the patient's relapse. Nevertheless, Longabaugh and his co-workers judged the potential iatrogenic effects of the relationally focused treatment in this study as so 'alarming' that individually focused treatment should be preferred. An implication of this study is that treatment providers should attend to the interaction between formal treatment and the efforts of family, friends, and the work environment to control drinking and support natural processes of healing.

Annis and Chan (1983) carried out a correctional study whose results have relevance for alcoholism treatment as well. The authors investigated the outcome of an intensive, highly confrontational group therapy programme and found a significant interaction with the self-image of offenders. Offenders with a positive self-image had fewer reconvictions and less serious offences, while those with a negative self-image had more reconvictions and more serious offences than a non-treatment control group during the year following release. A similar result was reported by McLellan and his co-workers (1984), who reported on a confrontational therapeutic community for drug addicts. While other patients improved as a result of the treatment, prognoses for patients with severe psychiatric problems worsened. The longer these patients remained in the programme, the poorer the posttreatment outcome was.

In a well-designed study of alcoholism treatment, Kadden and his co-workers (1989) also found that interactional treatment was less effective and probably too demanding for patients with severe psychiatric problems. It was, moreover, inappropriate for sociopathic alcoholics, who lack the social skills necessary to form meaningful relationships. These alcoholics and those with severe psychiatric problems gained more from a cognitive-behavioural relapse prevention programme. In contrast, alcoholics with personality characteristics indicating an ability to form rich and deep relationships benefited more from the interactional programme, which probably allowed them to experience success and self-efficacy. In summary, studies by Annis and Chan (1983), McLellan *et al.* (1984), and Kadden *et al.* (1989) underscore the need to stipulate personality-related contra-indications for different therapeutic procedures.

Recently, Annis and Davis (1988; 1989*b*) taught alcoholic clients appropriate coping responses in high-risk situations and provided mastery experiences so that their self-efficacy would be enhanced. This programme was found to be of benefit to clients who varied their drinking from one situation to another, but it was no more effective than traditional counselling for those whose drinking was similar across all types of situations. A Client Profile of drinking risk situations proved to be a useful indicator of who would profit from Annis and Davis's relapse prevention strategy.

The above discussion illustrates a type of consideration that takes into account the kind of treatment task and its 'psychological meaning' for the client. It is uncertain to what extent the results are generalizable to treatment situations other than the ones that have been studied. It is likely that indications for abstinence versus controlled drinking, inpatient versus outpatient treatment, and degree of structure and directiveness, must always be *supplemented* with specific indications and contra-indications that are related to the content of treatment, and that vary from one programme to another. Interaction effects should thus be investigated within each treatment organization for people with alcohol problems.

24.5   Implementing the systems approach

The body of research on client–treatment interactions can be utilized in a direct and immediate fashion in tailoring treatment to clients' needs. Cronbach (1975) emphasized, however, that in a complex and changing world, the contributions of the social sciences are largely of an indirect nature:

Though enduring systematic theories about man in society are not likely to be achieved, systematic inquiry can realistically hope to make two contributions. One reasonable aspiration is to assess local events accurately, to improve short-run control. The other reasonable aspiration is to develop explanatory concepts, concepts that will help people to use their heads. (p. 126)

Research on interaction can facilitate the interpretation of qualitative knowing gained from clinical experience. It offers a vocabulary (constructs) and a grammar (theoretical models) for various reflections upon treatment and human change. Thus, the fertility of the matching hypothesis cannot be measured solely in terms of the number of significant interaction effects observed. Its value will rather be judged by whether it is able to challenge traditional ways of thinking about alcoholism treatment. This is why I have taken pains not only to offer a comprehensive account of empirical findings, but also to discuss the matching hypothesis in the broader context of results and approaches within psychosocial treatment research, conceptions of alcoholism, and strategies for the treatment of alcoholics.

Research can also, however, provide impetus for local efforts to achieve a more efficient short-term utilization of treatment resources. In view of economic, political, cultural, and other differences between countries and periods, it cannot be taken for granted that interaction effects can be generalized from one treatment setting to another. In addition, shifts in the climate of opinion, population characteristics, personnel recruitment, administrative routines, etc. can change clinically relevant interactions even within one and the same programme.

Optimal matching therefore requires continuous research and development within the framework of a systems approach to alcoholism treatment. McLellan and his co-workers (1980c) have presented a feasible model by which they achieved a more effective matching of clients to interventions in alcoholism treatment. Dougherty (1976) had some success in testing a similar model for evaluation and differentiation of other psychologically oriented treatment. On a local level and in a short-term perspective, research on interaction will be as fertile for its methodology as for its results.

I will conclude this chapter by illustrating how a systems approach could be implemented to co-ordinate the treatment of alcoholism in a local community. The example is hypothetical; it does not predict what numerical proportion of each type of treatment is required for any existing population. Its purpose is to exemplify how local needs might be assessed by a systems-based model of what should be, rather than by a projection of what currently exists (cf. Rush 1990).

The illustration is inspired by the Core–Shell Treatment System, developed by Glaser and his colleagues in Toronto, Canada, in the late 1970s (see Chapter 15). In this system, treatment resources are organized so that they comprise a common core and a shell of specialized interventions (Fig. 24.1).

To recapitulate, clients enter the treatment organization through the core, which, in contrast to the shell, consists of services that are necessary for all kinds of clients. Here clients are interviewed by a person who will provide *continuity of care* for them throughout their contact with the treatment system. Each client then undergoes individual *assessment*. To enable the 'right' client to be assigned to the 'right' programme, repeated *follow-up* studies of selected samples will also be required.

Assignments to specialized interventions in the shell should be based on information from the individual assessment. The previous review suggests

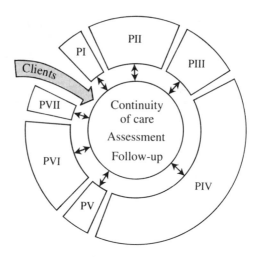

Fig. 24.1 A systems-based model of differential alcoholism treatment. P = programme. PI: relapse prevention, controlled drinking (5 per cent); PII: relapse prevention, abstinence (15 per cent); PIII: outpatient treatment, less structured (10 per cent); PIV: outpatient treatment, highly structured (45 per cent); PV: inpatient treatment, less structured (5 per cent); PVI: inpatient treatment, highly structured (15 per cent); PVII: sheltered living environment (5 per cent).

that the following client dimensions are critical for differential assignment, no matter what the specific treatment tasks are:

1. Psychiatric severity

McLellan *et al.* (1983*a*) found a highly significant relationship between a psychiatric severity score and treatment outcome. Alcoholics with no, or only minor, psychiatric symptoms (22 per cent of the clients) showed significant improvement regardless of which treatment programme they entered. However, the type of treatment selected did seem to matter for clients with recent symptoms of depression, anxiety, or cognitive confusion.

2. Social instability

In the study by McLellan *et al.* (1983*a*), alcoholics with moderately severe psychiatric problems showed better outcomes in inpatient than in outpatient treatment if the problems were *combined with* severe family-related problems, such as divorce or a family that is heavily involved in abuse, or severe work-related problems, such as unemployment or casual work. Psychiatric severity or social instability, each taken by itself, did not seem to constitute sufficient cause for inpatient treatment, however.

3. Need for structure

An impaired capacity for abstract thought, problem solving, analogical reasoning and learning is often found among alcoholics and problem drinkers. Erwin and Hunter (1984) showed that alcoholics with such problems tended to drop out of psychotherapy. Other studies suggest, however, that treatment modalities that provide a high degree of structure, active guidance, and concrete training may be helpful for these persons, as well as for clients who are at a low conceptual level, are field dependent, have an external locus of control, or who are sociopathic.

4. Severity of dependence

This dimension must be considered in deciding what drinking goal should be preferred. Controlled drinking is usually an unrealistic goal for alcohol-dependent persons, and may even increase the risk of relapse (Foy *et al.* 1984). For early-stage problem drinkers, however, controlled drinking can be an effective goal that is more acceptable than abstinence. Hence, in a system that provides a broad range of treatment options—from early intervention to specialized alcoholism treatment—a goal of controlled drinking may be feasible for some clients.

The model in Fig. 24.1 of how an optimal treatment system might be structured is based on research on interaction involving these four client

Table 24.1 A model of differential treatment selection

	Optimal client–treatment match	Psychiatric severity[a]	Social instability[b]	Need for structure[c]	Severity of dependence[d]
P I	Relapse prevention, controlled drinking	Low	Low/middle	Low	Low
P II	Relapse prevention, abstinence	Low	Low/middle	Low	High
P III	Outpatient treatment, less structured	Middle	Low/middle	Low	High
P IV	Outpatient treatment, highly structured	Middle	Low/middle	High	High
P V	Inpatient treatment, less structured	Middle	High	Low	High
P VI	Inpatient treatment, highly structured	Middle	High	High	High
P VII	Sheltered living environment	High	High	High	High

[a]Psychiatric severity is rated as low, middle, or high. [b]Social *in*stability is rated as low, middle, or high. [c]Need for structure is rated as low or high. [d]Severity of alcohol dependence is rated as low or high.

dimensions. It suggests how principal approaches, such as treatment settings, treatment modalities, and drinking goals, might be varied to increase cost-effectiveness and minimize the risk of harming clients. Table 24.1 summarizes criteria and typical combinations of scores that have been utilized in assessing the need for each type of treatment in the system's shell.

P I: *Relapse prevention, controlled drinking* (5 per cent of clients). That is, relapse prevention training directed towards a goal of moderation. For heavy drinkers with early symptoms of dependence but no, or only minor, psychiatric problems. Since the appropriate location for the effort directed at these drinkers should be community agencies, only a fraction of all clients in the specialized treatment sector will be eligible for this type of secondary prevention programme.

P II: *Relapse prevention, abstinence* (15 per cent of clients). That is, relapse prevention training directed towards a goal of abstinence. For heavy drinkers with symptoms of severe dependence but no, or only minor, psychiatric problems. These are probably the drinkers who, in Nordström's (1987) study, had 'the most favourable background characteristics in terms of personality and social stability', and who were sometimes able to resume social drinking after a prolonged period of abstinence (average, three years).

P III: *Outpatient treatment, less structured* (10 per cent of clients). For example relapse prevention training, biofeedback based on monthly Gamma-GT tests, and a supportive therapy encouraging self-expression and emphasizing the importance of the client's own efforts for successful treatment outcome. For alcoholics who have recent symptoms of depression, anxiety, or cognitive confusion, but have no, or only moderate, problems in terms of social stability, and low need for structure.

P IV: *Outpatient treatment, highly structured* (45 per cent of clients). For example relapse prevention training (emphasizing here behavioural rather than cognitive techniques, environmental contingencies rather than subjective states), supervised Antabuse/Temposil, and a supportive therapy providing guidance and reassurance. For alcoholics who have recent symptoms of depression, anxiety, or cognitive confusion, have only slight or moderate problems in terms of social stability, but have high need for structure. After several months of abstinence, some clients may well benefit from more abstract-symbolic tasks.

P V: *Inpatient treatment, less structured* (5 per cent of clients). For example a milieu therapy with social skills training, vocational rehabilitation, recommended AA attendance, check-up of posttreatment Gamma-GT values, etc. For alcoholics who have low need for structure, moderately severe psychiatric problems, but highly severe family-related problems, such as divorce or a family that is heavily involved in abuse, or highly severe work-related problems, such as unemployment or casual work.

P VI: *Inpatient treatment, highly structured* (15 per cent of clients). For example a programme similar to that described above, but with a sharper focus on instructional and behavioural approaches (e.g. education, advice, modelling, role playing, paradoxical intervention, promoting identification, behavioural rehearsal, task-assignment) and preparing for a highly structured aftercare programme, such as Azrin's (1976) community reinforcement approach. For alcoholics who have moderately severe psychiatric problems, highly severe family-related or work-related problems, and a high need for structure.

P VII: *Sheltered living environment* (5 per cent of clients). Many homeless and psychiatrically disabled alcoholics, who are making a living doing casual work at best, would benefit more from a long-term protective and supportive environment than from casual treatment interventions. Leach and Wing (1980), for example, have described an enabling model of rehabilitation, which would provide these 'destitute' individuals with a chain of housing and vocational opportunities.

25 Strategies of alcoholism treatment

25.1 The dynamics of treatment

Since client–treatment interactions are complex (Chapter 23), good theories are required for identifying them and developing effective approaches to treatment assignment. Without theoretical constructs, it is difficult or even impossible to detect higher-order interactions. Smart (1978b), in a study of the effects of alcoholism treatment against the background of 31 client characteristics and six treatment dimensions, was unable to find any significant effect of interaction. The study included 1100 persons, and he examined 186 possible interactions of the first order. If Smart had examined the occurrence of interaction effects of the second order, e.g. two client characteristics in interaction with one treatment dimension, he would have had to carry out more than 10 000 significance tests. This would have produced, through random variation, a considerable number of 'false' interaction effects, making the results virtually impossible to interpret.

Chen and Rossi's (1983) remark in their appeal for a more theory-driven approach to evaluation is justified:

The search for interactions should not be a matter of systematically testing out all possible interactions—a strategy that maximizes Type I errors [i.e. false positive findings]—but one which looks for those interactions that one has a good a priori reason to suspect exist. (p. 296)

In a review of the literature concerning effects of interaction, one is sometimes put in mind of the story of the man who lost his keys in a dark alley but went looking for them under the lamp-post—because the light was better there. Researchers have frequently investigated client characteristics and treatment dimensions that have been recorded for quite different purposes than analysing interactions. But these conventional factors have proved to a large extent to be irrelevant. Demographic predictors of treatment outcome such as gender, age, and social class and clinical predictors such as quantity of alcohol consumed and chronicity of dependence, seem to be of only indirect or negligible importance for the assignment to currently available treatment options.

An interesting phenomenon that has not been noticed in previous reviews is that all significant client–treatment interactions include *psychological* variables (including here the degree of alcohol dependence), sometimes in combination with demographic variables. This result may surprise readers who expect to find a direct link between aetiological variables and prognostic indicators. Indeed, this study (Chapter 8) refutes hypotheses that maintain that alcohol dependence is a symptom of underlying psychological problems. But if psychological-symptom theories are scientifically untenable, why is it then that psychological predictors seem to be of such relevance for differential treatment?

My interpretation of this finding is that psychosocial treatment has a dynamics of its own, which to a great extent is independent of the specific problem being treated or the specific treatment being applied to it. As was indicated in the preceding chapter, a treatment process can be understood in the light of:

1. The treatment goal, e.g. controlled drinking or abstinence.

2. The treatment approach, i.e. the task or procedure in which the client and the therapist are participating.

3. The therapeutic relationship. This can, for example, be highly or loosely structured, directive or non-directive.

4. The treatment setting, e.g. outpatient or inpatient treatment.

These characteristics can be integrated into a theoretical model for describing treatment processes (Fig. 25.1). The model reviews factors that should be taken into consideration in the selection of treatment for alcoholism. With its help, *clinical strategies* that must be employed for successful alcoholism treatment can be analysed.

The concept of clinical strategy has been borrowed from a review by Goldfried (1980) of commonalities among different treatment orientations. Goldfried contends that comparisons at the theoretical level are unlikely to reveal similarities, especially since little theoretical consensus exists within any given orientation. In the realm of specific therapeutic techniques (e.g. role playing, relaxation training), on the other hand, any similarities that may be found are likely to be trivial. Instead, the possibility of a meaningful

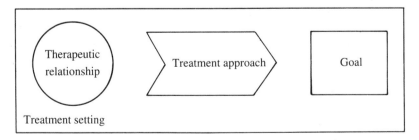

Fig. 25.1 Theoretical model for describing treatment processes.

dialogue across therapeutic orientations must be sought at a level of abstraction somewhere between theory and technique. At this level common clinical strategies or approaches to treatment are more likely to be revealed.

In the following I will interpret the results summarized in the preceding chapter. The line of reasoning is based on the theoretical model above and is oriented towards clinical strategies rather than towards individual theories or techniques. The empirical literature suggests that sucessful treatment for alcoholism should employ four strategies:

1. To assist the superego of the client by a consistent orientation towards a *treatment goal* of either abstinence or moderated drinking, depending on the client's wish and degree of alcohol dependence.

2. To select a *treatment approach* that makes the client avoid failures that may demoralize him and weaken his self-esteem.

3. To eliminate barriers to communication between the therapist and the client that might make the creation of a *therapeutic relationship* more difficult.

4. To select a *treatment setting* that provides a secure base from which the world of thoughts, feelings, and actions can be explored.

25.2 Supporting the superego

The *superego* is a Freudian term for the part of the mind that observes the self and makes it aware of what is right and wrong. It functions to approve as well as to disapprove of an individual's behaviour. Psychoanalytic writings, however, have often overlooked the very positive side of the superego as a source of love and self-esteem (Sandler 1987).

Normally, the superego is not distinguishable from the ego, because they work together harmoniously (Laufer and Alfie 1977). The judging and protective functions of the superego are prerequisites of *self-governance* or 'the sense of being and the power to be in charge of oneself' (Mack 1981, p. 133). In his writings on psychodynamic aspects of alcoholism, Mack (1981; Khantzian and Mack 1989) noted that self-governance is not a solitary process. The participation of the individual in a variety of group and institutional activities and affiliations has a powerful impact on his ability to regulate his life and drinking behaviour.

Thus, AA may be effective in so far as it becomes a part of the individual member's self-governance system (Khantzian and Mack 1989). This organization emphasizes the need to 'surrender' to the human reality of interdependence and to accept the 'powerlessness' to control one's drinking alone. Only by internalizing the care and controls of the group will the AA member be able to extend his domain of self-governance. The strategy of *superego support* implies a recognition of the fact that alcohol-dependent persons need help from the environment in controlling their own impulses to drink. The therapist must assume the role of a kind of external conscience so that the client is not left entirely to his own heavily strained conscience. In other words, the therapist must show that he cares whether the client drinks or not. Otherwise, the alcoholic will feel that he has to maintain control completely on his own, which experience has taught him he cannot manage. Once the client has accepted the therapist in this role, the therapist becomes an auxiliary superego. Gradually, when the client has internalized some of the support provided for him, the therapist can relax the external control of his drinking behaviour.

My term superego support bears some resemblance to both the vernacular 'moral support' and the broader technical term 'ego support'. None of these terms, however, focuses sharply on the impact of the generalized other on the individual's ability to regulate his life and drinking behaviour. The sociological term 'social control', on the other hand, does not explicitly emphasize the importance of *internalizing* the care and controls of significant others.

Supportive therapy (with or without Antabuse), behaviour therapy, and cognitive therapy are generally aimed directly and primarily at analysing and changing the drinking behaviour of alcoholics and helping them develop alternatives to drinking. Therapists of these orientations thus practise the clinical strategy described above. The same can be said of AA and peer group oriented programmes inspired by this organization, which incidentally is referred to by its members as a 'group conscience'. A cornerstone in the AA philosophy is the members' constantly reminding each other that 'there is one thing I cannot do'. Apparently, effective alcoholism treatment reminds the severely dependent drinker of the same simple fact, with firmness and consistency, but without reproach or moralizing.

The strategy of superego support may seem self-evident, but is often neglected nonetheless. George Vaillant has pointed out that the 'professional permissiveness' of many therapists constitutes a serious threat to substance abusers' precarious or deficient impulse control. In his essay 'Dangers of psychotherapy in the treatment of alcoholism' (1981), he warned of the tendency in dynamic psychotherapy to deflect attention away from the client's uncontrolled drinking, which is usually misinterpreted (see Chapter 8) as a symptom of underlying psychiatric disorder. Vaillant (1981) supported his criticism with data from a longitudinal study (Vaillant 1980*a*).

Freud himself, as well as Wolberg (1967), Ewing (1977), Saliba (1982), Levy (1987), Brickman (1988), and several other respected psychoanalysts, shared Vaillant's view that active alcoholism is a contra-indication for insight therapy. Gerard and Saenger (1966) found that the less outpatient clinics went into the 'causes' of the clients' drinking, the better was the outcome measured in terms of changed drinking behaviour. In a comparison between an 'insight-oriented' programme and a recreational programme, Levinson and Sereny (1969) showed that the latter setting was at least as effective as the former. The authors commented that 'the results of the present study should lend support to the ever-increasing reservation about the value of a psychiatrically-oriented approach to the treatment of alcoholism' (p. 146).

Later, Stinson *et al.* (1979) and Welte *et al.* (1979) reported in two large studies, one experimental and the other quasi-experimental, that severely alcohol-dependent clients reduced their drinking more effectively with peer-oriented programmes than with programmes of a traditional psychiatric nature. The former type of programme often has recovered alcoholics and paraprofessionals as therapists and adheres to the principles of AA. In a randomized controlled study, finally, Olson *et al.* (1981) showed that behavioural therapy was more effective than insight therapy. In fact, patients assigned to insight therapy did even worse than those in the control group, who were not given any therapy in addition to the milieu programme in which all patients participated.

These older and more recent studies, as well as the refutation of symptomatic theories in Chapter 8, corroborate Vaillant's (1981) warning against a clinical strategy that diverts attention from the client's drinking behaviour and from the exploration of alternatives to drinking.

Research on controlled drinking (Section 24.1) indicates that in the treatment of severely alcohol-dependent persons, therapists should advocate simple and unambiguous alcohol norms in order to provide effective support to the clients' superego functions. Normally, treatment should aim at abstinence, with the option of moderated drinking only for those clients who refuse to consider total abstinence. Owing to its methodological qualities, the study by Foy and colleagues (1984) is particularly instructive. The research team found that clients who had been trained in controlled drinking actually learned the necessary skills. But the result after discharge from the programme deflated the optimism of the clinical staff. It showed that alcoholics who had received special training in controlled drinking skills relapsed to a greater extent than others.

An orientation towards drinking behaviour as a primary problem must, however, be combined with a readiness to accept relapse. Vaillant (1983*b*) recalls the first step of Al-Anon, a self-help organization for spouses of alcoholics: 'And we admitted we were powerless over alcohol.' Only with this insight is it possible to maintain the firmness and consistency that are required to back up the alcoholics' own impulse control. Anyone who overestimates his or her ability to 'cure' will only too easily fall victim to despondency, promoting therapist burnout and blame of less successful clients.

In the first place, a single treatment episode weighs lightly against habits that have been developing for perhaps ten or twenty years. Rather than expecting immediate change, it might be appropriate to view the therapist's task as one of facilitating a process of long-term rehabilitation. In the second place, the prospects for a change in lifestyle are dependent on a great number of external circumstances which neither the clinician nor the client is capable of influencing alone—for example, cultural expectations and the availability of alcoholic beverages. And in the third place, the present-day state of knowledge is such that Vaillant (1983*b*) in his landmark study of the course of alcoholism had to admit: 'To a large extent relapse to and remission from alcoholism remain a mystery' (p. 303).

The principle of personifying the demand on abstention has been corroborated in work with alcohol-dependent persons, i.e. with clients of the type usually encountered in conventional alcoholism treatment. Secondary preventive programmes aimed at heavy drinkers who have not developed a dependence on alcohol should probably apply a non-problem drinking goal and a strategy that differs somewhat from that described here (cf. Sanchez-Craig *et al.* 1984; Babor *et al.* 1986; Kristenson 1987).

25.3 Natural healing processes

Except for treatment that deflects attention away from the client's drinking behaviour, all forms of treatment seem to do at least some good. It is true that the effects of alcoholism treatment tend to be weak and short-lived (Chapter 3), but it cannot be overemphasized that temporary and limited alleviation of a serious problem is better than no alleviation at all.

Moreover, stable remission is based in most cases on experience gained without the help of treatment. In an early study, Gerard, Saenger, and Wile (1962) found that only about 30 per cent of the men who had achieved abstinence took this crucial step in connection with treatment. The same result was obtained by Vaillant (1983*b*) twenty years later in his longitudinal study of a male community sample. In Knupfer's (1972) study of a sample of ex-alcoholics, no more than about 20 per cent had changed their drinking behaviour as a result of treatment. In Nordström and Berglund's (1986) long-term follow-up of a clinical sample, 19 per cent of the alcoholics chosen for good social adjustment reported treatment or probation as the main cause of improvement, while another 40 per cent stated that treatment or probation had been of contributory importance.

It is important to keep in mind that the therapeutic sessions arranged by alcoholism programmes represent only a minor fraction of the clients' encounters with other people. Room (1989) found that during one year, no less than one third of a US adult sample had engaged in informal efforts to control the drinking of family members or friends. He claimed that few people enter alcoholism treatment without having been pressured by others about their drinking. Moreover, results attributed to psychosocial treatment may in actuality have their basis in other concurrent events. It is, for example, very common that clients under treatment simultaneously seek support, advice, and guidance from persons other than the therapist, such as family members, friends, fellow-workers, physicians, and clergymen (Bergin and Lambert 1978, pp. 148–52). Therapy may also be given credit for improvement that is the result of a change in life circumstances, for example a change in work or family situation. Conversely, promising results of treatment can be nullified by severe personal setbacks suffered by the client.

However, the causal relationship between man and his environment works in both directions. As a result of treatment, people may choose, change, and create life circumstances that in turn contribute to transforming them. The symptomatic notion that most alcoholics, due to underlying personality disorder, create an unfavourable environment around themselves whether they drink or not has no scientific support (Moos, Finney, and Chan 1981). During a sober period, perhaps initiated by treatment, a client may, for example, find a new partner who refuses to accept his previous drinking behaviour, change to a 'drier' work setting, or acquire a new group affiliation that is incompatible with continued drinking, for example by joining AA or a church.

Saunders and Kershaw (1979), Vaillant (1983b), Nordström and Berglund (1986), Edwards et al. (1987), and others have presented findings that indicate that new social relations of this kind are a major precondition for the persistence of whatever the severely dependent drinker may have gained from treatment. Reduced alcohol tolerance and a serious deterioration of physical health are other common reasons why alcoholics—with or usually without treatment—achieve stable improvement. Direct intervention by family or friends, financial trouble, and legal complications may also persuade some alcoholics to change their style of life, although these consequences seem to have a greater impact on the less dependent drinker.

In view of what has been said here, it is essential to make a distinction between factors that *initiate* improvement and those that *maintain* it (cf. Atthowe 1973; Liberman 1978a; Brownell et al. 1986). As was pointed out in Chapter 3, one cannot expect to find, one year after discharge from an alcoholism programme, any significant difference in drinking outcome between a treatment group and a control group that has received no or minimal treatment. The interpretation of this result should not be that treatment of alcoholics is ineffective, but that any *long-term* remission is primarily due to circumstances over which the therapist has little or no control.

Consequently, the only theoretical problem which the present outcome research can shed light on is how to explain the short-term effects of alcoholism treatment, i.e. effects that can reasonably be attributed to the treatment. In other words, the question to which it is possible to provide an empirically founded answer must be restricted to the following:

What clinical strategies are effective in a time perspective of less than one year?

One such strategy was formulated in the previous section: a good therapist becomes an external superego, a living reminder of the disabling role played by alcohol in the client's life. The superego is the psychic agency that imposes moral demands and inhibits an alcoholic from yielding to his craving for alcohol. Successful treatment, however, seems to involve a *combination* of demands and empathy. The therapist, like the good parent, says Strupp (1982), needs to know how to love without spoiling and discipline without hurting. Hence the superego support appears to be truly effective only within the framework of what Lester Luborsky (1976) calls a *helping alliance*, that is, a human relationship which the client experiences as a help, or a possible help, in achieving his own goals.

According to Jerome Frank (1973), psychosocial treatment has in common the fact that a trained, socially sanctioned healer uses psychological means to *mobilize the help-seeker's natural healing powers*. Frank's transcultural model for describing and explaining how non-medical treatment contributes to the resistance of the help-seeker was summarized in Chapter 4. A basic thought is that treatment often manages to accelerate and facilitate healing processes that would have gone on more slowly in its absence. As evidenced by placebo studies, clients generally have a significantly greater capacity for self-healing than they are willing or prepared to recognize (Plotkin 1985).

To use a Socratic term, successful psychosocial treatment could be described as *maieutics* or midwifery, since it frees the help-seekers to exercise their self-healing competencies. Thus when Socrates in the *Theaetetus* describes his role as a teacher by analogy of a midwife who does nothing more than assist the pregnant mother to give birth with less pain and more assurance, his metaphor equally well applies to a modern therapist. The therapist may be of great help, but the impetus behind the 'natural' processes of healing is to be found in the help-seeker himself.

It is scarcely otherwise possible to explain the dominant role played by the selection of clients as compared with the choice of treatment for the outcome of alcoholism treatment (Conradsson and Holmgren 1974; Baekeland *et al.* 1975; Baekeland 1977). Adamson, Fostakowsky, and Chebib (1974) found that client variables that reflect a 'favourable view of self or others' predicted treatment outcome more reliably than, for example, level of education, social stability, or severity of drinking history. They concluded that the result had logical appeal in that 'it is obvious that the influence of previous life experience on behaviour is mediated by psychological set' (p. 333).

This conclusion is further supported by McLellan and his co-workers' (1983a) finding of a highly significant ($p < 0.001$) correlation between a global measure of psychiatric severity and treatment outcome. No other variable exhibited such high predictive power. According to these studies, the possibility of harnessing an alcoholic's will-power and coping ability appears to be more dependent on his *susceptibility to psychological influence* (cf. Strupp 1973, Ch. 5) than on such variations with respect to drinking history or demographic characteristics as are usually encountered within alcoholism treatment.

The situation is comparable to the predicament of medicine up until the breakthrough of the natural sciences at the end of the nineteenth century. Professional helpers faced with suffering for which no real cure was available were forced to rely on their ability to stimulate and mobilize the help-seeker's natural defences. Instead of merely combating isolated disturbances, skilled physicians, priests, and other helpers attempted with psychological means to induce people who were in a state of crisis to see themselves and to act as active subjects instead of as helpless victims.

In a previously quoted aphorism concerning the inadequacy of medical knowledge, Hippocrates pointed out that the physician must be prepared not only to discharge his own duties, but must also 'secure the cooperation of the patient, of the attendants and of externals' (Hippocrates 1923, Vol. 2, p. 99). Elsewhere in the Hippocratic Corpus, the author says: 'The art has three factors, the disease, the patient, the physician. The physician is the servant of the art. The patient must cooperate with the physician in combating the disease' (op. cit., Vol. 1, p. 165).

On the whole, the renaissance physician Paracelsus was probably right in that Hippocrates' fortune in his cures was not due to any extraordinary medical skill, but was rather the result of the great faith which common people had in his ability to restore their health (Osler 1910). That is, he was extraordinary successful in securing the co-operation of his fellow citizens in combating disease. However, given the lack of specific remedies, some Hippocratic recommendations, such as blood-letting in connection with lobar pneumonia, have the support of modern medical science as well (King 1982). The proposed measures could relieve symptoms temporarily and thus give the patient a chance to regain his strength and resistance.

In the last chapter of *The Republic*, Plato characterized the ancient art of medicine as an aid to self-help. In calamity, says Socrates in this dialogue, there are two opposite impulses in a man at the same time. Reason exhorts him to resist, while the bare feeling itself urges him to give way to his grief. However, no matter what are the underlying causes of distress, in order to lead his life with dignity, man must get in command of himself and his destiny. When asked what would be the best way to face misfortune and deal with it, Socrates answers:

[We need] to deliberate . . . about what has happened to us, and, as it were in the fall of the dice, to determine the movements of our affairs with reference to the numbers that turn up, in the way that reason indicates would be the best, and, instead of stumbling like children, clapping one's hands to the stricken spot and wasting the time in wailing, ever to accustom the soul to devote itself at once to the curing of the hurt and the raising up of what has fallen, banishing threnody by therapy. (Plato 1935, pp. 455–6)

Ultimately, psychosocial treatment aims at self-help of the kind Socrates is talking about here. Like the ancient art of medicine, it attempts to help sufferers to gain command of themselves and their destiny. Although the whims of fate may appear to be random as if dictated by the fall of the dice, man is free to choose how to deal with his lot, free to decide what conclusions to draw from it. No one is doomed to remain a helpless victim, no matter how distressing the circumstances may be, asserts Socrates in Plato's dialogue. It is from this insight and reliance on man's inherent powers of healing that a helping alliance can emerge.

25.4   Establishing a helping alliance

In analysing how a helping alliance can be created, it is helpful to regard what happens during treatment as the result of several interacting components, as was done in the theoretical model above (p. 289). So far, I have mainly concentrated on those aspects of alcoholism treatment that have to do with its goal. Below, I shall show how research on interaction effects and matching can also enrich our understanding of the importance of the treatment approach, the therapeutic relationship, and the treatment setting for the outcome of psychosocial treatment.

The treatment approach

The activities engaged in by therapists and clients within alcoholism treatment are of a highly diverse nature. Certain therapeutic procedures activate the help-seeker's powers of healing by means of physical agents, for example Antabuse treatment and modification of behaviour by regular feedback of values on a Gamma-GT test, which detects early signs of liver disorder. Other techniques, such as behaviour therapy and supportive psychotherapy, focus on human skills, cognitions, and emotive states related to drinking behaviour. Religious revivalist movements view alcoholism as a spiritual problem and therefore emphasize spiritual healing. Whether the symbolic interaction between helper and help-seeker takes place within a medical, cognitive-behavioural, or religious framework, however, the purpose is the same: to bring about, by appropriate means of persuasion, such a change in the patient's mental set and behaviour that he will be able to deal with his problems.

The feeling of being able to cope is usually rooted in success experiences. The professional helper usually only comes into contact with the minority of sufferers who have been unable to obtain effective help in their natural environment. Frank (1973, 1974*a*) describes persons seeking therapy as *demoralized*. They are aware that they have failed to live up to their own or their environment's expectations or that they have been unable to cope with some pressing problem in their lives. They feel powerless to change the situation or themselves. They have feelings of helplessness, isolation, and despair and are preoccupied with merely trying to survive.

According to Frank (1971, 1973), all psychosocial treatments employ procedures that *give the help-seeker an opportunity to experience success*. This experience is achieved in a large number of ways within alcoholism treatment. The daily Antabuse ritual, for example, verifies in symbolic form the alcohol-dependent person's victory over his craving for alcohol. This seems to be an effective method for certain persons, at least as long as other significant people convince them of the meaningfulness of their endeavours. With biofeedback according to Kristenson's (1987) method, the client can, by means of a monthly laboratory test (Gamma-GT test), determine how alcohol has affected his liver. This method of modifying behaviour also requires a good relationship between therapist and client (Blanchard and Young 1974).

As a consequence of supportive psychotherapy or participation in AA meetings, each day with activities other than drinking is experienced as a success. This takes on particular importance because the therapist or the fellow members of AA care about the progress of each individual. In a revivalist fellowship, the individual's way of life is also accorded religious meaning. Behaviour therapy focuses the client's attention on a few specific but essential problems, which he is given help in solving. The experience of some success in whatever area focused on, often activates self-healing processes which spread like ripples on a pond, eventually enabling the client to master his entire life situation more effectively than before (Bandura 1977, 1982, 1984).

Perceived self-efficacy operates as a common mechanism in personal change, says Bandura (1984). It partly determines how well people perform. For example, those who regard themselves as highly efficacious have been found to set themselves challenges and to intensify their efforts in the face of difficulties. Their accomplishments alter their self-percepts of efficacy in a mutually interactive way. If the performance is considered important, this process will affect their self-esteem or sense of self-worth.

Research has not demonstrated any superior method for the treatment of alcoholics. Yet studies of client–treatment interactions show that therapeutic procedures are not completely interchangeable. This does not, however, necessarily mean that the procedures are different in function. In his comparative study of psychologically oriented therapy, Frank (1973) said that

when therapies have a different effect [e.g., when one therapeutic technique is more successful than another with certain types of patients], it may depend on the differential ability of the technique to mobilize certain features common to all. For example, structured behaviour therapies may more readily engender success experiences than unstructured interview therapies in certain patients, while for others, unstructured interview therapies may be more effective. (pp. xvi–xvii)

Frank (1982) believed that the selection of psychotherapy is usually better guided by the personal characteristics and predilections of the therapist and the patient, and their accordance with each other and the type of therapy, than by the patient's symptoms.

Research on the interaction between client type, treatment approach, and outcome of alcoholism treatment confirms that the treatment task must be experienced as *meaningful* and *challenging*. A reasonable interpretation of the empirical findings summarized in the previous chapter is that specific types of clients find a meaning in and are able to profit from specific kinds of treatment tasks. What appears to be crucial for the outcome—in good agreement with modern theories of behaviour (Magnusson and Allen 1983)—is whether the client *perceives* the 'progress' made in the course of treatment as relevant, not whether it actually is related to his problem (cf. Liberman 1978b; Section 21.4 above).

Within the field of alcoholism, Wallerstein's (1957), Annis and Chan's (1983), Kadden and colleagues' (1989), and Longabaugh and colleagues' (in press) studies, in particular, indicate that the provision of success experiences and the mobilization of unexploited self-healing competencies will be hampered if the therapeutic task is construed as being irrelevant or too threatening. In the worst cases, as suggested by Annis and Chan and by Longabaugh *et al.*, clients can experience failures that damage their self-esteem and lead to a deterioration of their condition. The importance of strengthening the client's self-esteem is also highlighted by Sokolow and his colleagues' (1980) and Dahlgren and Willander's (1989) studies of women treated for alcohol problems.

The therapeutic relationship

A trusting relationship between client and therapist appears to be a necessary, though not sufficient, condition for hope-engendering experiences of success. Where such a relationship is lacking, the patient will not make the effort or will not listen to the therapist's interpretations, Freud pointed out in a letter to Carl Gustav Jung (published in Jones 1955). He went on to say that the therapeutic method that he had developed 'is in essence a cure through love' (p. 485). The importance of the client–therapist relationship for the effectiveness of psychoanalytic treatments was confirmed by Kernberg *et al.* (1972) in the Menninger Foundation's psychotherapy research project. It is probable, however, that favourable outcomes with other methods as well are essentially dependent on the therapist's ability to win the client's confidence (Strupp 1977; Strupp and Hadley 1979).

In a few early case studies of psychiatric patients who have benefited from psychotherapy, Blaine and McArthur (1958) drew attention to the fact that while the therapists tended to attribute patient improvements to the method (depth-psychological insights), patients themselves often emphasized the therapeutic relationship (the therapist's interest and concern) as the most important ingredient of the treatment received. The latter finding has been replicated by other and more comprehensive patient studies. Components such as 'getting reassurance and encouragement', and patients' notions regarding the therapist as an understanding person, have been rated as being of major therapeutic importance whether the therapy concerned was insight-oriented or behavioural (Llewelyn and Hume 1979; Cross, Sheehan, and Khan 1982). Research reviews have also shown that, at least with relatively unstructured treatments, variations in outcome typically have more to do with the therapist than with the type of treatment (Luborsky et al. 1986).

Some half-dozen teams of researchers have accepted Luborsky's (1976) challenge to develop reliable instruments for rating the helping alliance. Several investigators (see reviews by Luborsky et al. 1988; Gaston 1990) have observed that such ratings predict the outcome of psychotherapy. These findings have been reported across a diversity of treatment approaches, a variety of diagnostic categories, and various sources of information (patient, therapist, and clinical judges). Morgan, Luborsky, and their co-workers (1982) found, for example, that an early measure of the quality of the therapeutic relationship was a significant predictor in the treatment of non-psychotic patients at a psychiatric outpatient clinic. This measure explained about 25 per cent of the total variance in outcome at the end of treatment. Other theoretically relevant treatment variables (e.g. a measure of depth-psychological insights) were not significantly correlated with treatment outcome.

Gloria Litman (1982) reported on an interview survey of 25 patients who had been successful either in abstaining or controlling their drinking following treatment at the Maudsley and Bethlem Royal Hospitals in London. She was struck by the almost magical qualities attributed by these patients to the professional helper. Doctors, psychiatrists, social workers, etc. who may have been seen previously as being harsh, punitive, and unempathic now suddenly seemed to be endowed with almost supernatural powers. Litman assumed that it was scarcely the therapeutic skill of the helper that had increased, but rather the patient's perception of the helper that had changed. The helper was no longer regarded as the agent of denial, but rather as an ally in the struggle towards drinking goals and life values that gradually became the patient's own.

The realization that an open, honest, and trusting relationship is important in order for a given set of therapeutic techniques to be effective is by no means new. In his pioneering work on alcoholism, Thomas Trotter (1804) perceptively said: 'When the physician has once gained the full confidence of his patient, he will find little difficulty in beginning his plan of cure' (p. 173). Trotter was well aware, however, that obtaining this confidence 'is not accomplished at a first visit' (p. 172). A 'plan of cure' must involve establishing a trusting relationship. As Hans Strupp (1970; 1973, p. 119) pointed out, psychological methods of treatment can largely be regarded as means of *eliminating the barriers to a favourable interpersonal relationship.* One important function of the therapeutic procedure, for example, is to sustain the therapist's efforts long enough to establish a personal relationship with the client. Without any prescribed activities the therapist would 'run out of material' after a few sessions (Strupp 1986).

Frank (1973) also emphasized the ways in which the treatment method reinforces the therapeutic relationship:

Since [the procedure] requires active participation of both patient and therapist and is typically repetitive, it serves as the vehicle for maintaining the therapeutic relationship and transmitting the therapist's influence. It also enhances the therapist's self-confidence by enabling him to demonstrate mastery of a special set of skills. (p. 328)

Carl Rogers (1957) and Heinz Kohut (1971) in the US, and British object-relations analysts like W. R. D. Fairbairn, Donald Winnicott, and Harry Guntrip (e.g. Guntrip 1975), in particular, have emphasized the therapist's personal qualities and stressed the crucial importance of the therapeutic relationship. However, the significance of this relationship is now accepted by most therapeutic orientations. Hence fourteen American researchers, invited to consider key issues associated with psychotherapy integration, stated that it is 'probably the quintessential integrative variable' (Wolfe and Goldfried 1988).

The observation in alcoholism treatment that paraprofessional, peer-oriented programmes often are at least as successful as programmes of a traditional psychiatric kind (Stinson *et al.* 1979; Welte *et al.* 1979) confirms a general tendency within psychosocial treatment (see reviews by Smith and Glass 1977; Durlak 1979; Smith *et al.* 1980; Shapiro and Shapiro 1982; Hattie, Sharpley, and Rogers 1984). Paraprofessional helpers lack qualified training in the administration of specific therapeutic techniques. The results of the studies comparing paraprofessionals and professionals can therefore be interpreted as a support for theories that stress the role of the therapeutic relationship.

There is no satisfactory definition of a good human relationship. However, the literature on effects of interaction involving degree of treatment structure and directiveness (Section 24.3) may help us. It indicates that such a relationship can only be established if the therapist selects procedures adapted to the patient's ability to think abstractly and hypothetically. The predictive power of cognitive variables does not mean, however, that the emotive components of treatment are less important. What outcome research demonstrates is rather that effective communication is a prerequisite for an emotionally satisfying relationship. The dropout rate from many kinds of verbal approaches suggests that it is too easy to talk over people's heads, or else to talk down to them.

Of studies within alcoholism treatment, Karp *et al.* (1970), McLachlan (1972, 1974), and Erwin and Hunter (1984), in particular, indicate that persons with a limited capacity for abstract-verbal communication prefer, and do best with, a highly structured, concrete, and directive therapy. A therapeutic relationship characterized by these attributes appears to help such persons to feel secure and experience success during treatment. According to preliminary findings by Obitz (1978), Spoth (1983), and Hartman *et al.* (1988), a structured and directive approach may also facilitate communication in the treatment of alcoholics with an external locus of control. The same approach has been found effective with sociopathic alcoholics in studies by Wilbur *et al.* (1966), Norman and Schulze (1970), McLellan *et al.* (1983a; p. 164), and Kadden *et al.* (1989).

The treatment setting

Bruce Jones (1983) and John Bowlby (1988) draw upon the latter's well-known attachment theory (Bowlby 1969) to explain how the relationship between therapist and help-seeker can mobilize self-healing forces. Bowlby maintains that the capacity to form affectional bonds is inherited and is of the same primary importance for the survival of the human race as hunger and sex drives. It develops in the relationship to the mother, who in the life of the small child becomes a *secure base*. As long as the mother is available and responsive, the child feels secure in exploring its environment and its own capabilities. If danger threatens, it instinctively returns to her proximity.

Adolescents extend their excursions to weeks or months. But for them, too, a secure home base within access in emergency is indispensable for their well-being. In fact, throughout the life cycle we need someone to lean on when problems become too much for us. Whatever our age, anxiety tends to be relieved when we know that someone cares about us and accepts us as we are.

According to Jones (1983) and Bowlby (1988), the role of the professional helper is to provide such a secure base for people in a state of alarm. With an interested and concerned helper by their side, help-seeking persons obtain the strength to attack their problems and try new solutions. In the same spirit, Frank (1973) described the treatment setting as

a temporary refuge from the demands and distractions of daily life. . . . Protected by the setting, the patient can concentrate on the prescribed therapeutic activities. He can participate in complex, emotionally charged rituals, suspend his critical faculties, freely express his emotions, indulge in leisurely self-exploration, daydream, or do whatever else the therapy prescribes, secure in the knowledge that no harm will come to him during the session and that he will not be held accountable in his daily life for whatever he says or does during it. By thus freeing him to experiment, the combination of healer and setting create favourable conditions for change. (pp. 326–7)

The studies of interaction effects that were summarized in the previous chapter indicate that a favourable relationship and a secure base can generally develop just as well in outpatient as in inpatient care. However, there appears to be a small group of alcoholics who, owing to psychiatric problems and social instability, do better in inpatient care (Kissin *et al.* 1970; Welte *et al.* 1981; McLellan *et al.* 1983*a*, 1983*c*). To feel secure and to be able to concentrate their energies on the treatment, these persons must spend some time in an environment that provides a certain measure of protection and structure. Inpatient care can thus be warranted under special circumstances by the principle of *creating a secure base that enables a therapeutic process to take place.*

References

Abbott, M. W. (1984). Locus of control and treatment outcome in alcoholics, *Journal of Studies on Alcohol*, **45**, 46–52.

Abramowitz, C. V., Abramowitz, S. I., Roback, H. B., and Jackson, C. (1974). Differential effectiveness of directive and nondirective group therapies as a function of client internal–external control, *Journal of Consulting and Clinical Psychology*, **42**, 849–53.

Abrams, D. B. and Niaura, R. S. (1987). Social learning theory. In *Psychological theories of drinking and alcoholism* (ed. H. T. Blane and K. E. Leonard) pp. 131–78. Guilford Press, New York.

ACP. *See* American College of Physicians.

Adamson, J. D., Fostakowsky, R. T., and Chebib, F. S. (1974). Measures associated with outcome on one year follow-up of male alcoholics, *British Journal of Addiction*, **69**, 325–37.

Adler, M. J. (1988). Teaching, learning, and their counterfeits. In M. J. Adler *Reforming education: The opening of the American mind*, pp. 167–75. Macmillan, New York.

Aiken, M., Dewar R., DiTomaso, N., Hage, J., and Zeitz, G. (1975). *Co-ordinating human services*, Jossey-Bass, San Francisco.

Albrecht, G. L. (1973). The alcoholism process: A social learning viewpoint. In *Alcoholism: Progress in research and treatment* (ed. P. G. Bourne and R. Fox) pp. 11–42. Academic Press, New York.

Alcoholics Anonymous (1939). *The story of how more than 1000 men have recovered from alcoholism*, Works Publishing Company, New York.

Alcoholics Anonymous (1957). *Alcoholics Anonymous comes of age*, Harper and Brothers, New York.

Allman, L. R., Taylor, H. A., and Nathan, P. E (1972). Group drinking during stress: Effects on drinking behavior, affect, and psychopathology, *American Journal of Psychiatry*, **129**, 669–78.

Almond, R. (1983). Concepts and new developments in milieu treatment. In *Principles and practice of milieu therapy* (ed. J. G. Gunderson, O. A. Will, Jr., and L. R. Mosher) pp. 127–40. Jason Aronson, New York.

Alterman, A. I. and Tarter, R. E. (1986). An examination of selected typologies: Hyperactivity, familial, and antisocial alcoholism. In *Recent developments in alcoholism, Vol. 4* (ed. M. Galanter) pp. 169–89. Plenum Press, New York.

AMA. *See* American Medical Association.

Åmark, C. (1951). A study in alcoholism: Clinical, social-psychiatric and genetic investigations, *Acta Psychiatrica et Neurologica Scandinavia*, Supplementum 70.

American College of Physicians, ACP (1989). Disulfiram treatment of alcoholism, *Annals of Internal Medicine*, **111**, 943–5.

American Medical Association, AMA (1961). *Standard nomenclature of diseases and operations*, 5th edn., Blakiston, New York.

American Medical Association, AMA (1987). Council on scientific affairs. Aversion therapy, *The Journal of the American Medical Association*, **258**, 2562–6.

American Psychiatric Association, APA. Committee on nomenclature and statistics (1968, 1980, 1987). *Diagnostic and statistical manual of mental disorders*. DSM-II, 1968; DSM-III, 1980; DSM-III-R, 1987. APA, Washington, DC.

Anastasi, A. (1968). *Psychological testing*, 3rd edn., Macmillan, New York.

Anderson, J. G. and Gilbert, F. S. (1989). Communication skills training with alcoholics for improving performance of the Alcoholics Anonymous recovery steps, *Journal of Studies on Alcohol*, **50**, 361–7.

Andrews, G. and Harvey, R. (1981). Does psychotherapy benefit neurotic patients? *Archives of General Psychiatry*, **38**, 1203–8.

Annis, H. M. (1979). Group treatment of incarcerated offenders with alcohol and drug problems: A controlled evaluation, *Canadian Journal of Criminology*, **21**, 3–15.

Annis, H. M. (1980). Treatment of alcoholic women. In *Alcoholism treatment in transition* (ed. G. Edwards and M. Grant) pp. 128–39. Croom Helm, London.

Annis, H. M. (1986). Is inpatient rehabilitation of the alcoholic cost effective? Con position, *Advances in Alcohol and Substance Abuse*, **5** (1/2), 175–90.

Annis, H. M. (1987). Effective treatment for drug and alcohol problems: What do we know? Invited address presented at the Annual Meeting of the Institute of Medicine. National Academy of Sciences, Washington, DC, October 21.

Annis, H. M. (1988). Patient–treatment matching in the management of alcoholism. In *Problems of drug dependence* (ed. L. S. Harris) pp. 152–61. NIDA Research Monograph No. 90, National Institute on Drug Abuse, Rockville, Md.

Annis, H. M. and Chan, D. (1983). The differential treatment model: Empirical evidence from a personality typology of adult offenders, *Criminal Justice and Behavior*, **10**, 159–73.

Annis, H. M. and Davis, C. S. (1988). Self-efficacy and the prevention of alcoholic relapse: Initial findings from a treatment trial. In *Assessment and treatment of addictive disorders* (ed. T. B. Baker and D. S. Cannon) pp. 88–112. Praeger, New York.

Annis, H. M. and Davis, C. S. (1989*a*). Relapse prevention. In *Handbook of alcoholism treatment approaches* (ed. R. K. Hester and W. R. Miller) pp. 170–82. Pergamon Press, New York.

Annis, H. M. and Davis, C. S. (1989*b*). Relapse prevention training: A cognitive-behavioral approach based on self-efficacy theory, *Journal of Chemical Dependency Treatment*, **2** (2), 81–103.

Annis, H. M. and Liban, C. B. (1980). Alcoholism in women: Treatment modalities and outcomes. In *Research advances in alcohol and drug problems, Vol. 5* (ed. O. J. Kalant) pp. 385–422. Plenum Press, New York.

APA. *See* American Psychiatric Association.

Aristotle (1925). Ethica Nicomachea. In *The works of Aristotle, Vol. 9* (ed. W. D. Ross), Oxford University Press, Oxford.

Armor, D. J. (1980). The Rand reports and the analysis of relapse. In *Alcoholism treatment in transition* (ed. G. Edwards and M. Grant) pp. 81–94. Croom Helm, London.

Armor, D. J., Polich, J. M., and Stambul, H. B. (1978). *Alcoholism and treatment*, Wiley, New York.

Armstrong, J. D. (1958). The search for the alcoholic personality, *Annals of the American Academy of Political and Social Science,* **315**, 40–7.

Ashem, B. and Donner, L. (1968). Covert sensitization with alcoholics: A controlled replication, *Behavioral Research and Therapy*, **6**, 7–12.

ASIST. *See* Assessment Handbook.

Assessment Handbook (1989). A Handbook on Procedures for Addictions Assessment/Referral Services including ASIST, Addiction Research Foundation, Toronto.

Atthowe, J. M. (1973). Behavior innovation and persistence, *American Psychologist*, 28, 34–41.

Attia, P. R. (1988). Dual diagnosis: Definition and treatment, *Alcoholism Treatment Quarterly*, 5 (3/4), 53–63.

Austrian, R. W. and Goldbergèr, L. (1982). Field dependence–independence and performance in therapy: Analogue interview. Lund University, Psychological Research Bulletin 22:5, Lund, Sw.

Ausubel, D. P. (1961). Personality disorder is disease, *American Psychologist*, 16, 69–74.

Azrin, N. H. (1976). Improvements in the community-reinforcement approach to alcoholism, *Behavior Research and Therapy*, 14, 339–48.

Azrin, N. H. (1978). A strategy for applied research: Learning based but outcome oriented. In *Annual review of behavior therapy theory and practice, Vol. 6* (ed. C. M. Franks and G. T. Wilson) pp. 29–48. Brunner/Mazel, New York.

Azrin, N. H., Sisson, R. W., Meyers, R., and Godley, M. (1982). Alcoholism treatment by disulfiram and community reinforcement therapy, *Journal of Behavior Therapy and Experimental Psychiatry*, 13, 105–12.

Babor, T. F., Dolinsky, Z., Rounsaville, B., and Jaffe, J. (1988). Unitary versus multidimensional models of alcoholism treatment outcome: An empirical study, *Journal of Studies on Alcohol*, 49, 167–77.

Babor, T. F., Ritson, E. B., and Hodgson, R. J. (1986). Alcohol-related problems in the primary health care setting: A review of early intervention strategies, *British Journal of Addiction*, 81, 23–46.

Babor, T. F., Treffardier, M., Weill, J., Fegueur, L., and Ferrant, J. P. (1983). The early detection and secondary prevention of alcoholism in France, *Journal of Studies on Alcohol*, 44, 600–16.

Babow, I. (1975). The treatment monopoly in alcoholism and drug dependence: A sociological critique, *Journal of Drug Issues*, 5, 120–8.

Bacon, F. (1620). *The works, Vol. 4: The new organon; or, True directions concerning the interpretation of nature.* (Reprinted in London, 1883)

Bacon, S. D. (1973). The problems of alcoholism in American society. In D. Malikin *Social disability: Alcoholism, drug addiction, crime and social disadvantage*, pp. 8–30. New York University Press, New York.

Baekeland, F. (1977). Evaluation of treatment methods in chronic alcoholism. In *The biology of alcoholism, Vol. 5: Treatment and rehabilitation of the chronic alcoholic* (ed. B. Kissin and H. Begleiter) pp. 385–440. Plenum Press, New York.

Baekeland, F., Lundwall, L., and Kissin, B. (1975). Methods for the treatment of chronic alcoholism: A critical appraisal. In *Research advances in alcohol and drug problems, Vol. 2* (ed. R. J. Gibbins, Y. Israel, H. Kalant, R. E. Popham, W. Schmidt, and R. G. Smart) pp. 247–327. Wiley, New York.

Bakan, D. (1970). The test of significance in psychological research. In *The significance test controversy: A reader* (ed. D. E. Morrison and R. E. Henkel) pp. 231–51. Aldine, Chicago.

Balch, P. and Ross, A. W. (1975). Predicting success in weight reduction as a function of locus of control: A unidimensional and multidimensional approach, *Journal of Consulting and Clinical Psychology*, 43, 119.

Bandura, A. (1977). Self-efficacy: Toward a unifying theory of behavior change, *Psychological Review*, **84**, 191–215.

Bandura, A. (1982). Self-efficacy mechanism in human agency, *American Psychologist*, **37**, 122–47.

Bandura, A. (1984). Recycling misconceptions of perceived self-efficacy, *Cognitive Therapy and Research*, **8**, 231–55.

Barlow, D. H., Hayes, S. C., and Nelson, R. O. (1984) *The scientist practitioner: Research and accountability in clinical and educational settings*, Pergamon Press, New York.

Barlow, D. H. and Hersen, M. (1984). *Single case experimental designs: Strategies for studying behavior change*, 2nd edn., Pergamon Press, New York.

Barnes, G. E. (1979). The alcoholic personality: A reanalysis of the literature, *Journal of Studies on Alcohol*, **40**, 571–634.

Barnes, G. E. (1983). Clinical and prealcoholic characteristics. In *The biology of alcoholism, Vol. 6: The pathogenesis of alcoholism—psychosocial factors* (ed. B. Kissin and H. Begleiter) pp. 113–95. Plenum Press, New York.

Barry, H. III (1974). Psychological factors in alcoholism. In *The biology of alcoholism, Vol. 3: Clinical pathology* (ed. B. Kissin and H. Begleiter) pp. 53–107. Plenum Press, New York.

Bateson, G. (1971). The cybernetics of 'self': A theory of alcoholism. *Psychiatry*, **34**, 1–18.

Bean-Bayog, M. (1985) Alcoholism treatment as an alternative to psychiatric hospitalization, *Psychiatric Clinics of North America*, **8**, 501–12.

Bean-Bayog, M. (1986). Psychopathology produced by alcoholism. In *Psychopathology and addictive disorders* (ed. R. E. Meyer) pp. 334–45. Guilford Press, New York.

Beardslee, W. R., Son, L., and Vaillant, G. E. (1986). Exposure to parental alcoholism during childhood and outcome in adulthood: A prospective longitudinal study, *British Journal of Psychiatry*, **149**, 584–91.

Beardslee, W. R. and Vaillant, G. E. (1984). Prospective prediction of alcoholism and psychopathology, *Journal of Studies on Alcohol*, **45**, 500–3.

Beaubrun, M. H. (1967). Treatment of alcoholism in Trinidad and Tobago, *British Journal of Psychiatry*, **113**, 643–58.

Beauchamp, D. E. (1981). *Beyond alcoholism: Alcohol and public health policy*, Temple University Press, Philadelphia.

Beigel, A. and Ghertner, S. (1977). Toward a social model: An assessment of social factors which influence problem drinking and its treatment. In *The biology of alcoholism, Vol. 5: Treatment and rehabilitation of the chronic alcoholic* (ed. B. Kissin and H. Begleiter) pp. 197–233. Plenum Press, New York.

Bejerot, N. (1972a). *Addiction: An artificially induced drive*, Charles C Thomas, Springfield, Ill.

Bejerot, N. (1972b). A theory of addiction as an artificially induced drive, *American Journal of Psychiatry*, **128**, 842–6.

Bejerot, N. (1975). The biological and social character of drug dependence. In *Psychiatrie der Gegenwart, Vol. 3*, 2nd edn. (ed. K. P. Kisker, J.-E. Meyer, C. Müller, and E. Strömgren) pp. 468–518. Springer, Berlin.

Bejerot, N. (1977). The nature of addiction. In *Drug dependence: Current problems and issues* (ed. M. M. Glatt) pp. 69–96. MTP Press, Lancaster, England.

Bejerot, N. (1980). Addiction to pleasure: A biological and social-psychological theory of addiction. In *Theories on drug abuse: Selected contemporary perspectives* (ed.

D. J. Lettieri, M. Sayers, and H. Wallenstein Pearson) pp. 246–55. NIDA Research Monograph No. 30, National Institute on Drug Abuse, Rockville, Md.

Bellak, A. S. and Hersen, M. (1988). *Behavioral assessment: A practical handbook*, 3d edn., Pergamon Press, New York.

Bem, D. J. and Funder, D. C. (1978). Predicting more of the people more of the time: Assessing the personality of situations, *Psychological Review*, **85**, 485–501.

Bergin, A. E. (1971). The evaluation of therapeutic outcomes. In *Handbook of psychotherapy and behavior change: An empirical analysis*, 1st edn. (ed. A. E. Bergin and S. L. Garfield) pp. 217–70. Wiley, New York.

Bergin, A. E. and Lambert, M. J. (1978). The evaluation of therapeutic outcomes. In *Handbook of psychotherapy and behavior change: An empirical analysis*, 2nd edn. (ed. S. L. Garfield and A. E. Bergin) pp. 139–89. Wiley, New York.

Bergin, A. E. and Strupp, H. H. (1972). *Changing frontiers in the science of psychotherapy*, Aldine-Atherton, Chicago.

Bergman, H. (1985). Cognitive deficits and morphological cerebral changes in a random sample of social drinkers. In *Recent developments in alcoholism, Vol. 3* (ed. M. Galanter) pp. 265–76. Plenum Press, New York.

Bergman, H. (1987). Brain dysfunction related to alcoholism: Some results from the KARTAD project. In *Neuropsychology of alcoholism: implications for diagnosis and treatment* (ed. O. A. Parsons, N. Butters, and P. E. Nathan) pp. 21–44. Guilford Press, New York.

Berzins, J. I. (1977). Therapist–patient matching. In *Effective psychotherapy: A handbook of research* (ed. A. S. Gurman and A. M. Razin) pp. 222–51. Pergamon Press, Oxford.

Best, J. A. (1975). Tailoring smoking withdrawal procedures to personality and motivational differences, *Journal of Consulting and Clinical Psychology*, **43**, 1–8.

Best, J. A. and Steffy, R. A. (1975). Smoking modification procedures for internal and external locus of control clients, *Canadian Journal of Behavioral Science*, **7**, 155–65.

Beutler, L. E. (1979). Toward specific psychological therapies for specific conditions, *Journal of Consulting and Clinical Psychology*, **47**, 882–97.

Beutler, L. E. (1983). *Eclectic psychotherapy: A systematic approach*, Pergamon Press, New York.

Beutler, L. E. (1989). Differential treatment selection: The role of diagnosis in psychotherapy, *Psychotherapy*, **26**, 271–81.

Billings, A. G. and Moos, R. H. (1983). Psychosocial processes of recovery among alcoholics and their families: Implications for clinicians and program evaluators, *Addictive Behaviors*, **8**, 205–18.

Bittner, E. (1967). The police in Skid-Row: A study of peace keeping, *American Sociological Review*, **32**, 699–715.

Bjerver, K. (1972). An evaluation of compulsive treatment programs for alcoholic patients in Stockholm with particular reference to longitudinal development, epidemiological aspects and patient morbidity, *Opuscula Medica*, Supplementum 25, Stockholm.

Blaine, G. B. and McArthur, C. C. (1958). What happened in therapy as seen by the patient and his psychiatrist, *The Journal of Nervous and Mental Disease*, **127**, 344–50.

Blanchard, E. B. and Young, L. D. (1974). Clinical application of biofeedback training, *Archives of General Psychiatry*, **30**, 573–89.

Blane, H. T. (1968). *The personality of the alcoholic: Guises of dependency*, Harper and Row, New York.

Blane, H. T. (1977). Issues in the evaluation of alcoholism treatment, *Professional Psychology*, **8**, 593–608.

Bloch, S., Bond, G., Qualls, B., Yalom, I., and Zimmerman, E. (1977). Outcome in psychotherapy evaluated by independent judges, *British Journal of Psychiatry*, **131**, 410–14.

Blumberg, L., Shipley, T. E., and Shandler, I. W. (1973). *Skid Row and its alternatives: Research and recommendations from Philadelphia*, Temple University Press, Philadelphia.

Blume, S. B. (1986). Women and alcohol: A review, *The Journal of the American Medical Association*, **256**, 1467–70.

Bohman, M., Cloninger, R., Sigvardsson, S., and von Knorring, A.-L. (1982). Predisposition to petty criminality in Swedish adoptees, 1: Genetic and environmental heterogeneity, *Archives of General Psychiatry*, **39**, 1233–41.

Bootzin, R. B. and Lick, J. R. (1979). Expectancies in therapy research: Interpretive artifact or mediating mechanism, *Journal of Consulting and Clinical Psychology*, **47**, 852–5.

Bowlby, J. (1969). *Attachment and loss, Vol. 1: Attachment*, Basic Books, New York.

Bowlby, J. (1988). *A secure base: Clinical applications of attachment theory*, Routledge, London.

Bowman, K. M. and Jellinek, E. M. (1941). Alcohol addiction and its treatment, *Quarterly Journal of Studies on Alcohol*, **2**, 98–176.

Bratt, I. (1953). *Alkoholismen—en sjukdom?* (Alcoholism—a disease?), Bonniers, Stockholm.

Brewer, C. (1987). Fact, fiction, finance and effectiveness in alcoholism treatment, *The British Journal of Clinical Practice*, **41** (Suppl. 51), 39–44.

Brickman, B. (1988). Psychoanalysis and substance abuse: Toward a more effective approach, *Journal of The American Academy of Psychoanalysis*, **16**, 359–79.

Brill, R. (1977). Effects of Residential Program Structure and Conceptual Level in the Treatment of Delinquent Boys. University of Toronto. (Doctoral dissertation)

Brill, R. (1978). Implications of the Conceptual Level matching model for the treatment of delinquents, *Journal of Research in Crime and Delinquency*, **15**, 229–46.

Bromet, E. and Moos, R. H. (1977). Environmental resources and the post-treatment functioning of alcoholic patients, *Journal of Health and Social Behavior*, **18**, 326–38.

Bromet, E. J., Moos, R., Bliss, F., and Wuthmann, C. (1977). Posttreatment functioning of alcoholic patients: Its relation to program participation, *Journal of Consulting and Clinical Psychology*, **45**, 829–42.

Brook, R. R. (1962). Personality Correlates Associated with Differential Success of Affiliation with Alcoholics Anonymous. University of Colorado. (Doctoral dissertation) (University Microfilms No. 62-6262)

Brooks, M., Fusco, E., and Grennon, J. (1983). Cognitive levels matching, *Educational Leadership*, **40** (8), 4–8.

Brophy, J. E. and Good, T. L. (1974). *Teacher–student relationships: Causes and consequences*, Holt, Rinehart and Winston, New York.

Brower, K. J., Blow, F. C., and Beresford, T. P. (1989). Treatment implications of chemical dependency models: An integrative approach, *Journal of Substance Abuse Treatment*, **6**, 147–57.

Brown, S. (1985). *Treating the alcoholic: A developmental model of recovery*, Wiley, New York.

Brown, S. A., Irwin, M., and Schuckit, M. A. (1991). Changes in anxiety among abstinent male alcoholics, *Journal of Studies on Alcohol*, **52**, 55–61.

Brown, S. A. and Schuckit, M. A. (1988). Changes in depression among abstinent alcoholics, *Journal of Studies on Alcohol*, **49**, 412–17.

Brownell, K. D., Marlatt, G. A., Lichtenstein, E., and Wilson, G. T. (1986). Understanding and preventing relapse, *American Psychologist*, **41**, 765–82.

Bruun, K., Edwards, G., Lumio, M., Mäkelä, K., Pan, L., Popham, R. E., Room, R., Schmidt, W., Skog, O.-J., Sulkunen, P., and Österberg, E. (1975). *Alcohol control policies in public health perspective*, The Finnish Foundation for Alcohol Studies, Vol. 25. Aurasen Kirjapaino, Forssa.

Butcher, J. N. and Koss, M. P. (1978). Research on brief and crises-oriented therapies. In *Handbook of psychotherapy and behavior change: An empirical analysis*, 2nd edn. (ed. S. L. Garfield and A. E. Bergin) pp. 725–67. Wiley, New York.

Butler, S. F. and Strupp, H. H. (1986). Specific and nonspecific factors in psychotherapy: A problematic paradigm for psychotherapy research, *Psychotherapy*, **23**, 30–40.

Caddy, G. R. (1978). Toward a multivariate analysis of alcohol abuse. In *Alcoholism: New directions in behavioral research and treatment* (ed. P. E. Nathan, G. A. Marlatt, and T. Løberg) pp. 71–117. Plenum Press, New York.

Caddy, G. R. (1980). Problems in conducting alcohol treatment outcome studies: A review. In *Evaluating alcohol and drug abuse treatment effectiveness: Recent advances* (ed. L. C. Sobell, M. B. Sobell, and E. Ward) pp. 151–76. Pergamon Press, New York.

Caddy, G. R., Goldman, R. D., and Huebner, R. (1976*a*). Group differences in attitudes towards alcoholism, *Addictive Behaviors*, **1**, 281–6.

Caddy, G. R., Goldman, R. D., and Huebner, R. (1976*b*). Relationships among different domains of attitudes towards alcoholism: Model, cost and treatment, *Addictive Behaviors*, **1**, 159–67.

Cadogan, D. A. (1973). Marital group therapy in the treatment of alcoholism, *Quarterly Journal of Studies on Alcohol*, **34**, 1187–94.

Cadoret, R. J. (1986). Adoption studies: Historical and methodological critique, *Journal of Psychiatric Developments*, **1**, 45–64.

Cadoret, R. J., O'Gorman, T. W., Troughton, E., and Heywood, E. (1985). Alcoholism and antisocial personality: Interrelationships, genetic and environmental factors, *Archives of General Psychiatry*, **42**, 161–7.

Cahalan, D. (1970). *Problem drinkers: A national survey*, Jossey-Bass, San Francisco.

Cahalan, D. (1988). Implications of the disease concept of alcoholism. *Drugs and Society*, **2** (3/4), 49–68.

Campbell, D. T. (1984). Hospital and landsting as continuously monitoring social polygrams: Advocacy and warning. In *Evaluation of mental health services programs* (ed. B. Cronholm and L. von Knorring) pp. 13–39. The Swedish Medical Research Council, Stockholm.

Campbell, D. T. and Erlebacher, A. (1970). How regression artifacts in quasi-experimental evaluations can mistakenly make compensatory education look harmful. In *The disadvantaged child, Vol. 3* (ed. J. Hellmuth) pp. 185–210. Brunner/Mazel, New York.

Campbell, D. T. and Stanley, J. C. (1963). *Experimental and quasi-experimental designs for research*, Rand McNally, Chicago.

Cappell, H. (1975). An evaluation of tension models of alcohol consumption. In *Research advances in alcohol and drug problems, Vol. 2* (ed. R. J. Gibbons, Y. Israel, H. Kalant, R. E. Popham, W. Schmidt, and R. G. Smart) pp. 177–209. Wiley, New York.

Cappell, H. and Greeley, J. (1987). Alcohol and tension reduction: An update on research and theory. In *Psychological theories of drinking and alcoholism* (ed. H. T. Blane and K. E. Leonard) pp. 15–54. Guilford Press, New York.

Cappell, H. and Herman, C. P. (1972). Alcohol and tension reduction: A review, *Quarterly Journal of Studies on Alcohol*, **33**, 33–64.

Carr, J. E. (1965). The role of conceptual organization in interpersonal discrimination, *Journal of Psychology*, **59**, 159–76.

Carr, J. E. (1970). Differentiation similarity of patient and therapist and the outcome of psychotherapy, *Journal of Abnormal Psychology*, **76**, 361–9.

Carr, J. E. (1980). Personal construct theory and psychotherapy research. In *Personal construct psychology: Psychotherapy and personality* (ed. A. W. Landfield and L. M. Leitner) pp. 233–70. Wiley, New York.

Carr, J. E. and Posthuma, A. B. (1975). The role of cognitive process in social interaction, *The International Journal of Social Psychiatry*, **21**, 157–65.

Caudill, B. D. and Marlatt, G. A. (1975). Modeling influences in social drinking: An experimental analogue, *Journal of Consulting and Clinical Psychology*, **43**, 405–15.

Chafetz, M. E. (1965). Is compulsory treatment of the alcoholic effective? *Northwest Medicine*, **64**, 932–7.

Chan, R. M. (1975). The Effect of Group Learning on Performance and Satisfaction Change as a Function of Need for Affiliation. University of Toronto. (Doctoral dissertation)

Chan, R. M. (1980). The effect of student need for affiliation on performance and satisfaction in group learning, *Interchange*, **11** (1), 39–46.

Chen, H.-T. and Rossi, P. H. (1983). Evaluating with sense: The theory-driven approach, *Evaluation Review*, **7**, 283–302.

Chertok, L. and Stengers, I. (1988). From Lavoisier to Freud: A historical epistemological note with contemporary significance, *The Journal of Nervous and Mental Disease*, **176**, 645–7.

Chick, J. (1984). Secondary prevention of alcoholism and the Centres d'Hygiène Alimentaire, *British Journal of Addiction*, **79**, 221–5.

Chick, J. (1987). Two empirical questions, *British Journal of Addictions*, **82**, 240–3.

Chick, J. D. and Ritson, E. B. (1989). Alcoholism: Advice versus extended treatment, *British Journal of Addiction*, **84**, 817–19.

Chick, J., Ritson, B., Connaughton, J., Stewart, A., and Chick, J. (1988). Advice versus extended treatment for alcoholism: A controlled study. *British Journal of Addiction*, **83**, 159–70.

Chipperfield, B. and Vogel-Sprott, M. (1988). Family history of problem drinking among young male social drinkers: Modeling effects on alcohol consumption, *Journal of Abnormal Psychology*, **97**, 423–8.

Clancy, J., Vanderhoof, E., and Campbell, P. (1967). Evaluation of an aversive technique as a treatment for alcoholism: Controlled trial with succinylcholine-induced apnea, *Quarterly Journal of Studies on Alcohol*, **28**, 476–85.

Clark, D. C. and Fawcett, J. (1989). Does lithium carbonate therapy for alcoholism deter relapse drinking? In *Recent developments in alcoholism, Vol. 7* (ed. M. Galanter) pp. 315–28. Plenum Press, New York.

Clark, S. (1984). The scientific status of demonology. In *Occult and scientific mentalities in the Renaissance* (ed. B. Vickers) pp. 351–74. Cambridge University Press, Cambridge.

Clark, W. B. (1976). Loss of control, heavy drinking and drinking problems in a longitudinal study, *Journal of Studies on Alcohol*, **37**, 1256–90.

Clark, W. B. and Cahalan, D. (1976). Changes in problem drinking over a four-year span, *Addictive Behaviors*, **1**, 251–9.

Cloninger, C. R. (1987). Neurogenetic adaptive mechanisms in alcoholism, *Science*, **236**, 410–16.

Cloninger, C. R., Bohman, M., and Sigvardsson, S. (1981). Inheritance of alcohol abuse: Cross-fostering analysis of adopted men, *Archives of General Psychiatry*, **38**, 861–8.

Cloninger, C. R., Sigvardsson, S., and Bohman, M. (1988a). Childhood personality predicts alcohol abuse in young adults, *Alcoholism: Clinical and Experimental Research*, **12**, 494–505.

Cloninger, C. R., Sigvardsson, S., Gilligan, S. B., von Knorring, A.-L., Reich, T., and Bohman, M. (1988b). Genetic heterogeneity and the classification of alcoholism, *Advances in Alcohol and Substance Abuse*, **7** (3/4), 3–16.

Cloninger, C. R., Sigvardsson, S., von Knorring, A.-L., and Bohman, M. (1988c). The Swedish studies of the adopted children of alcoholics: A reply to Littrell, *Journal of Studies on Alcohol*, **49**, 500–9.

Clopton, J. R. (1978). Alcoholism and the MMPI: A review, *Journal of Studies on Alcohol*, **39**, 1540–58.

Cohen, M., Liebson, I. A., and Faillace, L. A. (1971). The modification of drinking in chronic alcoholics. In *Recent advances in studies of alcoholism* (ed. N. K. Mello and J. H. Mendelson) pp. 745–66. Publication No. /HSM/ 71-9045, US Government Printing Office, Washington DC.

Cohen, S. (1985). Foreword to Second Edition. In *Practical approaches to alcoholism psychotherapy* (ed. S. Zimberg, J. Wallace, and S. B. Blume) pp. vii–viii. Plenum Press, New York.

Cole, S. G., Lehman, W. E., Cole, E. A., and Jones, A. (1981). Inpatient versus outpatient treatment of alcohol and drug abusers, *American Journal of Drug and Alcohol Abuse*, **8**, 329–45.

Collins, R. L. and Marlatt, G. A. (1981). Social modeling as a determinant of drinking behavior: Implications for prevention and treatment, *Addictive Behaviors*, **6**, 233–40.

Colón, I., Cutter, H. S. G., and Jones, W. C. (1982). Prediction of alcoholism from alcohol availability, alcohol consumption and demographic data, *Journal of Studies on Alcohol*, **43**, 1199–213.

Conger, J. J. (1951). The effects of alcohol on conflict behavior in the albino rat, *Quarterly Journal of Studies on Alcohol*, **12**, 1–29.

Conger, J. J. (1956). Alcoholism: Theory, problem and challenge, 2: Reinforcement theory and the dynamics of alcoholism, *Quarterly Journal of Studies on Alcohol*, **17**, 296–305.

Conrad, P. and Schneider, J. W. (1980). *Deviance and medicalization: From badness to sickness*, C. V. Mosby, St. Louis.

Conradsson, C. and Holmgren, S. (1974). Behandlingsmetoder vid alkoholmissbruk— översikt och kritisk granskning (Treatment methods for alcoholism: A critical review). Umeå University, Department of Psychology, Umeå, Sw. (Master's thesis)

Cook, C. C. H. (1988). The Minnesota Model in the management of drug and alcohol dependency: Miracle, method or myth? Part II: Evidence and conclusions, *British Journal of Addiction*, **83**, 735–48.

Cook, T. D. and Campbell, D. T. (1979). *Quasi-experimentation: Design and analysis issues for field settings*, Houghton Mifflin, Boston.

Cooney, N. L., Kadden, R. M., and Litt, M. D. (1990). A comparison of methods for assessing sociopathy in male and female alcoholics, *Journal of Studies on Alcohol*, **51**, 42–8.

Cooper, H. M. (1982). Scientific guidelines for conducting integrative research reviews, *Review of Educational Research*, **52**, 291–302.

Cooper, H. M. (1984). *The integrative research review: A systematic approach*, Sage, Beverly Hills, Calif.

Cooper, M. L., Russell, M., and George, W. H. (1988). Coping, expectancies, and alcohol abuse: A test of social learning formulations, *Journal of Abnormal Psychology*, **97**, 218–30.

Coppen, A. (1980). Lithium in the treatment of alcoholism. In *Psychopharmacology of alcohol* (ed. M. Sandler) pp. 209–14. Raven Press, New York.

Cosper, R. (1979). Drinking as conformity: A critique of sociological literature on occupational differences in drinking, *Journal of Studies on Alcohol*, **40**, 868–91.

Costello, R. M. (1975a). Alcoholism treatment and evaluation, 1: In search of methods, *The International Journal of the Addictions*, **10**, 251–75.

Costello, R. M. (1975b). Alcoholism treatment and evaluation, 2: Collation of two year follow-up studies, *The International Journal of the Addictions*, **10**, 857–68.

Costello, R. M. (1980). Alcoholism treatment effectiveness: Slicing the outcome variance pie. In *Alcoholism treatment in transition* (ed. G. Edwards and M. Grant) pp. 113–127. Croom Helm, London.

Cox, W. M. (1987). Personality theory and research. In *Psychological theories of drinking and alcoholism* (ed. H. T. Blane and K. E. Leonard) pp. 55–89. Guilford Press, New York.

Crawford, A., Plant, M. A., Kreitman, N., and Latcham, R. W. (1987). Unemployment and drinking behaviour: Some data from a general population survey of alcohol use, *British Journal of Addiction*, **82**, 1007–16.

Crawford, J. J. and Chalupsky, A. B. (1977). The reported evaluation of alcoholism treatment, 1968–71: A methodological review, *Addictive Behaviors*, **2**, 63–74.

Crawford, J. R. and Heather, N. (1987). Public attitudes to the disease concept of alcoholism, *The International Journal of the Addictions*, **22**, 1129–38.

Crawford, J. R., Thomson, N. A., Gullion, F. E., and Garthwaite, P. (1989). Does endorsement of the disease concept of alcoholism predict humanitarian attitudes to alcoholics? *The International Journal of the Addictions*, **24**, 71–7.

Critchlow Leigh, B. (1989). In search of the Seven Dwarves: Issues of measurement and meaning in alcohol expectancy research, *Psychological Bulletin*, **105**, 361–73.

Cronbach, L. J. (1957). The two disciplines of scientific psychology, *American Psychologist*, **12**, 671–84.

Cronbach, L. J. (1975). Beyond the two disciplines of scientific psychology, *American Psychologist*, **30**, 116–27.

Cronbach, L. J. and Snow, R. E. (1977). *Aptitudes and instructional methods: A handbook for research on interactions*, Irvington, New York.

Cronbach, L. J. and Webb, N. (1975). Between-class and within-class effects in a reported aptitude X treatment interaction: Reanalysis of a study by G. L. Anderson, *Journal of Educational Psychology*, **67**, 717–24.

Cronkite, R. C. and Moos, R. H. (1978). Evaluating alcoholism treatment programs: An integrated approach, *Journal of Consulting and Clinical Psychology*, **46**, 1105–19.

Cronkite, R. C. and Moos, R. H. (1980). Determinants of the posttreatment functioning of alcoholic patients: A conceptual framework, *Journal of Consulting and Clinical Psychology*, **48**, 305–16.

Cross, D. G., Sheehan, P. W., and Khan, J. A. (1982). Short- and long-term follow-up of clients receiving insight-oriented therapy and behavior therapy, *Journal of Consulting and Clinical Psychology*, **50**, 103–12.

Cross, G. M., Morgan, C. W., Mooney, A. J. III, Martin, C. A., and Rafter, J. A. (1990). Alcoholism treatment: A ten-year follow-up study, *Alcoholism: Clinical and Experimental Research*, **14**, 169–73.

Crowe, L. C. and George, W. H. (1989). Alcohol and human sexuality: Review and integration, *Psychological Bulletin*, **105**, 374–86.

Cunningham, W. G. (1975). The impact of student–teacher pairings on teacher effectiveness, *American Educational Research Journal*, **12**, 169–89.

Cushing, H. (1925). *The life of Sir William Osler*, Clarendon, Oxford.

Dahlgren, L. and Willander, A. (1989). Are special treatment facilities for female alcoholics needed? A controlled 2-year follow-up study from a specialized female unit (EWA) versus a mixed male/female treatment facility, *Alcoholism: Clinical and Experimental Research*, **13**, 499–504.

Davies, D. L. (1962). Normal drinking in recovered alcohol addicts, *Quarterly Journal of Studies on Alcohol*, **23**, 94–104.

Davies, D. L. (1974). Is alcoholism really a disease? *Contemporary Drug Problems*, **3**, 197–212.

Davis, D. I., Berenson, D., Steinglass, P., and Davis, S. (1974). The adaptive consequences of drinking, *Psychiatry*, **37**, 209–15.

Dawes, R. M. and Corrigan, B. (1974). Linear models in decision making, *Psychological Bulletin*, **81**, 95–106.

Deever, S. G. (1968). Ratings of task-oriented expectancy for success as a function of internal control and field independence, *Dissertation Abstracts, Section B*, **29** (1), 365.

Dickerson, M. (1977). The role of the betting shop environment in the training of 'compulsive' gamblers, *Bulletin of the British Association for Behavioural Psychotherapy*, **5**, 3–8.

Dobson, K. S. (ed.) (1988). *Handbook of cognitive-behavioral therapies*, Guilford, New York.

Dodes, L. M. (1988). The psychology of combining dynamic psychotherapy and Alcoholics Anonymous, *Bulletin of the Menninger Clinic*, **52**, 283–93.

Donovan, D. M. and O'Leary, M. R. (1978). The Drinking-Related Locus of Control Scale: Reliability, factor structure and validity, *Journal of Studies on Alcohol*, **39**, 759–84.

Donovan, D. M. and O'Leary, M. R. (1979). Control orientation among alcoholics: A cognitive social learning perspective, *American Journal of Drug and Alcohol Abuse*, **6**, 487–99.

Donovan, D. M., Walker, R. D., and Kivlahan, D. R. (1987). Recovery and remediation of neuropsychological functions: Implications for alcoholism rehabilitation process and outcome. In *Neuropsychology of alcoholism: Implications for diagnosis and treatment* (ed. O. A. Parsons, N. Butters, and P. E. Nathan) pp. 339–60. Guilford, New York.

Dougherty, F. E. (1976). Patient–therapist matching for prediction of optimal and minimal therapeutic outcome, *Journal of Consulting and Clinical Psychology*, **44**, 889–97.

Dowds, B. N., Fontana, A. F., Russakoff, L. M., and Harris, M. (1977). Cognitive mediators between patients' social class and therapists' evaluations, *Archives of General Psychiatry*, **34**, 917–20.

Drake, R. E. and Vaillant, G. E. (1988). Predicting alcoholism and personality disorder in a 33-year longitudinal study of children of alcoholics, *British Journal of Addiction*, **83**, 799–807.

Drew, L. R. H. (1968). Alcoholism as a self-limiting disease, *Quarterly Journal of Studies on Alcohol*, **29**, 956–67.

Dua, P. S. (1970). Comparison of the effects of behaviorally oriented action and psychotherapy reeducation on introversion, emotionality, and internal–external control, *Journal of Counseling Psychology*, **17**, 567–72.

Dukta, C., Colangelo, M., Lounsbury, N., Palmer, P., and Peltz, S. (1976). *ADAPT: The Alcoholism and Drug Addiction Project Community-Based Treatment in Halton Region*, Substudy No. 770, Addiction Research Foundation, Toronto.

Dunham, R. G. and Mauss, A. L. (1982). Reluctant referrals: The effectiveness of legal coercion in outpatient treatment for problem drinkers, *Journal of Drug Issues*, **12**, 5–20.

Dunn, R. (1984). Learning style: State of the science, *Theory into Practice*, **23**, 10–19.

Durlak, J. A. (1979). Comparative effectiveness of paraprofessional and professional helpers, *Psychological Bulletin*, **86**, 80–92.

Dwyer, D. and Ogborne, A. C. (1984). *An Examination of Alternative Models for Delivering Assessment/Referral Services in Ontario*. ARF Internal Document No. 26, Addiction Research Foundation, Regional Research Centre, London, Ontario.

Eddy, N. B., Halbach, H., Isbell, H., and Seevers, M. H. (1965). Drug dependence: Its significance and characteristics, *Bulletin of the World Health Organization*, **32**, 721–33.

Edwards, G. (1970*a*). Alcoholism: The analysis of treatment. In *Alcohol and alcoholism* (ed. R. E. Popham) pp. 173–8. University of Toronto Press, Toronto.

Edwards, G. (1970*b*). The status of alcoholism as a disease. In *Modern trends in drug dependence and alcoholism* (ed. R. V. Phillipson) pp. 140–63. Appleton-Century-Crofts, New York.

Edwards, G. (1974). Drugs, drug dependence, and the concept of plasticity, *Quarterly Journal of Studies on Alcohol*, **35**, 176–95.

Edwards, G. (1977). The alcohol dependence syndrome: Usefulness of an idea. In *Alcoholism: New knowledge and new responses* (ed. G. Edwards and M. Grant) pp. 136–56. Croom Helm, London.

Edwards, G. (1980). Alcoholism treatment: Between guesswork and certainty. In *Alcoholism treatment in transition* (ed. G. Edwards and M. Grant) pp. 307–20. Croom Helm, London.

Edwards, G. (1984). Drinking in longitudinal perspective: Career and natural history, *British Journal of Addiction*, **79**, 175–83.

Edwards, G. (1986). The alcohol dependence syndrome: A concept as stimulus to enquiry, *British Journal of Addiction*, **81**, 171–83.

Edwards, G. (1987). Review of G. A. Marlatt and J. R. Gordon (ed.) 'Relapse Prevention', New York, 1985, *British Journal of Addiction*, **82**, 319.

Edwards, G. (1989). As the years go rolling by: Drinking problems in the time dimension, *British Journal of Psychiatry*, **154**, 18–26.

Edwards, G., Brown, D., Duckitt, A., Oppenheimer, E., Sheehan, M., and Taylor, C. (1987). Outcome of alcoholism: The structure of patient attributions as to what causes change, *British Journal of Addiction*, **82**, 533–45.

Edwards, G., Duckitt, A., Oppenheimer, E., Sheehan, M., and Taylor, C. (1983). What happens to alcoholics? *Lancet*, **ii**, 269–71.

Edwards, G. and Gross, M. M. (1976). Alcohol dependence: Provisional description of a clinical syndrome, *British Medical Journal*, **i**, 1058–61.

Edwards, G., Gross, M. M., Keller, M., and Moser, J. (1976). Alcohol-related problems in the disability perspective: A summary of the consensus of the WHO group of investigators on criteria for identifying and classifying disabilities related to alcohol consumption, *Journal of Studies on Alcohol*, 37, 1360–82.

Edwards, G., Gross, M. M., Keller, M., Moser, J., and Room, R. (1977*b*). *Alcohol-related disabilities*, Offset Publication No. 32, World Health Organization, Geneva.

Edwards, G. and Guthrie, S. (1966). A comparison of inpatient and outpatient treatment of alcohol dependence, *Lancet*, i, 467–8.

Edwards, G. and Guthrie, S. (1967). A controlled trial of inpatient and outpatient treatment of alcohol dependence, *Lancet*, i, 555–9.

Edwards, G., Kyle, E., and Nicholls, P. (1974). Alcoholics admitted to four hospitals in England, *Quarterly Journal of Studies on Alcohol*, 35, 499–522.

Edwards, G. and Orford, J. (1977). A plain treatment for alcoholism, *Proceedings of the Royal Society of Medicine*, 70, 344–8.

Edwards, G., Orford, J., Egert, S., Guthrie, S., Hawker, A., Hensman, C., Mitcheson, M., Oppenheimer, E., and Taylor, C. (1977*a*). Alcoholism: A controlled trial of 'treatment' and 'advice', *Journal of Studies on Alcohol*, 38, 1004–31.

Einstein, S., Wolfson E., and Gecht, D. (1970). What matters in treatment: Relevant variables in alcoholism, *The International Journal of the Addictions*, 5, 43–67.

Elal-Lawrence, G., Slade, P. D., and Dewey, M. E. (1986). Predictors of outcome type in treated problem drinkers, *Journal of Studies on Alcohol*, 47, 41–7.

Emrick, C. D. (1974). A review of psychologically oriented treatment of alcoholism, 1: The use and interrelationships of outcome criteria and drinking behavior following treatment, *Quarterly Journal of Studies on Alcohol*, 35, 523–49.

Emrick, C. D. (1975). A review of psychologically oriented treatment of alcoholism, 2: The relative effectiveness of different treatment approaches and the effectiveness of treatment versus no treatment, *Journal of Studies on Alcohol*, 36, 88–108.

Emrick, C. D. (1979). Perspectives in clinical research: Relative effectiveness of alcohol abuse treatment, *Family and Community Health*, 2, 71–88.

Emrick, C. D. (1982). Evaluation of alcoholism psychotherapy methods. In *Encyclopedic handbook of alcoholism* (ed. E. M. Pattison and E. Kaufman) pp. 1152–69. Gardner Press, New York.

Emrick, C. D. (1987). Alcoholics Anonymous: Affiliation processes and effectiveness as treatment, *Alcoholism: Clinical and Experimental Research*, 11, 416–23.

Emrick, C. D. (1989). Overview of 'Alcoholics Anonymous: Emerging concepts'. In *Recent developments in alcoholism, Vol. 7* (ed. M. Galanter) pp. 3–10. Plenum Press, New York.

Emrick, C. D. and Hansen, J. (1983). Assertions regarding effectiveness of treatment for alcoholism: Fact or fantasy? *American Psychologist*, 38, 1078–88.

Ends, E. J. and Page, C. W. (1957). A study of three types of group psychotherapy with hospitalized male inebriates, *Quarterly Journal of Studies on Alcohol*, 18, 263–77.

English, G. E. and Curtin, M. E. (1975). Personality differences in patients at three alcoholism treatment agencies, *Journal of Studies on Alcohol*, 36, 52–68.

Eriksen, L. (1986). The effect of waiting for inpatient alcoholism treatment after detoxification: An experimental comparison between inpatient treatment and advice only, *Addictive Behaviors*, 11, 389–97.

Eriksen, L., Björnstad, S., and Götestam, K. G. (1986). Social skills training in groups for alcoholics: One-year treatment outcome for groups and individuals, *Addictive Behaviors*, 11, 309–29.

Erwin, J. E. and Hunter, J. J. (1984). Prediction of attrition in alcoholic aftercare by scores on the Embedded Figures Test and two Piagetian tasks, *Journal of Consulting and Clinical Psychology*, **52**, 354–8.

Evans, G. D. (1979). Commentary on Dr. Ogborne's article, *Canadian Journal of Public Health*, **70**, 125–8.

Evans, K. and Sullivan, J. M. (1990). *Dual diagnosis: Counseling the mentally ill substance abuser*. Guilford Press, Hove, East Sussex.

Ewing, J. A. (1977). Different approaches to the treatment of alcoholism. In *Recent advances in the study of alcoholism* (ed. C.-M. Ideström) pp. 23–31. Excerpta Medica, Amsterdam.

Eysenck, H. J. (1980). A unified theory of psychotherapy, behaviour therapy and spontaneous remission, *Zeitschrift für Psychologie*, **188**, 43–56.

Eysenck, H. J. (1983). Special review, *Behaviour Research and Therapy*, **21**, 315–20.

Fabrega, H., Jr. (1979). Disease and illness from a biocultural standpoint. In *Toward new definition of health: Psychosocial dimensions* (ed. P. I. Ahmed and G. V. Coelho) pp. 23–51. Plenum Press, New York.

Fagan, R. W. and Mauss, A. L. (1978). Padding the revolving door: An initial assessment of the uniform alcoholism and intoxication treatment act in practice, *Social Problems*, **26**, 232–46.

Farrington, B. (1953). *Greek science: Its meaning for us*, Penguin, London.

Feuerlein, W. and Küfner, H. (1989). A prospective multicentre study of in-patient treatment for alcoholics: 18- and 48-month follow-up (Munich Evaluation for Alcoholism Treatment, MEAT), *European Archives of Psychiatry and Neurological Sciences*, **239**, 144–57.

Fillmore, K. M. (1988). *Alcohol use across the life course: A critical review of 70 years of international longitudinal research*, Addiction Research Foundation, Toronto.

Fingarette, H. (1988). *Heavy drinking: The myth of alcoholism as a disease*, University of California Press, Berkeley, Calif.

Fink, E. B., Longabaugh, R., McCrady, B. S., Stout, R. L., Beattie, M., Ruggieri-Authelet, A., and McNeil, D. (1987). Effectiveness of alcoholism treatment in partial versus inpatient settings: Twenty-four month outcomes, *Addictive Behaviors*, **10**, 235–48.

Finney, J. W. and Moos, R. H. (1979). Treatment and outcome for empirical subtypes of alcoholic patients, *Journal of Consulting and Clinical Psychology*, **47**, 25–38.

Finney, J. W. and Moos, R. H. (1981). Characteristics and prognoses of alcoholics who become moderate drinkers and abstainers after treatment, *Journal of Studies on Alcohol*, **42**, 94–105.

Finney, J. W. and Moos, R. H. (1986). Matching patients with treatments: Conceptual and methodological issues, *Journal of Studies on Alcohol*, **47**, 122–34.

Finney, J. W., Moos, R., and Mewborn, C. R. (1980). Post-treatment experience and treatment outcome of alcoholic patients six and two years after hospitalization, *Journal of Consulting and Clinical Psychology*, **48**, 134–41.

Flores, P. J. (1988). Alcoholics Anonymous: A phenomenological and existential perspective, *Alcoholism Treatment Quarterly*, **5** (1/2), 73–94.

Foon, A. E. (1987). Locus of control as a predictor of outcome of psychotherapy, *British Journal of Medical Psychology*, **60**, 99–107.

Foy, D. W., Nunn, L. B., and Rychtarik, R. G. (1984). Broad-spectrum behavioral treatment for chronic alcoholics: Effects of training controlled drinking skills, *Journal of Consulting and Clinical Psychology*, **52**, 218–30.

Foy, D. W. and Rychtarik, R. G. (1987). Practical issues in selecting and using treatment goals with severely dependent alcohol abusers. In *Moderation as a goal or outcome of treatment for alcohol problems: A dialogue* (ed. M. B. Sobell and L. C. Sobell) pp. 69–81. Drugs and Society Series, Vol. 1, Nos. 2/3, Haworth Press, New York.

Frances, A. and Clarkin, J. (1981). Differential therapeutics: A guide to treatment selection, *Hospital and Community Psychiatry*, **32**, 537–46.

Frank, A. F. and Gunderson, J. G. (1984). Matching therapists and milieus: Effects on engagement and continuance in psychotherapy, *Psychiatry*, **47**, 201–10.

Frank, J. D. (1961). *Persuasion and healing: A comparative study of psychotherapy*, 1st edn., Johns Hopkins University Press, Baltimore.

Frank, J. D. (1968). The role of hope in psychotherapy, *The International Journal of Psychiatry*, **5**, 383–95.

Frank, J. D. (1971). Therapeutic factors in psychotherapy, *American Journal of Psychotherapy*, **25**, 350–61.

Frank J. D. (1973). *Persuasion and healing: A comparative study of psychotherapy*, 2nd edn., Johns Hopkins University Press, Baltimore.

Frank, J. D. (1974*a*). Psychotherapy: The restoration of morale, *American Journal of Psychiatry*, **131**, 271–4.

Frank, J. D. (1974*b*). Therapeutic components of psychotherapy, *The Journal of Nervous and Mental Disease*, **159**, 325–42.

Frank, J. D. (1976). Psychotherapy and the sense of mastery. In *Evaluation of psychological therapies* (ed. R. L. Spitzer and D. F. Klein) pp. 47–56. Johns Hopkins University Press, Baltimore.

Frank, J. D. (1978). *Psychotherapy and the human predicament: A psychosocial approach*, Schocken Books, New York.

Frank, J. D. (1979). The present status of outcome studies, *Journal of Consulting and Clinical Psychology*, **47**, 310–16.

Frank, J. D. (1981). Reply to Telch, *Journal of Consulting and Clinical Psychology*, **49**, 476–7.

Frank, J. D. (1982). Therapeutic components shared by all psychotherapies. In *Psychotherapy research and behavior change* (ed. J. H. Harvey and M. M. Parks) pp. 5–37. Master Lecture Series, Vol. 1, American Psychological Association, Washington, DC.

Frederiksen, N. (1972). Toward a taxonomy of situations, *American Psychologist*, **27**, 114–23.

Freed, E. X. (1979). *An Alcoholic personality?* Slack, Thorofare, NJ.

Friedman, M. L. and Dies, R. R. (1974). Reactions of internal and external test-anxious students to counselling and behavior therapies, *Journal of Consulting and Clinical Psychology*, **42**, 921.

Fries, J. F. (1976). A data bank for the clinician? *New England Journal of Medicine*, **294**, 1400–2.

Galanter, M. (1981). Sociobiology and informal social controls of drinking: Findings from two charismatic sects, *Journal of Studies on Alcohol*, **42**, 64–79.

Galanter, M. (1982). Overview: Charismatic religious sects and psychiatry, *American Journal of Psychiatry*, **139**, 1539–48.

Galanter, M. (1983). Engaged members of the Unification Church: The impact of a charismatic group on adaptation and behavior, *Archives of General Psychiatry*, **40**, 1197–203.

Galanter, M. (1986). Treating substance abusers: Why therapists fail, *Hospital and Community Psychiatry*, **37**, 769.

Galanter, M., Castaneda, R., and Salamon, I. (1987). Institutional self-help therapy for alcoholism: Clinical outcome, *Alcoholism: Clinical and Experimental Research*, **11**, 424–9.

Galanter, M. and Sperber, J. (1982). General hospitals in the alcoholism treatment system. In *Encyclopedic handbook of alcoholism* (ed. E. M. Pattison and E. Kaufman) pp. 828–36. Gardner Press, New York.

Gallant, D. M. (1971). Evaluation of compulsory treatment of the alcoholic municipal court offender. In *Recent advances in studies of alcoholism* (ed. N. K. Mello and J. H. Mendelson) pp. 730–44. Publication No. /HSM/ 71-9045, US Government Printing Office, Washington, DC.

Gallant, D. M., Faulkner, M., Stoy, B., Bishop, M. P., and Langdon, D. (1968). Enforced clinic treatment of paroled criminal alcoholics: A pilot evaluation, *Quarterly Journal of Studies on Alcohol*, **29**, 77–83.

Gallo, P. S. (1978). Meta-analysis—A mixed meta-phor? *American Psychologist*, **33**, 515–17.

Garfield, S. L. (1981*a*). Evaluating the psychotherapies, *Behavior Therapy*, **12**, 295–307.

Garfield, S. L. (1981*b*). Psychotherapy: A 40-year appraisal, *American Psychologist*, **36**, 174–83.

Garfield, S. L. (1983). Effectiveness of psychotherapy: The perennial controversy, *Professional Psychology*, **14**, 35–43.

Gaston, L. (1990). The concept of the alliance and its role in psychotherapy: Theoretical and empirical considerations, *Psychotherapy*, **27**, 143–53.

Gazda, P. (1984). The benefits of computerization. In F. B. Glaser *et al. A system of health care delivery, Vol. 1*, pp. 183–93. Addiction Research Foundation, Toronto.

George, W. H. and Marlatt, G. A. (1983). Alcoholism: The evolution of a behavioral perspective. In *Recent developments in alcoholism, Vol. 1* (ed. M. Galanter) pp. 105–38. Plenum Press, New York.

Gerard, D. L. and Saenger, G. (1966). *Out-patient treatment of alcoholism: A study of outcome and its determinants*, Brookside Monograph No. 4, University of Toronto Press, Toronto.

Gerard, D. L., Saenger, G., and Wile, R. (1962). The abstinent alcoholic, *Archives of General Psychiatry*, **6**, 83–95.

Gergen, K. J. (1973). Social psychology as history, *Journal of Personality and Social Psychology*, **26**, 309–20.

Gibbs, L. E. (1980). A classification of alcoholics relevant to type-specific treatment, *The International Journal of the Addictions*, **15**, 461–88.

Gibbs, L. E. (1981). The need for a new design for evaluating alcoholism treatment programs, *Drug and Alcohol Dependence*, **8**, 287–99.

Gibbs, L. E. and Flanagan, J. (1977). Prognostic indicators of alcoholism treatment outcome, *The International Journal of the Addictions*, **12**, 1097–141.

Giesbrecht, N. (1983). Stakes in conformity and the 'normalization' of deviants: Accounts by former and current skid row inebriates, *Journal of Drug Issues*, **13**, 299–322.

Giesbrecht, N. A., Giffen, P. J., Lambert, S., and Oki, G. (1981). Changes in the social control of Skid Row inebriates in Toronto: Assessments by Skid Row informants, *Canadian Journal of Public Health*, **72**, 101–4.

Giffen, P.J. and Lambert, S. (1978). Decriminalization of public drunkenness. In *Research advances in alcohol and drug problems, Vol. 4* (ed. Y. Israel, F. B. Glaser, H. Kalant, R. E. Popham, W. Schmidt, and G. Smart) pp. 395–440. Plenum Press, New York.

Gillespie, D. G. (1967). The fate of alcoholics: An evaluation of alcoholism follow-up studies. In *Alcoholism* (ed. D. J. Pittman) pp. 159–73. Harper and Row, New York.

Gillis, J. S. and Jessor, R. (1970). Effects of brief psychotherapy on belief in internal control: An exploratory study, *Psychotherapy: Theory, Research, and Practice*, **7**, 135–7.

Gitlow, S. E. (1973). Alcoholism: A disease. In *Alcoholism: Progress in research and treatment* (ed. P. G. Bourne and R. Fox) pp. 1–9. Academic Press, New York.

Glad, D. D. (1947). Attitudes and experiences of American–Jewish and American–Irish male youths as related to differences in adult rates of inebriety, *Quarterly Journal of Studies on Alcohol*, **8**, 406–72.

Glaser, F. B. (1977). Comments on 'Alcoholism: A controlled trial of "treatment" and "advice"', *Journal of Studies on Alcohol*, **38**, 1819–27.

Glaser, F. B. (1980). Anybody got a match? Treatment research and the matching hypothesis. In *Alcoholism treatment in transition* (ed. G. Edwards and M. Grant) pp. 178–96. Croom Helm, London.

Glaser, F. B. (1984*a*). The nature and utility of assessment. In *A system of health care delivery, Vol. 2*, (ed. F. B. Glaser *et al.*) pp. 73–106. Addiction Research Foundation, Toronto.

Glaser, F. B. (1984*b*). The nature of primary care. In *A system of health care delivery, Vol. 2*, (ed. F. B. Glaser *et al.*) pp. 3–34. Addiction Research Foundation, Toronto.

Glaser, F. B. (1984*c*). Problem—Indicator—Intervention Matrix: An attempt. In *A system of health care delivery, Vol. 3*, (ed. F. B. Glaser *et al.*) pp. 109–13. Addiction Research Foundation, Toronto.

Glaser, F. B. (1984*d*). A systems approach to treatment and treatment research. In *Alcohol related problems* (ed. N. Krasner, J. S. Madden, and R. J. Walker) pp. 279–91. Wiley, New York.

Glaser, F. B. (1990). From theory to practice: The planned treatment of drug users. Interview by S. Einstein, *The International Journal of the Addictions*, **25**, 307–43.

Glaser, F. B., Annis, H. M., Pearlman, S., Segal, R. L., and Skinner, H. A. (1985). The differential therapy of alcoholism: A systems approach. In *Alcoholism and substance abuse: Strategies for intervention* (ed. T. E. Bratter and G. G. Forrest) pp. 431–50. Free Press/Macmillan, New York.

Glaser, F. B., Annis, H. M., Skinner, H. A., Pearlman, S., Segal, R. L., Sisson, B., Ogborne, A. C., Bohnen, E., Gazda, P., and Zimmerman, T. (1984). *A system of health care delivery*, 3 vols. Addiction Research Foundation, Toronto.

Glaser, F. B., Greenberg, S. W., and Barrett, M. (1978). *A systems approach to alcohol treatment*, Addiction Research Foundation, Toronto.

Glaser, F. B. and Hubbard, R. N. (1985). Application of a treatment system model in rural Alberta. Paper presented at the 34th International Congress on Alcoholism and Drug Dependence, Calgary, Alberta.

Glaser, F. B. and Skinner, H. A. (1981). Matching in the real world: A practical approach. In *Matching patient needs and treatment methods in alcoholism and drug abuse* (ed. E. Gottheil, A. T. McLellan, and K. A. Druley) pp. 295–324. Charles C Thomas, Springfield, Ill.

Glass, G. V. (1976). Primary, secondary, and meta-analysis of research, *Educational Researcher*, **5** (10), 3–8.

Glass, G. V. (1979). Policy for the unpredictable (Uncertainty research and policy), *Educational Researcher*, **8** (9), 12–14.

Glass, G. V., McGaw, B., and Smith, M. L. (1981). *Meta-analysis in social research*, Sage, Beverly Hills, Calif.

Glassner, B. and Berg, B. (1980). How Jews avoid alcohol problems, *American Sociological Review*, **45**, 647–64.

Glatt, M. (1972). *The alcoholic and the help he needs*, 2nd edn., Priory Press, London.

Glueck, S. and Glueck, E. (1950). *Unravelling juvenile delinquency*, The Commonwealth Fund, New York.

Glueck, S. and Glueck, E. (1968). *Delinquents and nondelinquents in perspective*, Harvard University Press, Cambridge, Mass.

Goldberg, L. R. (1968). Seer over sign: The first 'good' example? *Journal of Experimental Research in Personality*, **3**, 168–71.

Goldberg, L. R. (1970). Man versus model of man: A rationale, plus some evidence, for a method of improving on clinical inferences, *Psychological Bulletin*, **73**, 422–32.

Goldfried, M. R. (1980). Toward the delineation of therapeutic change principles, *American Psychologist*, **35**, 991–9.

Goldfried, M. R., (ed.) (1982). *Converging themes in psychotherapy: Trends in psychodynamic, humanistic, and behavioral practice*, Springer, New York.

Goldfried, M. R., Greenberg, L. S., and Marmar, C. (1990). Individual psychotherapy: Process and outcome, *Annual Review of Psychology*, **41**, 659–88.

Goldfried, M. R. and Padawer, W. (1982). Current status and future directions in psychotherapy. In *Converging themes in psychotherapy: Trends in psychodynamic, humanistic, and behavioral practice* (ed. M. R. Goldfried) pp. 3–49. Springer, New York.

Goldman, M. S. (1983). Cognitive impairment in chronic alcoholics: Some cause for optimism, *American Psychologist*, **38**, 1045–54.

Goldman, M. S. (1986). Neuropsychological recovery in alcoholics: Endogenous and exogenous processes, *Alcoholism: Clinical and Experimental Research*, **10**, 136–44.

Goldman, M. S., Brown, S. A., and Christiansen, B. A. (1987). Expectancy theory: Thinking about drinking. In *Psychological theories of drinking and alcoholism* (ed. H. T. Blane and K. E. Leonard) pp. 181–226. Guilford Press, New York.

Goldstein, M. S., Surber, M., and Wilner, D. M. (1984). Outcome evaluations in substance abuse: A comparison of alcoholism, drug abuse, and other mental health interventions, *The International Journal of the Addictions*, **19**, 479–502.

Goldstein, S. G. and Linden, J. D. (1969). Multivariate classification of alcoholics by means of the MMPI, *Journal of Abnormal Psychology*, **74**, 661–9.

Gomes-Schwartz, B., Hadley, S. W., and Strupp, H. H. (1978). Individual psychotherapy and behavior therapy, *Annual Review of Psychology*, **29**, 435–71.

Goodwin, D. W. (1979). Alcoholism and heredity: A review and hypothesis, *Archives of General Psychiatry*, **36**, 57–61.

Goodwin, D. W. (1985). Alcoholism and genetics: The sins of fathers, *Archives of General Psychiatry*, **42**, 171–4.

Goodwin, D. W. (1988). *Alcohol and the writer*, Andrews and McMeel, Kansas City.

Goodwin, D. W. and Guze, S. B. (1981). *Psychiatric diagnosis*, Oxford University Press, New York.

Gordis, E. (1976). What is alcoholism research? *Annals of Internal Medicine*, **85**, 821–3.

Gottheil, E., McLellan, A. T., and Druley, K. A. (1981). Reasonable and unreasonable methodological standards for the evaluation of alcoholism treatment. In *Matching patient needs and treatment methods in alcoholism and drug abuse* (ed. E. Gottheil, A. T. McLellan, and K. A. Druley) pp. 371–89. Charles C Thomas, Springfield, Ill.

Gottlieb, B. H. (1983). Social support as a focus for integrative research in psychology, *American Psychologist*, **38**, 278–87.

Graham, J. R. and Strenger, V. E. (1988). MMPI characteristics of alcoholics: A review, *Journal of Consulting and Clinical Psychology*, **56**, 197–205.

Greenwald, A. G. (1975). Consequences of prejudice against the null hypothesis, *Psychological Bulletin*, **82**, 1–20.

Gunderson, J. G. (1978). Patient–therapist matching: A research evaluation, *American Journal of Psychiatry*, **135**, 1193–7.

Guntrip, H. (1975). My experience of analysis with Fairbairn and Winnicott, *International Review of Psycho-Analysis*, **2**, 145–56.

Guthrie, A. and Elliott, W.A. (1980). The nature and reversibility of cerebral impairment in alcoholism: Treatment implications, *Journal of Studies on Alcohol*, **41**, 147-55.

Halikas, J. A. (1980). A clinical prognostic scale for Skid Row male alcoholics. In *Currents in alcoholism, Vol. 7: Recent advances in research and treatment* (ed. M. Galanter) pp. 321–30. Grune and Stratton, New York.

Halleck. S. L. (1982). The concept of responsibility in psychotherapy, *American Journal of Psychotherapy*, **36**, 292–303.

Harding, G. T. (1975). Psychotherapy in the treatment of drug dependence: A survey of the scientific literature. In *Drug dependence: Treatment and treatment evaluation* (ed. H. Boström, T. Larsson, and N. Ljungstedt) pp. 59–78. Almqvist and Wiksell International, Stockholm.

Hare, F. (1924). Treatment of alcoholism, *Practitioner*, **113**, 295–316.

Hartman, L., Krywonis, M., and Morrison, E. (1988). Psychological factors and health-related behaviour change: Preliminary findings from a controlled clinical trial, *Canadian Family Physician*, **34**, 1045–50.

Harvey, O. J., Hunt, D. E., and Schroder, H. M. (1961). *Conceptual systems and personality organization*, Wiley, New York.

Hattie, J. A., Sharpley, C. F., and Rogers, H. J. (1984). Comparative effectiveness of professional and paraprofessional helpers, *Psychological Bulletin*, **95**, 534–41.

Hayman, M. (1956). Current attitudes to alcoholism of psychiatrists in Southern California, *American Journal of Psychiatry*, **112**, 485–93.

Heather, N. (1987). Misleading confusion, *British Journal of Addiction*, **82**, 253–5.

Heather, N. (1989*a*). Controlled drinking treatment: Where do we stand today? In *Addictive behaviors: Prevention and early intervention* (ed. T. Løberg, W. R. Miller, and G. A. Marlatt) pp. 31–50. Swets and Zeitlinger, Amsterdam.

Heather, N. (1989*b*). Disulfiram treatment for alcoholism: Deserves re-examination, *British Medical Journal*, **299**, 471–2.

Heather, N. and Robertson, I. (1981). *Controlled drinking*, Methuen, London.

Heather, N., Whitton, B., and Robertson, I. (1986). Evaluation of a self-help manual for media-recruited problem drinkers: Six-month follow-up results, *British Journal of Clinical Psychology*, **25**, 19–34.

Helzer, J. E., Robins, L. N., Taylor, J. R., Carey, K., Miller, R. H., Combs-Orme, T., and Farmer, A. (1985). The extent of long-term moderate drinking among alcoholics discharged from medical and psychiatric treatment facilities, *New England Journal of Medicine*, **312**, 1678–82.

Hendriks, V. M., Kaplan, C. D., van Limbeek, J., and Geerlings, P. (1989). The Addiction Severity Index: Reliability and validity in a Dutch addict population, *Journal of Substance Abuse Treatment*, **6**, 133–41.

Hershon, H. (1974). Alcoholism and the concept of disease, *British Journal of Addiction*, **69**, 123–31.

Hesselbrock, M. N. (1986). Alcoholic typologies: A review of empirical evaluations of common classification schemes. In *Recent developments in alcoholism, Vol. 4* (ed. M. Galanter) pp. 191–206. Plenum Press, New York.

Hester, R. K., Miller, W. R., Delaney, H. D., and Meyers, R. J. (1990). Effectiveness of the community reinforcement approach. Paper presented at the 24th Annual Meeting of the Association for Advancement of Behavior Therapy, San Francisco, November 2.

Hiatt, H. H. (1975). Protecting the medical commons: Who is responsible? *New England Journal of Medicine*, **293**, 235-41.

Hill, M. J. and Blane, H. T. (1967). Evaluation of psychotherapy with alcoholics: A critical review, *Quarterly Journal of Studies on Alcohol*, **28**, 76-104.

Hill, S. Y. (1985). The disease concept of alcoholism, *Drug and Alcohol Dependence*, **16**, 193-214.

Hingson, R., Mangione, T., Meyers, A., and Scotch, N. (1982). Seeking help for drinking problems: A study in the Boston Metropolitan Area, *Journal of Studies on Alcohol*, **43**, 273-88.

Hinrichsen, J. J. (1976). Locus of control among alcoholics: Some empirical and conceptual issues, *Journal of Studies on Alcohol*, **37**, 908-16.

Hippocrates, 4 vols. (1923). Ed. and trans. W. H. S. Jones. Harvard University Press (Loeb Classical Library), Cambridge, Mass.

Hodgson, R. J. (1980*a*). The alcohol dependence syndrome: A step in the wrong direction? *British Journal of Addiction*, **75**, 255-63.

Hodgson, R. J. (1980*b*). Editorial note on 'The course of alcoholism: Four years after treatment', *British Journal of Addiction*, **75**, 343.

Hodgson, R. J., Rankin, H. J., and Stockwell, T. R. (1979). Alcohol dependence and the priming effect, *Behaviour Research and Therapy*, **17**, 379-87.

Hodgson, R. and Stockwell, T. (1985). The theoretical and empirical basis of the alcohol dependence model: A social learning perspective. In *The misuse of alcohol: Crucial issues in dependence, treatment and prevention* (ed. N. Heather, I. Robertson, and P. Davies) pp. 17-34. Croom Helm, Beckenham.

Hodgson, R. J., Stockwell, T. R., Rankin, H. J., and Edwards, G. (1978). Alcohol dependence: The concept, its utility and measurement, *British Journal of Addiction*, **73**, 339-42.

Hoffmann, H. (1976). Personality measurement for the evaluation and prediction of alcoholism. In *Alcoholism: Interdisciplinary approaches to an enduring problem* (ed. R. E. Tarter and A. A. Sugerman) pp. 309-58. Addison-Wesley, Reading, Mass.

Holder, H. D. and Blose, J. O. (1986). Alcoholism treatment and total health care utilization and costs: A four-year longitudinal analysis of federal employees, *Journal of the American Medical Association*, **256**, 1456-60.

Holder, H. D. and Stratas, N. E. (1972). A systems approach to alcoholism programming, *American Journal of Psychiatry*, **129**, 64-9.

Holt, R. R. (1958). Clinical *and* statistical prediction: A reformulation and some new data, *Journal of Abnormal and Social Psychology*, **56**, 1-12.

Holt, S., Steward, I. C., Dixon, J. M. J., Elton, R. A., Taylor, T. V., and Little, K. (1980). Alcohol and the emergency service patient, *British Medical Journal*, **281**, 638-40.

Howden Chapman, P. L. and Huygens, I. (1988). An evaluation of three treatment programmes for alcoholism: An experimental study with 6- and 18-month follow-ups, *British Journal of Addiction*, **83**, 67-81.

Hulbert, R. J. and Lens, W. (1988). Time perspective, time attitude, and time orientation in alcoholism: A review, *The International Journal of the Addictions*, **23**, 279-98.

Hull, J. G. and Bond, C. F. (1986). Social and behavioral consequences of alcohol consumption and expectancy: A meta-analysis, *Psychological Bulletin*, **99**, 347–60.

Hunt, D. D., Carr, J. E., Dagadakis, C. S., and Walker, E. A. (1985). Cognitive match as a predictor of psychotherapy outcome, *Psychotherapy*, **22**, 718–21.

Hunt, D. E. (1971). *Matching models in education: The coordination of teaching models with student characteristics*, Monograph Series No. 10, Ontario Institute for Studies in Education, Toronto.

Hunt, D. E. (1975). Person–environment interaction: A challenge found wanting before it was tried, *Review of Educational Research*, **45**, 209–30.

Hunt, D. E. (1978). Conceptual level theory and research as guides to educational practice, *Interchange*, **8** (4), 78–90.

Hunt, D. E. (1979). Learning style and student needs: An introduction to conceptual level. In W. R. Anderson *et al. Student learning styles: Diagnosing and prescribing programs*, pp. 27–38. National Association of Secondary School Principals, Reston, Virginia.

Hunt, D. E. (1980). How to be your own best theorist, *Theory in Practice*, **19**, 287–93.

Hunt, D. E., Butler, L. F., Noy, J. E., and Rosser, M. E. (1978). Assessing Conceptual Level by the Paragraph Completion Method. Ontario Institute for Studies in Education, Toronto.

Hunt, D. E. and Gow, J. (1984). How to be your own best theorist, 2. *Theory in Practice*, **23**, 64–71.

Hunt, D. E. and Joyce, B. R. (1967). Teacher trainee personality and initial teaching style, *American Educational Research Journal*, **4**, 253–9.

Hunt, G. H. and Azrin, N. H. (1973). A community-reinforcement approach to alcoholism, *Behavior Research and Therapy*, **11**, 91–104.

Huss, M. (1849–51). *Alcoholismus chronicus eller Chronisk alkoholsjukdom* (Alcoholismus chronicus or Chronic alcohol disease), 2 vols. Stockholm.—German edn.: Chronische Alkoholkrankheit oder Alcoholismus chronicus. Stockholm and Leipzig, 1852.

Hyman, H., Wright, C. R., and Hopkins, T. K. (1962). *Applications of methods of evaluation*, University of California Press, Berkeley.

Ingram, J. A. and Salzberg, H. C. (1988). Cognitive-behavioral approaches to the treatment of alcoholic behavior. In *Progress in behavior modification, Vol. 23* (ed. M. Hersen, R. M. Eisler, and P. M. Miller) pp. 62–95. Sage, Newbury Park, Calif.

Institute of Medicine, IOM (1988). *Homelessness, health, and human needs*, National Academy Press, Washington, DC.

Institute of Medicine, IOM (1989). *Prevention and treatment of alcohol problems: Research opportunities*, National Academy Press, Washington, DC.

Institute of Medicine, IOM (1990). *Broadening the base of treatment for alcohol problems*, National Academy Press, Washington, DC.

Intagliata, J. C. (1978). Increasing the interpersonal problem-solving skills of an alcoholic population, *Journal of Consulting and Clinical Psychology*, **46**, 489–98.

IOM. *See* Institute of Medicine.

Ito, J. R., Donovan, D. M., and Hall, J. J. (1988). Relapse prevention in alcohol aftercare: Effects on drinking outcome, change process, and aftercare attendance, *British Journal of Addiction*, **83**, 171–81.

Iversen, L. and Klausen, H. (1986). Alcohol consumption among laid-off workers before and after closure of a Danish ship-yard: A 2-year follow-up study, *Social Science and Medicine*, **22**, 107–9.

Jeffrey, D. B. (1975). Treatment evaluation issues in research on addictive behaviors, *Addictive Behaviors*, **1**, 23–36.

Jellinek, E. M. (1946). Phases in the drinking history of alcoholics, *Quarterly Journal of Studies on Alcohol*, **7**, 1–88.

Jellinek, E. M. (1952). Phases of alcohol addiction, *Quarterly Journal of Studies on Alcohol*, **13**, 673–84.

Jellinek, E. M. (1960). *The disease concept of alcoholism*, Hillhouse Press, New Haven, Conn.

Jellinek, E. M. (1962). Cultural differences in the meaning of alcoholism. In *Society, culture, and drinking patterns* (ed. D. J. Pittman and C. R. Snyder) pp. 382–8. Wiley, New York.

Joe, V. C. (1971). Review of the internal–external control construct as a personality variable, *Psychological Reports*, Monograph Supplement 3-V28, 619–40.

Johnson, D. H. and Gelso, C. J. (1980). The effectiveness of time limits in counseling and psychotherapy: A critical review, *The Counseling Psychologist*, **9**, 70–83.

Johnson, R. K. and Meyer, R. G. (1974). The locus of control construct in EEG alpha rhythm feedback, *Journal of Consulting and Clinical Psychology*, **42**, 913.

Jones, B. A. (1983). Healing factors of psychiatry in light of attachment theory, *American Journal of Psychotherapy*, **37**, 235–44.

Jones, E. (1955). *Sigmund Freud: Life and work, Vol. 2*, Hogarth Press, London.

Jones, W. H. S. (1946). Philosophy and medicine in ancient Greece, *Bulletin of the History of Medicine*, Suppl. 8. Johns Hopkins Press, Baltimore.

Jyrkämä, J. (1980). *Arbetslöshet och bruk av rusmedel. Översikt och utvärdering av nordisk forskning om förhållandet mellan arbetslöshet och rusmedelsdryck* (Unemployment and the use of alcohol and drugs: A critical review of Nordic research). NU Series A 1980: 16. Nordic Council/Nordic Council of Ministers, Stockholm.

Kadden, R. M., Cooney, N. L., Getter, H., and Litt, M. D. (1989). Matching alcoholics to coping skills or interactional therapies: Posttreatment results, *Journal of Consulting and Clinical Psychology*, **57**, 698–704.

Kahneman, D., Slovic, P., and Tversky, A., (ed.) (1982). *Judgment under uncertainty: Heuristics and biases*. Cambridge University Press, Cambridge.

Kammeier, M. L., Hoffmann, H., and Loper, R. G. (1973). Personality characteristics of alcoholics as college freshmen and at time of treatment, *Quarterly Journal of Studies on Alcohol*, **34**, 390–9.

Karasu, T. B. (1986). The specificity versus nonspecificity dilemma: Toward identifying therapeutic change agents, *American Journal of Psychiatry*, **143**, 687–95.

Karp, S. A., Kissin, B., and Hustmyer, F. E. (1970). Field dependence as a predictor of alcoholic therapy dropouts, *The Journal of Nervous and Mental Disease*, **150**, 77–83.

Kazdin, A. E. (1979). Nonspecific treatment factors in psychotherapy outcome research, *Journal of Consulting and Clinical Psychology*, **47**, 846–51.

Kazdin, A. E. (1981). Drawing valid inferences from case studies, *Journal of Consulting and Clinical Psychology*, **49**, 183–92.

Kazdin, A. E. (1982). *Single-case research designs: Methods for clinical and applied settings*. Oxford University Press, New York.

Kazdin, A. E. and Wilson, G. T. (1978). *Evaluation of behavior therapy: Issues, evidence, and research strategies*, Ballinger, Cambridge, Mass.

Keller, M. (1962). The definition of alcoholism and the estimation of its prevalence. In *Society, culture and drinking patterns* (ed. D. J. Pittman and C. R. Snyder) pp. 310–29. Wiley, New York.

Keller, M. (1969). Some views on the nature of addiction. Invited address presented to the 15th International Institute on the Prevention and Treatment of Alcoholism, Budapest, Hungary, June 9–18.

Keller, M. (1972). The oddities of alcoholics, *Quarterly Journal of Studies on Alcohol*, **33**, 1147–8.

Keller, M. (1976). The disease concept of alcoholism revisited, *Journal of Studies on Alcohol*, **37**, 1694–717.

Kelly, G. A. (1955). *The psychology of personal constructs, Vol. 1: A theory of personality*, Norton, New York.

Kendall, P. C. and Norton-Ford, J. D. (1982). Therapy outcome research methods. In *Handbook of research methods in clinical psychology* (ed. P. C. Kendall and J. N. Butcher) pp. 429–60. Wiley, New York.

Kendell, R. E. (1979). Alcoholism: A medical or a political problem? *British Medical Journal*, **i**, 367–71.

Kendell, R. E., de Roumanie, M., and Ritson, E. B. (1983). Influence of an increase in excise duty on alcohol consumption and its adverse effects, *British Medical Journal*, **ii**, 809–11.

Kendell, R. E. and Staton, M. C. (1966). The fate of untreated alcoholics, *Quarterly Journal of Studies on Alcohol*, **27**, 30–41.

Kernberg, O. F., Burstein, E. D., Coyne, L., Appelbaum, A., Horwitz, L., and Voth, H. (1972). Psychotherapy and psychoanalysis: Final report of the Menninger Foundation's psychotherapy research project, *Bulletin of the Menninger Clinic*, **36**, 1–276.

Keso, L. (1988). Inpatient Treatment of Employed Alcoholics: A Randomized Clinical Trial on Hazelden and Traditional Treatment. Helsinki University Central Hospital, Research Unit of Alcohol Diseases, Helsinki, Fin. (Doctoral dissertation)

Keso, L. and Salaspuro, M. (1990). Inpatient treatment of employed alcoholics: A randomized clinical trial on Hazelden-type and traditional treatment, *Alcoholism: Clinical and Experimental Research*, **14**, 584–9.

Khantzian, E. J. and Mack, J. E. (1989). Alcoholics Anonymous and contemporary psychodynamic theory. In *Recent developments in alcoholism, Vol. 7* (ed. M. Galanter) pp. 67–89. Plenum Press, New York.

Kiesler, D. J. (1966). Some myths of psychotherapy, research and the search for a paradigm, *Psychological Bulletin*, **65**, 110–36.

Kiesler, D. J. (1971). Experimental designs in psychotherapy research. In *Handbook of psychotherapy and behavior change: An empirical analysis* (ed. A. E. Bergin and S. L. Garfield) pp. 36–74. Wiley, New York.

Kilmann, P. R., Albert, B. M., and Sotile, W. M. (1975). Relationship between locus of control, structure of therapy and outcome, *Journal of Consulting and Clinical Psychology*, **43**, 588.

Kilmann, P. R. and Howell, R. J. (1974). Effects of structure of marathon group therapy and locus of control on therapeutic outcome, *Journal of Consulting and Clinical Psychology*, **42**, 912.

King, L. S. (1982). *Medical thinking: A historical preface*, Princeton University Press, Princeton, NJ.

Kish, G. B., Ellsworth, R. B., and Woody, M. M. (1980). Effectiveness of an 84-day and 60-day alcoholism treatment program, *Journal of Studies on Alcohol*, **40**, 81–5.

Kissin, B. (1977a). Comments on 'Alcoholism: A controlled trial of "treatment" and "advice"', *Journal of Studies on Alcohol*, **38**, 1804–8.

Kissin, B. (1977b). Patient characteristics and treatment specificity in alcoholism.

In *Recent advances in the study of alcoholism* (ed. C.-M. Ideström) pp. 110–22. Excerpta Medica, Amsterdam.

Kissin, B. (1977c). Theory and practice in the treatment of alcoholism. In *The biology of alcoholism, Vol. 5: Treatment and rehabilitation of the chronic alcoholic* (ed. B. Kissin and H. Begleiter) pp. 1–51. Plenum Press, New York.

Kissin, B. and Hanson, M. (1982). The bio-psycho-social perspective in alcoholism. In *Alcoholism and clinical psychiatry* (ed. J. Solomon) pp. 1–19. Plenum Press, New York.

Kissin, B., Platz, A., and Su, W. H. (1970). Social and psychological factors in the treatment of chronic alcoholism, *Journal of Psychiatric Research*, **8**, 13–27.

Kissin, B., Platz, A., and Su, W. H. (1971). Selective factors in treatment choice and outcome in alcoholics. In *Recent advances in studies of alcoholism* (ed. N. K. Mello and J. H. Mendelson) pp. 781–802. Publication No. /HSM/ 71-9045, US Government Printing Office, Washington, DC.

Kissin, B., Rosenblatt, S. M., and Machover, S. (1968). Prognostic factors in alcoholism, *Psychiatric Research Reports*, **24**, 22–43.

Klajner, F., Hartman, L. M., and Sobell, M. B. (1984). Treatment of substance abuse by relaxation training: A review of its rationale, efficacy, and mechanisms, *Addictive Behaviors*, **9**, 41–55.

Kline, N. S., Wren, J. C., Cooper, T. B., Varga, F., and Cannel, O. (1974). Evaluation of lithium therapy in chronic and periodic alcoholism, *American Journal of Medical Science*, **268**, 15–22.

Knight, R. P. (1937). The dynamics and treatment of chronic alcohol addiction, *Bulletin of the Menninger Clinic*, **1**, 233–50.

Knupfer, G. (1972). Ex-problem drinkers. In *Life history research in psychopathology, Vol. 2* (ed. M. Roff, L. N. Robins, and M. Pollack) pp. 256–80. The University of Minnesota Press, Minneapolis.

Knupfer, G. (1989). The prevalence in various social groups of eight different drinking patterns, from abstaining to frequent drunkenness: Analysis of 10 U.S. surveys combined, *British Journal of Addiction*, **84**, 1305–18.

Kohut, H. (1971). *The analysis of the self*, International Universities Press, New York.

Kraepelin, E. (1883). *Compendium der Psychiatrie* (Compendium of psychiatry), Leipzig, Germany.

Kratochwill, T. R., ed. (1978). *Single subject research: Strategies for evaluating change*, Academic Press, New York.

Kristenson, H. (1987). Methods of intervention to modify drinking patterns in heavy drinkers. In *Recent developments in alcoholism, Vol. 5* (ed. M. Galanter) pp. 403–23. Plenum Press, New York.

Kristenson, H., Öhlin, H., Hultén-Nosslin, M.-B., Trell, E., and Hood, B. (1983). Identification and intervention of heavy drinking in middle-aged men: Results and follow-up of 24–60 months of long-term study with randomized controls, *Alcoholism: Clinical and Experimental Research*, **7**, 203–9.

Kurosawa, K. (1984). Meta-analysis and selective publication bias, *American Psychologist*, **39**, 73–4.

Kurtz, N. R. and Regier, M. (1975). The Uniform Alcoholism and Intoxication Treatment Act: The compromising process of social policy formulation, *Journal of Studies on Alcohol*, **36**, 1421–41.

Laberg, J. C. (1986). Alcohol and expectancy: Subjective, psychophysiological and behavioral responses to alcohol stimuli in severely, moderately and non-dependent drinkers, *British Journal of Addiction*, **81**, 797–808.

Lambert, M. J., Bergin, A. E., and Collins, J. L. (1977). Therapist-induced deterioration in psychotherapy. In *Effective psychotherapy: A handbook of research* (ed. A. S. Gurman and A. M. Razin) pp. 452–81. Pergamon Press, Oxford.

Lambert, M. J., Shapiro, D. A., and Bergin, A. E. (1986). The effectiveness of psychotherapy. In *Handbook of psychotherapy and behavior change*, 3rd edn. (ed. S. L. Garfield and A. E. Bergin) pp. 157–211. Wiley, New York.

Landfield, A. W. (1971). *Personal construct systems in psychology*, Rand McNally, Chicago.

Landman, J. T. and Dawes, R. M. (1982). Psychotherapy outcome: Smith and Glass' conclusions stand up under scrutiny, *American Psychologist*, 37, 504–16.

LaPorte, D. J., MacGahan, J. A., and McLellan, A. T. (1979). One year experience with combined treatment of drug and alcohol abusers. In *Addiction research and treatment: Converging trends* (ed. E. L. Gottheil, A. T. McLellan, K. A. Druley, and A. I. Alterman) pp. 79–90. Pergamon Press, New York.

LaPorte, D. J., McLellan, A. T., Erdlen, F. R., and Parente, R. J. (1981). Treatment outcome as a function of follow-up difficulty in substance abusers, *Journal of Consulting and Clinical Psychology*, 49, 112–19.

Laufer, M. W. and Alfie, S. (1977). Superego: Its functions. In *International Encyclopedia of Psychiatry, Psychology, Psychoanalysis, and Neurology, Vol. 11* (ed. B. B. Wolman) pp. 41–4. Aesculapius, New York.

Laundergan, J. C. (1982). *Easy does it: Alcoholism treatment outcomes, Hazelden and the Minnesota Model*. Hazelden Foundation, Center City, Minn.

Lazarus, A. A. (1977). Has behavior therapy outlived its usefulness? *American Psychologist*, 32, 550–4.

Leach, J. and Wing, J. (1980). *Helping destitute men*. Tavistock, London.

Lefcourt, H. M. (1966). Internal versus external control of reinforcement: A review, *Psychological Bulletin*, 65, 206–20.

Lefcourt, H. M. (1972). Recent developments in the study of locus of control. In *Progress in experimental personality research, Vol. 6* (ed. B. A. Maher) pp. 1–39. Academic Press, New York.

Lefcourt, H. M. and Telegdi, M. (1971). Perceived locus of control and field dependence as predictors of cognitive activity, *Journal of Consulting and Clinical Psychology*, 37, 53–6.

Leigh, H. and Reiser, M. F. (1980). *The patient: Biological, psychological, and social dimensions of medical practice*, Plenum Press, New York.

Leitner, L. M. (1982). Literalism, perspectivism, chaotic fragmentalism and psychotherapy techniques, *British Journal of Medical Psychology*, 55, 307–17.

Lesyk, J. J. (1969). Effects of intensive operant conditioning on belief in personal control in schizophrenic women. *Dissertation Abstracts, Section B*, 29 (12), 4849.

Lettieri, D. J., ed. (1988). *Research strategies in alcoholism treatment assessment*. Drugs and Society Series, Vol. 2, No. 2, 1987/88. Haworth Press, New York.

Levinson, T. and Sereny, G. (1969). An experimental evaluation of 'insight therapy' for the chronic alcoholic, *Canadian Psychiatric Association Journal*, 14, 143–6.

Levy, M. (1987). A change in orientation: Therapeutic strategies for the treatment of alcoholism, *Psychotherapy*, 24, 786–93.

Lewin, K. (1935). *A dynamic theory of personality*, McGraw-Hill, New York.

Lewin, K. (1936). *Principles of topological psychology*, McGraw-Hill, New York.

Lewinsohn, P. M. and Rosenbaum, M. (1987). Recall of parental behavior by acute depressives, remitted depressives, and nondepressives, *Journal of Personality and Social Psychology*, 52, 611–19.

Liberman, B. L. (1978*a*). The maintenance and persistence of change: Long-term follow-up investigations of psychotherapy. In *Effective ingredients of successful psychotherapy* (ed. J. D. Frank, R. Hoehn-Saric, S. C. Imber, B. L. Liberman, and A. R. Stone) pp. 107–29. Brunner/Mazel, New York.

Liberman, B. L. (1978*b*). The role of mastery in psychotherapy: Maintenance of improvement and prescriptive change. In *Effective ingredients of successful psychotherapy* (ed. J. D. Frank, R. Hoehn-Saric, S. C. Imber, B. L. Liberman, and A. R. Stone) pp. 35–72. Brunner/Mazel, New York.

Light, R. J. and Smith, P. V. (1971). Accumulating evidence: Procedures for resolving contradictions among different research studies, *Harvard Educational Review*, **41**, 429–71.

Lindberg, S. and Ågren, G. (1988). Mortality among male and female hospitalized alcoholics in Stockholm 1962–1983, *British Journal of Addiction*, **83**, 1193–200.

Lindman, R. (1980). Anxiety and Alcohol: Limitations of Tension Reduction Theory in Nonalcoholics. Reports from the Department of psychology at Åbo akademi, Monograph Supplement No. 1. Åbo, Finland. (Doctoral dissertation)

Liskow, B. I. and Goodwin, D. W. (1987). Pharmacological treatment of alcohol intoxication, withdrawal and dependence: A critical review, *Journal of Studies on Alcohol*, **48**, 356–70.

Litman, G. K. (1982). Personal meanings and alcoholism survival: Translating subjective experience into empirical data. In *Personal meanings* (ed. J. Watson and E. Shepherd). Wiley, New York.

Llewelyn, S. P. and Hume, W. I. (1979). The patient's view of therapy, *British Journal of Medical Psychology*, **52**, 29–35.

Logue, P. E., Gentry, W. D., Linnoila, M., and Erwin, C. W. (1978). Effect of alcohol consumption on state anxiety changes in male and female nonalcoholics, *American Journal of Psychiatry*, **135**, 1079–81.

Longabaugh, R. (1986). The matching hypothesis: Theoretical and empirical status. Paper presented at the Annual Meeting of the American Psychological Association, Washington, DC, August 24.

Longabaugh, R. and Beattie, M. (1985). Optimizing the cost effectiveness of treatment for alcohol abusers. In *Future directions in alcohol abuse treatment research* (ed. B. S. McCrady, N. E. Noel, and T. D. Nirenberg) pp. 104–36. Research Monograph No. 15, National Institute on Alcohol Abuse and Alcoholism, Rockville, Md.

Longabaugh, R., Beattie, M., Noel, N., Stout, R., and Malloy, P. The effect of social investment on treatment outcome, *Journal of Studies on Alcohol*, in press.

Longabaugh, R., McCrady, B. S., Fink, E. B., Stout, R. L., McAuley, T., Doyle, C., and McNeill, D. (1983). Cost effectiveness of alcoholism treatment in partial vs inpatient settings: Six-month outcomes, *Journal of Studies on Alcohol*, **44**, 1049–71.

Lovibond, S. H. (1977). Behavioral control of excessive drinking. In *Progress in behavior modification, Vol. 5.* (ed. M. Hersen, R. M. Eisler, and P. M. Miller) pp. 63–109. Academic Press, New York.

Luborsky, L. (1976). Helping alliances in psychotherapy: The groundwork for a study of their relationship to its outcome. In *Successful psychotherapy* (ed. J. L. Claghorn) pp. 92–116. Brunner/Mazel, New York.

Luborsky, L., Chandler, M., Aurbach, A., and Cohen, J. (1971). Factors influencing the outcome of psychotherapy: A review of quantitative research, *Psychological Bulletin*, **75**, 145–85.

Luborsky, L., Crits-Christoph, P., McLellan, T., Woody, G., Piper, W., Liberman, B., Imber, S., and Pilkonis, P. (1986). Do therapists vary much in their success?

Findings from four outcome studies, *American Journal of Orthopsychiatry*, **56**, 501–12.

Luborsky, L., Crits-Christoph, P., Mintz, J., and Auerbach, A. (1988). *Who will benefit from psychotherapy? Predicting therapeutic outcomes*, Basic Books, New York.

Luborsky, L. and McLellan, A. T. (1981). Optimal matching of patients with types of psychotherapy: What is known and some designs for knowing more. In *Matching patient needs and treatment methods in alcoholism and drug abuse* (ed. E. Gottheil, A. T. McLellan, and K. A. Druley) pp. 51–71. Charles C Thomas, Springfield, Ill.

Luborsky, L., Singer, B., and Luborsky, L. (1975). Comparative studies of psychotherapies: Is it true that 'Everyone has won and all must have prizes'? *Archives of General Psychiatry*, **32**, 995–1008.

Ludwig, A. M. (1985). Cognitive processes associated with 'spontaneous' recovery from alcoholism, *Journal of Studies on Alcohol*, **46**, 53–8.

Ludwig, A. M., Levine, J., and Stark, L. H. (1970). *LSD and alcoholism: A clinical study of treatment efficacy*, Charles C Thomas, Springfield, Ill.

Ludwig, A. M. and Wikler, A. (1974). 'Craving' and relapse to drink, *Quarterly Journal of Studies on Alcohol*, **35**, 108–30.

Ludwig, A. M., Wikler, A., and Stark, L. H. (1974). The first drink: Psychobiological aspects of craving, *Archives of General Psychiatry*, **30**, 539–47.

Lyons, J. P., Welte, J. W., Brown, J., Sokolow, L., and Hynes, G. (1982). Variation in alcoholism treatment orientation: Differential impact upon specific subpopulations, *Alcoholism: Clinical and Experimental Research*, **6**, 333–43.

MacAndrew, C. and Edgerton, R. B. (1969). *Drunken comportment: A social explanation*, Aldine, Chicago.

McCabe, R. J. R. (1986). Alcohol-dependent individuals sixteen years on, *Alcohol and Alcoholism*, **21**, 85–91.

McCance, C. and McCance, P. F. (1969). Alcoholism in North-East Scotland: Its treatment and outcome, *British Journal of Psychiatry*, **115**, 189–98.

McCord, J. (1988). Identifying developmental paradigms leading to alcoholism, *Journal of Studies on Alcohol*, **49**, 357–62.

McCord, W. and McCord, J. (1960). *Origins of psychiatry*, Stanford University Press, Stanford, Calif.

McCrady, B.S. (1987). Implications of neuropsychological research findings for the treatment and rehabilitation of alcoholics. In *Neuropsychology of alcoholism: Implications for diagnosis and treatment* (ed. O. A. Parsons, N. Butters, and P. E. Nathan) pp. 381–91. Guilford, New York.

McCrady, B. S. (1989). Outcomes of family-involved alcoholism treatment. In *Recent developments in alcoholism, Vol. 7* (ed. M. Galanter) pp. 165–82. Plenum Press, New York.

McCrady, B. S., Fink, E. B., Longabaugh, R., and Stout, R. L. (1983). Behavioral alcoholism treatment in the partial hospital, *International Journal of Partial Hospitalization*, **2**, 83–95.

McCrady, B., Longabaugh, R., Fink, E., Stout, R., Beattie, M., and Ruggieri-Authelet, A. (1986). Cost effectiveness of alcoholism treatment in partial hospital versus inpatient settings after brief inpatient treatment: 12-month outcomes, *Journal of Consulting and Clinical Psychology*, **54**, 708–13.

McCrady, B. S. and Smith, D. E. (1986). Implications of cognitive impairment for the treatment of alcoholism, *Alcoholism: Clinical and Experimental Research*, **10**, 145–9.

McLachlan, J. F. C. (1972). Benefit from group therapy as a function of patient-therapist match on conceptual level, *Psychotherapy: Theory, Research and Practice*, **9**, 317–23.

McLachlan, J. F. C. (1974). Therapy strategies, personality orientation and recovery from alcoholism, *Canadian Psychiatric Association Journal*, **19**, 25–30.

McLachlan, J. F. C. and Hunt, D. E. (1973). Differential effects of discovery learning as a function of conceptual level, *Canadian Journal of Behavioural Science*, **5**, 152–60.

McLachlan, J. F. C. and Stein, R. L. (1982). Evaluation of a day clinic for alcoholics, *Journal of Studies on Alcohol*, **43**, 261–72.

McLachlan, J. F. C., Walderman, R. L., Birchmore, D. F., and Marsden, L. R. (1979). Self-evaluation, role satisfaction, and anxiety in the woman alcoholic, *The International Journal of the Addictions*, **14**, 809–32.

McLatchie, B. H. and Lomp, K. G. E. (1988*a*). Alcoholics Anonymous affiliation and treatment outcome among a clinical sample of problem drinkers, *The American Journal of Drug and Alcohol Abuse*, **14**, 309–24.

McLatchie, B. H. and Lomp, K. G. E. (1988*b*). An experimental investigation of the influence of aftercare on alcoholic relapse, *British Journal of Addiction*, **83**, 1045–54.

McLean, P. D. (1981). Matching treatment to patient characteristics in an outpatient setting. In *Behavior therapy for depression: Present status and future directions* (ed. L. P. Rehm) pp. 197–207. Academic Press, New York.

McLellan, A. T. and Childress, A. R. (1985). Aversive therapies for substance abuse: Do they work? *Journal of Substance Abuse Treatment*, **2**, 187–91.

McLellan, A. T., Childress, A. R., Griffith, J., and Woody, G. E. (1984). The psychiatrically severe drug abuse patient: Methadone maintenance or therapeutic community? *American Journal of Drug and Alcohol Abuse*, **10**, 77–95.

McLellan, A. T., Erdlen, F. R., Erdlen, D. L., and O'Brien, C. P. (1981*a*). Psychological severity and response to alcoholism rehabilitation, *Drug and Alcohol Dependence*, **8**, 23–35.

McLellan, A. T., Luborsky, L., Cacciola, J., Griffith, J., Evans, F., Barr, H. L., and O'Brien, C. P. (1985*a*). New data from the Addiction Severity Index: Reliability and validity in three centers, *The Journal of Nervous and Mental Disease*, **173**, 412–23.

McLellan, A. T., Luborsky, L., Cacciola, J., Griffith, J., McGahan, P., and O'Brien, C. P. (1985*b*). Guide to the Addiction Severity Index: Background, Administration, and Field Testing Results. DHHS Publication No. (ADM) 85-1419, US Department of Health and Human Services, National Institute on Drug Abuse, Rockville, Md.

McLellan, A. T., Luborsky, L., Erdlen, F. R., LaPorte, D. J., and Intintolo, V. (1980*a*). The Addiction Severity Index: A diagnostic/evaluative profile of substance abuse patients. In *Substance abuse and psychiatric illness* (ed. E. Gottheil, A. T. McLellan, and K. A. Druley) pp. 151–9. Pergamon Press, New York.

McLellan, A. T., Luborsky, L., O'Brien, C. P., Barr, H. L., and Evans, F. (1986). Alcohol and drug abuse treatment in three different populations: Is there improvement and is it predictable? *American Journal of Drug and Alcohol Abuse*, **12**, 101–20.

McLellan, A. T., Luborsky, L., O'Brien, C. P., Woody, G. E., and Druley, K. A. (1982). Is treatment for substance abuse effective? *The Journal of the American Medical Association*, **247**, 1423–8.

McLellan, A. T., Luborsky, L., Woody, G. E., and O'Brien, C. P. (1980*b*). An improved diagnostic evaluation instrument for substance abuse patients: The Addiction Severity Index, *The Journal of Nervous and Mental Disease*, **168**, 26–33.

McLellan, A. T., Luborsky, L., Woody, G. E., and O'Brien, C. P. (1981*b*). The generality of benefits from alcohol and drug abuse treatments. In *Problems of drug dependence, 1980*, pp. 373–9. NIDA Research Monograph No. 34, National Institute on Drug Abuse, Rockville, Md.

McLellan, A. T., Luborsky, L., Woody, G. E., O'Brien, C. P., and Druley, K. A. (1983*a*). Predicting response to alcohol and drug abuse treatments: The role of psychiatric severity, *Archives of General Psychiatry*, **40**, 620–5.

McLellan, A. T., Luborsky, L., Woody, G. E., O'Brien, C. P., and Kron, R. (1981*c*). Are the 'addiction-related' problems of substance abusers really related? *The Journal of Nervous and Mental Disease*, **169**, 232–9.

McLellan, A. T., O'Brien, C. P., Kron, R., Alterman, A. I., and Druley, K. A. (1980*c*). Matching substance abuse patients to appropriate treatments: A conceptual and methodological approach, *Drug and Alcohol Dependence*, **5**, 189–95.

McLellan, A. T., O'Brien, C. P., Luborsky, L., Druley, K. A., and Woody, G. E. (1981*d*). Certain types of substance abuse patients do better in certain kinds of treatments: Evidence for patient–program matching. In *Problems of drug dependence, 1980*, pp. 123–30. NIDA Research Monograph No. 34, National Institute on Drug Abuse, Rockville, Md.

McLellan, A. T., Woody, G. E., Luborsky, L., O'Brien, C. P., and Druley, K. A. (1983*b*). Increased effectiveness of drug abuse treatment from patient–program matching. In *Problems of drug dependence, 1982*, pp. 335–41. NIDA Research Monograph No. 43, National Institute on Drug Abuse, Rockville, Md.

McLellan, A. T., Woody, G. E., Luborsky, L., O'Brien, C. P., and Druley, K. A. (1983*c*). Increased effectiveness of substance abuse treatment: A prospective study of patient–treatment 'matching', *The Journal of Nervous and Mental Disease*, **171**, 597–605.

McNamee, H. B., Mendelson, J. H., and Mello, N. K. (1968). Experimental analysis of drinking patterns of alcoholics, concurrent psychiatric observations, *American Journal of Psychiatry*, **124**, 1063–9.

Mack, J. E. (1981). Alcoholism, A.A. and the governance of the self. In *Dynamic approaches to the understanding and treatment of alcoholism* (ed. M. H. Bean and N. E. Zinberg) pp. 128–62. The Free Press, New York.

Magaro, P. A. and DeSisto, M. (1981). A developmental treatment program for the chronic patient, *American Journal of Psychotherapy*, **35**, 47–60.

Magaro, P. A., Gripp, R., and McDowell, D. J. (1978). *The mental health industry: A cultural phenomenon*, Wiley, New York.

Magnusson, D. (1988). *Individual development from an interactional perspective: A longitudinal study*, Lawrence Erlbaum, Hillsdale, NJ.

Magnusson, D. and Allen, V. L. (1983). An interactional perspective for human development. In *Human development: An interactional perspective* (ed. D. Magnusson and V. L. Allen) pp. 3–31. Academic Press, New York.

Maher, B. A. (1978). A reader's, writer's, and reviewer's guide to assessing research reports in clinical psychology, *Journal of Consulting and Clinical Psychology*, **46**, 835–8.

Maier, S. F. and Seligman, M. E. (1976). Learned helplessness: Theory and evidence, *Journal of Experimental Psychology*, **105**, 3–46.

Maisto, S. A. and Carey, K. B. (1987). Treatment of alcohol abuse. In *Developments in the assessment and treatment of addictive behaviors* (ed. T. D. Nirenberg and S. A. Maisto) pp. 173–211. Ablex, Norwood, New Jersey.

Maisto, S. A. and Schefft, B. K. (1977). The construct of craving for alcohol and loss of control drinking: Help or hindrance to research, *Addictive Behaviors*, 2, 207–17.

Mäkelä, K. (1980). What can medicine properly take on? In *Alcoholism treatment in transition* (ed. G. Edwards and M. Grant) pp. 225–33. Croom Helm, London.

Mäkelä, K., Room, R., Single, E., Sulkunen, P., and Walsh, B. (1981). *Alcohol, society, and the state, Vol. 1: A comparative study of alcohol control*, Addiction Research Foundation, Toronto.

Malikin, D. (1973). *Social disability: Alcoholism, drug addiction, crime and social disadvantage*, New York University Press, New York.

Mallams, J. H., Godley, M. D., Hall, G. M., and Meyers, R. J. (1982). A social-systems approach to resocializing alcoholics in the community, *Journal of Studies on Alcohol*, 43, 1115–23.

Mandell, W. (1979). A critical overview of evaluation of alcoholism treatment, *Alcoholism: Clinical and Experimental Research*, 3, 315–23.

Mann, M. (1968). *New primer on alcoholism*, Holt, Rinehart and Winston, New York.

Marlatt, G. A. (1976). Alcohol, stress and cognitive control. In *Stress and anxiety, Vol. 3* (ed. I. G. Sarason and C. D. Spielberger) pp. 271–96. Hemisphere/Wiley, Washington, DC.

Marlatt, G. A. (1978). Craving for alcohol, loss of control and relapse: A cognitive-behavioral analysis. In *Alcoholism: New directions in behavioral research and treatment* (ed. P. E. Nathan, G. A. Marlatt, and T. Løberg) pp. 271–314. Plenum Press, New York.

Marlatt, G. A. (1979). Alcohol use and problem drinking: A cognitive-behavioral analysis. In *Cognitive-behavioral interventions: Theory, research, and procedures* (ed. P. C. Kendall and S. D. Hollon) pp. 319–55. Academic Press, New York.

Marlatt, G. A. (1985). Cognitive assessment and intervention procedures for relapse prevention. In *Relapse prevention: Maintenance strategies in the treatment of addictive behaviors* (ed. G. A. Marlatt and J. R. Gordon) pp. 201–79. Guilford Press, New York.

Marlatt, G. A. (1988). Matching clients to treatment: Treatment models and stages of change. In *Assessment of addictive behaviors* (ed. D. M. Donovan and G. A. Marlatt) pp. 474–83. Guilford Press, New York.

Marlatt, G. A., Demming, B., and Reid, J. B. (1973). Loss of control drinking in alcoholics: An experimental analogue, *Journal of Abnormal Psychology*, 81, 233–41.

Marlatt, G. A. and Donovan, D. M. (1981). Alcoholism and drug dependence: Cognitive social learning factors in addictive behaviors. In *Behavior modification: Principles, issues, and applications*, 2nd edn. (ed. W. E. Craighead, A. E. Kazdin, and M. J. Mahoney) pp. 264–85. Houghton Mifflin, Boston.

Marlatt, G. A. and Donovan, D. M. (1982). Behavioral psychology approaches to alcoholism. In *Encyclopedic handbook of alcoholism* (ed. E. M. Pattison and E. Kaufman) pp. 560–77. Gardner Press, New York.

Marlatt, G. A. and George, W. H. (1984). Relapse prevention: Introduction and overview of the model, *British Journal of Addiction*, 79, 261–73.

Marlatt, G. A. and Gordon, J. R. (1980). Determinants of relapse: Implications for the maintenance of behavior change. In *Behavioral medicine: Changing health lifestyles* (ed. P. O. Davidson and S. M. Davidson) pp. 410–52. Brunner/Mazel, New York.

Marlatt, G. A. and Gordon, J. R., ed. (1985). *Relapse prevention: Maintenance strategies in the treatment of addictive behaviors.* Guilford Press, New York.

Marlatt, G. A. and Rohsenow, D. J. (1980). Cognitive processes in alcohol use: Expectancy and the balanced placebo design. In *Advances in substance abuse: Behavioral and biological research, Vol. 1* (ed. N. K. Mello) pp. 159–200. JAI Press, Greenwich, Conn.

Matakas, F., Koester, H., and Leidner, B. (1978). Welche Behandlung für welche Alkoholiker? *Psychiatrische Praxis*, **5**, 143–52.

May, S. J. and Kuller, L. H. (1975). Methodological approaches in the evaluation of alcoholism treatment: A critical review, *Preventive Medicine*, **4**, 464–81.

Mayer, J. and Myerson, D. J. (1971). Outpatient treatment of alcoholics: Effects of status, stability and nature of treatment, *Quarterly Journal of Studies on Alcohol*, **32**, 620–7.

Meehl, P. E. (1954). *Clinical versus statistical prediction: A theoretical analysis and a review of the evidence*, University of Minnesota Press, Minneapolis.

Meehl, P. E. (1965). Seer over sign: The first good example, *Journal of Experimental Research in Personality*, **1**, 27–32.

Megargee, E. I. (1972). *The California Psychological Inventory handbook*, Jossey-Bass, San Francisco.

Mello, N. K. (1972). Behavioral studies of alcoholism. In *The biology of alcoholism, Vol. 2: Physiology and behavior* (ed. B. Kissin and H. Begleiter) pp. 219–91. Plenum Press, New York.

Mello, N. K. and Mendelson, J. H. (1971). Drinking patterns during work contingent and non-contingent alcohol acquisition. In *Recent advances in studies of alcoholism* (ed. N. K. Mello and J. H. Mendelson) pp. 647–86. Publication No. /HSM/ 71-9045, US Government Printing Office, Washington, DC.

Meltzoff, J. and Kornreich, M. (1970). *Research in psychotherapy*, Atherton Press, New York.

Merry, J., Reynolds, C. M., Bailey, J., and Coppen, A. (1976). Prophylactic treatment of alcoholism by lithium carbonate: A controlled study, *Lancet*, **ii**, 481–2.

Meyer, R. E. and Babor, T. F. (1989). Explanatory models of alcoholism. In *American Psychiatric Press review of psychiatry, Vol. 8* (ed. A. Tasman, R. E. Hales, and A. J. Frances) pp. 273–91. American Psychiatric Press, Washington, DC.

Meyer, R. E., Babor, T. F., and Mirkin, P. M. (1983). Typologies in alcoholism: An overview, *The International Journal of the Addictions*, **18**, 235–49.

Miller, A. (1978). Conceptual systems theory: A critical review, *Genetic Psychology Monographs*, **97**, 77–126.

Miller, A. (1981). Conceptual matching models and interactional research in education, *Review of Educational Research*, **51**, 33–84.

Miller, B. A., Pokorny, A. D., Valles, J., and Cleveland, S. E. (1970). Biased sampling in alcoholism treatment research, *Quarterly Journal of Studies on Alcohol*, **31**, 97–107.

Miller, P. M. (1975). A behavioral intervention program for chronic public drunkenness offenders, *Archives of General Psychiatry*, **32**, 915–18.

Miller, P. M. (1976). *Behavioral treatment of alcoholism*, Pergamon Press, Oxford.

Miller, P. M. and Eisler, R. M. (1975). Alcohol and drug abuse. In *Behavior modification: Principles, issues, and applications* (ed. W. E. Craighead, A. E. Kazdin, and M. J. Mahoney) pp. 376–93. Houghton Mifflin, Boston.

Miller, S., Helmick, E., Berg, L., Nutting, P., and Schorr, G. (1974). Alcoholism: A statewide program evaluation, *American Journal of Psychiatry*, **131**, 210–14.

Miller, S. I. and Frances, R. (1986). Psychiatrists and the treatment of addictions: Perceptions and practices, *The American Journal of Drug and Alcohol Abuse*, **12**, 187–97.

Miller, W. R. (1983). Controlled drinking: A history and a critical review, *Journal of Studies on Alcohol*, **44**, 68–83.

Miller, W. R. (1986). Haunted by the *Zeitgeist*: Reflections on contrasting treatment goals and concepts of alcoholism in Europe and the United States, *Annals of the New York Academy of Sciences*, **472**, 110–29.

Miller, W. R. (1988). The effectiveness of treatment for alcohol problems: Reasons for optimism. Paper presented at a conference on Drug Abuse and Alcohol: New Prospects for Recovery, London, England, May 10.

Miller, W. R. and Hester, R. K. (1980). Treating the problem drinker: Modern approaches. In *The addictive behaviors: Treatment of alcoholism, drug abuse, smoking, and obesity* (ed. W. R. Miller) pp. 11–141. Pergamon Press, Oxford.

Miller, W. R. and Hester, R. K. (1986*a*). The effectiveness of alcoholism treatment: What research reveals. In *Treating addictive behaviors: Processes of change* (ed. W. R. Miller and N. Heather) pp. 121–74. Plenum Press, New York.

Miller, W. R. and Hester, R. K. (1986*b*). Inpatient alcoholism treatment: Who benefits? *American Psychologist*, **41**, 794–805.

Miller, W. R. and Hester, R. K. (1986*c*). Matching problem drinkers with optimal treatments. In *Treating addictive behaviors: Processes of change* (ed. W. R. Miller and N. Heather) pp. 175–203. Plenum Press, New York.

Mintz, J., Luborsky, L., and Cristoph, P. (1979). Measuring the outcomes of psychotherapy: Findings of the Penn Psychotherapy Project, *Journal of Consulting and Clinical Psychology*, **47**, 319–34.

Mischel, W. (1973). Toward a cognitive social learning reconceptualization of personality, *Psychological Review*, **80**, 252–83.

Mischel, W. (1981). *Introduction to personality*, 3rd edn., Holt, Rinehart and Winston, New York.

Moll, J. K. and Narin, F. (1977). Characterization of the alcohol research literature, *Journal of Studies on Alcohol*, **38**, 2165–80.

Moore, M. H. and Gerstein, D. R. (1981). *Alcohol and public policy: Beyond the shadow of prohibition*, National Academy Press, Washington, DC.

Moore, R. A. and Buchanan, T. K. (1966). State hospitals and alcoholism: A national-wide survey of treatment techniques and results, *Quarterly Journal of Studies on Alcohol*, **27**, 459–68.

Moore, R. D., Bone, L. R., Geller, G., Mamon, J. A., Stokes, E. J., and Levine, D. M. (1989). Prevalence, detection, and treatment of alcoholism in hospitalized patients, *The Journal of the American Medical Association*, **261**, 403–7.

Moos, R. H. (1973). Conceptualizations of human environments, *American Psychologist*, **28**, 652–65.

Moos, R. H., Cronkite, R. C., and Finney, J. W. (1982). A conceptual framework for alcoholism treatment evaluation. In *Encyclopedic handbook of alcoholism* (ed. E. M. Pattison and E. Kaufman) pp. 1120–39. Gardner Press, New York.

Moos, R. H. and Finney, J. W. (1983). The expanding scope of alcoholism treatment evaluation, *American Psychologist*, **38**, 1036–44.

Moos, R. H., Finney, J. W., and Chan, D. A. (1981). The process of recovery from alcoholism, 1: Comparing alcoholic patients and matched community controls, *Journal of Studies on Alcohol*, **42**, 383–402.

Moos, R. H., Finney, J. W., and Cronkite, R. C. (1990). *Alcoholism treatment: Context, process, and outcome*, Oxford University Press, New York.

Morey, L. C. and Skinner, H. A. (1986). Empirically derived classifications of alcohol-related problems. In *Recent developments in alcoholism, Vol. 4* (ed. M. Galanter) pp. 145–68. Plenum Press, New York.

Morey, L. C., Skinner, H. A., and Blashfield, R. K. (1984). A typology of alcohol abusers: Correlates and implications, *Journal of Abnormal Psychology*, **93**, 408–417.

Morgan, R., Luborsky, L., Crits-Christoph, P., Curtis, H., and Solomon, J. (1982). Predicting the outcomes of psychotherapy by the Penn Helping Alliance Rating Method, *Archives of General Psychiatry*, **39**, 397–402.

Mosher, V., Davis, J., Mulligan, D., and Iber, F. L. (1975). Comparison of outcome in a 9-day and 30-day alcoholism treatment program, *Journal of Studies on Alcohol*, **36**, 1277–81.

Moskowitz, J. M. (1989). The primary prevention of alcohol problems: A critical review of the research literature, *Journal of Studies on Alcohol*, **50**, 54–88.

Mumford, E., Schlesinger, H. J., and Glass, G. V. (1978). A critical review and indexed bibliography of the literature up to 1978 on the effects of psychotherapy on medical utilization. Department of Psychiatry, University of Colorado Medical Center, Denver.

Murray, R. M. (1975). Alcoholism and employment, *Journal of Alcoholism*, **10**, 23–6.

Muuronen, A., Bergman, H., Hindmarsh, T., and Telakivi, T. (1989). Influence of improved drinking habits on brain atrophy and cognitive performance in alcoholic patients: A 5-year follow-up study, *Alcoholism: Clinical and Experimental Research*, **13**, 137–41.

Myers, J. L. (1972). *Fundamentals of experimental design*, 2nd edn., Allyn and Bacon, Boston.

Nace, E. P. (1989). The natural history of alcoholism versus treatment effectiveness: Methodological problems, *American Journal of Drug and Alcohol Abuse*, **15**, 55–60.

Naroll, R. (1983). *The moral order: An introduction to the human situation*, Sage, Beverly Hills, Calif.

Nathan, P. E. (1988). The addictive personality is the behavior of the addict, *Journal of Consulting and Clinical Psychology*, **56**, 183–8.

Nathan, P. E. (1990). Integration of biological and psychosocial research on alcoholism, *Alcoholism: Clinical and Experimental Research*, **14**, 368–74.

Nathan, P. E. and Lansky, D. (1978*a*). Common methodological problems in research on the addictions, *Journal of Consulting and Clinical Psychology*, **46**, 713–26.

Nathan, P. E. and Lansky, D. (1978*b*). Management of the chronic alcoholic: A behavioral viewpoint. In *Controversy in psychiatry* (ed. J. P. Brady and H. K. H. Brodie) pp. 326–49. Saunders, Philadelphia.

Nathan, P. E., Lipson, A. G., Vettraino, A. P., and Solomon, P. (1968). The social ecology of an urban clinic for alcoholism, *International Journal of Addictions*, **3**, 55–64.

Nathan, P. E. and Lisman, S. A. (1976). Behavioral and motivational patterns of chronic alcoholics. In *Alcoholism: Interdisciplinary approaches to an enduring problem* (ed. R. E. Tarter and A. A. Sugerman) pp. 479–522. Addison-Wesley, Reading, Mass.

Nathan, P. E. and Skinstad, A.-H. (1987). Outcomes of treatment for alcohol problems: Current methods, problems, and results, *Journal of Consulting and Clinical Psychology*, **55**, 332–40.

Nathan, P. E., Titler, N. A., Lowenstein, L. M., Solomon, P., and Rossi, A. M. (1970). Behavioral analysis of chronic alcoholism, *Archives of General Psychiatry*, **22**, 419–30.

Nerviano, V. J. and Gross, H. W. (1983). Personality types of alcoholics on objective inventories: A review, *Journal of Studies on Alcohol*, **44**, 837–51.

Neuringer, C. (1982). Alcohol addiction: Psychological tests and measurements. In *Encyclopedic handbook of alcoholism* (ed. E. M. Pattison and E. Kaufman) pp. 517–28. Gardner Press, New York.

New Encyclopaedia Britannica, Vol. 13 (1989). 15th edn. Encyclopaedia Britannica, Chicago.

Newcomb, M. D., Bentler, P. M., and Collins, C. (1986). Alcohol use and dissatisfaction with self and life: A longitudinal analysis of young adults, *The Journal of Drug Issues*, **16**, 479–94.

Newton, J. R. and Stein, L. I. (1972). Implosive therapy. In *Proceedings of the First Annual Meeting of the National Institute on Alcohol Abuse and Alcoholism (NIAAA)*. NIAAA, Rockville, Md.

Nicholson, R. A. and Berman, J. S. (1983). Is follow-up necessary in evaluating psychotherapy? *Psychological Bulletin*, **93**, 261–78.

Nisbett, R. and Ross, L. (1980). *Human inference: Strategies and shortcomings of social judgment*, Prentice-Hall, Englewood Cliffs, NJ.

Norcross, J. C., ed. (1986). *Handbook of eclectic psychotherapy*, Brunner/Mazel, New York.

Nordström, G. (1987). Successful Outcome in Alcoholism: A Prospective Long-term Follow-up Study. University of Lund, Department of Psychiatry I, Lund, Sw. (Doctoral dissertation)

Nordström, G. and Berglund, M. (1986). Successful adjustment in alcoholism: Relationships between causes of improvement, personality, and social factors, *The Journal of Nervous and Mental Disease*, **174**, 664–8.

Nordström, G. and Berglund, M. (1987*a*). Ageing and recovery from alcoholism, *British Journal of Psychiatry*, **151**, 382–8.

Nordström, G. and Berglund, M. (1987*b*). A prospective study of successful long-term adjustment in alcohol dependence: Social drinking versus abstinence, *Journal of Studies on Alcohol*, **48**, 95–103.

Nordström, G. and Berglund, M. (1987*c*). Type 1 and type 2 alcoholics (Cloninger and Bohman) have different patterns of successful long-term adjustment, *British Journal of Addiction*, **82**, 761–9.

Norman, J. (1979). Socialmedicinska studier av hemlösa män i Stockholm (Social Medical Studies of Homeless Men in Stockholm). University of Gothenburg, Department of Social Medicine, Gothenburg, Sw. (Doctoral dissertation; English summary: pp. 199–213)

Norman, J. and Schulze, R. (1970). Hemlösa män i Stockholm (Homeless Men in Stockholm). Reports and Memorials of the Municipal Board, Appendix 1970: 99, Stockholm.

Norton, G. R., Dinardo, P. A., and Barlow, D. H. (1983). Predicting phobics' response to therapy: A consideration of subjective, physiological and behavioral measures, *Canadian Psychologist*, **24**, 50–8.

Obitz, F. W. (1978). Control orientation and disulfiram, *Journal of Studies on Alcohol*, **39**, 1297–8.

O'Brien, C. P., Woody, G. E., and McLellan, A. T. (1983). Modern treatment of substance abuse, *Drug and Alcohol Dependence*, **11**, 95-7.

O'Brien, C. P., Woody, G. E., McLellan, A. T., Driscoll, G., Childress, A. R., Alterman, A. I., Ehrman, R., and Pomerantz, B. (1988). Substance Abuse Treatment Research Center Philadelphia VA Medical Center and The University of Pennsylvania, *British Journal of Addiction*, **83**, 1261-70.

O'Doherty, F. and Davies, J. B. (1987). Life events and addiction: A critical review, *British Journal of Addiction*, **82**, 127-37.

Ogborne, A. C. (1978). Patient characteristics as predictors of treatment outcomes for alcohol and drug abusers. In *Research advances in alcohol and drug problems, Vol. 4* (ed. Y. Israel, F. B. Glaser, H. Kalant, R. E. Popham, W. Schmidt, and R. G. Smart) pp. 177-223. Plenum Press, New York.

Ogborne, A. C. (1979). Toward a systematic approach to helping people with drinking problems, *Canadian Journal of Public Health*, **70**, 120-4.

Ogborne, A. C. (1984). A brief history of treatment and of treatment research at the Addiction Research Foundation of Ontario, 1949-1983. Addiction Research Foundation, Regional Research Centre, London, Ontario. (Unpublished manuscript)

Ogborne, A. C. (1988). Bridging the gap between the two cultures of alcoholism research and treatment, *British Journal of Addiction*, **83**, 729-33.

Ogborne, A. C. (1989). Some limitations of Alcoholics Anonymous. In *Recent developments in alcoholism, Vol. 7* (ed. M. Galanter) pp 55-65. Plenum Press, New York.

Ogborne, A. C. and Dwyer, D. (1986). A survey of assessment/referral services for alcohol and drug abusers in Ontario, *Canadian Journal of Community Mental Health*, **5**, 89-97.

Ogborne, A. C. and Glaser, F. B. (1981). Characteristics of affiliates of Alcoholics Anonymous: A review of the literature, *Journal of Studies on Alcohol*, **42**, 661-75.

Ogborne, A. C. and Rush, B. R. (1983). The coordination of treatment services for problem drinkers: Problems and prospects, *British Journal of Addiction*, **78**, 131-8.

Ogborne, A. C. and Rush, B. R. (1990). Specialized addictions assessment/referral services in Ontario: A review of their characteristics and roles in the addiction treatment system, *British Journal of Addiction*, **85**, 197-204.

Ogborne, A. C., Sobell, M. B., and Sobell, L. C. (1985). The significance of environmental factors for the design and the evaluation of alcohol treatment programs. In *Determinants of substance abuse: Biological, psychological, and environmental factors* (ed. M. Galizio and S. A. Maisto) pp. 363-82. Plenum Press, New York.

Öjehagen, A. and Berglund, M. (1986). To keep the alcoholic in out-patient treatment: A differentiated approach through treatment contracts, *Acta Psychiatrica Scandinavica*, **73**, 68-75.

Öjesjö, L. (1981). Long-term outcome in alcohol abuse and alcoholism among males in the Lundby general population, Sweden, *British Journal of Addiction*, **76**, 391-400.

Okpaku, S. O. (1986). Psychoanalytically oriented psychotherapy of substance abuse, *Advances in Alcohol and Substance Abuse*, **6** (1), 17-33.

O'Leary, D. E., O'Leary, M. R., and Donovan, D. M. (1976). Social skill acquisition and psychosocial development of alcoholics: A review, *Addictive Behaviors*, **1**, 111-20.

Olson, R. P., Ganley, R., Devine, V. T., and Dorsey, G. C., Jr. (1981). Long-term effects of behavioral versus insight-oriented therapy with inpatient alcoholics, *Journal of Consulting and Clinical Psychology*, **49**, 866-77.

Oltman, P. K. (1968). A portable rod and frame apparatus, *Perceptual and Motor Skills*, **26**, 503–6.

Omer, H. (1987). Therapeutic impact: A nonspecific major factor in directive psychotherapies, *Psychotherapy*, **24**, 52–7.

Omer, H. (1989). Specifics and nonspecifics in psychotherapy, *American Journal of Psychotherapy*, **43**, 181–92.

Omer, H. and London, P. (1988). Metamorphosis in psychotherapy: End of the systems era, *Psychotherapy*, **25**, 171–84.

Omer, H. and London, P. (1989). Signal and noise in psychotherapy: The role and control of non-specific factors, *British Journal of Psychiatry*, **155**, 239–45.

Orford, J. (1980). Understanding treatment: Controlled trials and other strategies. In *Alcoholism treatment in transition* (ed. G. Edwards and M. Grant) pp. 143–61. Croom Helm, London.

Orford, J. and Edwards, G. (1977). *Alcoholism: A comparison of treatment and advice, with a study of the influence of marriage*, Oxford University Press, Oxford.

Orford, J. and Keddie, A. (1986a). Abstinence or controlled drinking in clinical practice: Indications at initial assessment, *Addictive Behaviors*, **11**, 71–86.

Orford, J. and Keddie, A. (1986b). Abstinence or controlled drinking in clinical practice: A test of the dependence and persuasion hypotheses. *British Journal of Addiction*, **81**, 495–504.

Orford, J., Oppenheimer, E., and Edwards, G. (1976). Abstinence or control: The outcome for excessive drinkers two years after consultation, *Behavior Research and Therapy*, **14**, 409–18.

Orlinsky, D. E. and Howard, K. I. (1986). Process and outcome in psychotherapy. In *Handbook of psychotherapy and behavior change*, 3rd edn. (ed. S. L. Garfield and A. E. Bergin) pp. 311–81. Wiley, New York.

Osler, W. (1910). The faith that heals, *The British Medical Journal*, **1**, 1470–2.

Öst, L-G., Jerremalm, A., and Johansson, J. (1981). Individual response patterns and the efforts of different behavioral methods in the treatment of social phobia, *Behavior Research and Therapy*, **19**, 1–16.

Öst, L-G., Johansson, J., and Jerremalm, A. (1982). Individual response patterns and the effect of different behavioral methods in the treatment of claustrophobia, *Behavior Research and Therapy*, **20**, 445–60.

Oxford English Dictionary, Vol. 17 (1989). 2nd edn. Oxford University Press, Oxford.

Page, R. D. and Schaub, L. H. (1979). Efficacy of a three- versus a five-week alcohol treatment program, *International Journal of the Addictions*, **14**, 697–714.

Pardes, H., Papernik, D. S., and Winston, A. (1974). Field differentiation in inpatient psychotherapy, *Archives of General Psychiatry*, **31**, 311–15.

Park, P. (1983). Social-class factors in alcoholism. In *The biology of alcoholism, Vol. 6: The pathogenesis of alcoholism—psychosocial factors* (ed. B. Kissin and H. Begleiter) pp. 365–404. Plenum Press, New York.

Parloff, M. B. (1986). Frank's 'common elements' in psychotherapy: Nonspecific factors and placebos, *American Journal of Orthopsychiatry*, **56**, 521–30.

Parsons, O. A. and Leber, W. R. (1982). Alcohol, cognitive dysfunction, and brain damage. In *Biomedical processes and consequences of alcohol use*. Alcohol and Health Monograph No. 2, National Institute on Alcohol Abuse and Alcoholism, Rockville, Md., pp. 213–53.

Parsons, T. (1952). *The social system*, Tavistock, London.

Pattison, E. M. (1966). A critique of alcoholism treatment concepts, with special reference to abstinence, *Quarterly Journal of Studies on Alcohol*, **27**, 49–71.

Pattison, E. M. (1967). Morality and the treatment of the character disorders, *Journal of Religion and Health*, **4**, 290-316.

Pattison, E. M. (1969). Morality, guilt, and forgiveness in psychotherapy. In *Clinical psychiatry and religion* (ed. E. M. Pattison) pp. 93-115. Little, Brown and Company, Boston.

Pattison, E. M. (1974). Rehabilitation of the chronic alcoholic. In *The biology of alcoholism, Vol. 3: Clinical pathology* (ed. B. Kissin and H. Begleiter) pp. 587-658. Plenum Press, New York.

Pattison, E. M. (1976). A conceptual approach to alcoholism treatment goals, *Addictive Behaviors*, **1**, 177-92.

Pattison, E. M. (1977). Ten years of change in alcoholism treatment and delivery systems, *American Journal of Psychiatry*, **134**, 261-6.

Pattison, E. M. (1978). The Jack Donovan memorial lecture—1978: Differential approaches to multiple problems associated with alcoholism, *Contemporary Drug Problems*, **7**, 265-309.

Pattison, E. M. (1979). The selection of treatment modalities for the alcoholic patient. In *The diagnosis and treatment of alcoholism* (ed. J. H. Mendelson and N. K. Mello) pp. 125-227. McGraw-Hill, New York.

Pattison, E. M. (1982*a*). Diagnosis of alcoholism in relation to treatment and outcome. In *Prevention, intervention and treatment: Concerns and models*. Alcohol and Health Monograph No. 3, National Institute on Alcohol Abuse and Alcoholism, Rockville, Md., pp. 89-123.

Pattison, E. M., ed. (1982*b*). *Selection of treatment for alcoholics*. NIAAA-RUCAS Alcoholism Treatment Series, No. 1, Rutgers Center of Alcohol Studies, New Brunswick, NJ.

Pattison, E. M. (1982*c*). A systems approach to alcoholism treatment. In *Encyclopedic handbook of alcoholism* (ed. E. M. Pattison and E. Kaufman) pp. 1089-108. Gardner Press, New York.

Pattison, E. M., Coe, R., and Doerr, H. O. (1973). Population variation between alcoholism treatment facilities, *International Journal of the Addictions*, **8**, 199-229.

Pattison, E. M., Coe, R., and Rhodes, R. J. (1969). Evaluation of alcoholism treatment: A comparison of three facilities, *Archives of General Psychiatry*, **20**, 478-88.

Pattison, E. M., Headley, E. B., Gleser, G. C., and Gottschalk, L. A. (1968). Abstinence and normal drinking: An assessment of changes in drinking patterns in alcoholics after treatment, *Quarterly Journal of Studies on Alcohol*, **29**, 610-33.

Pattison, E. M., Sobell, M. B., and Sobell, L. C., ed. (1977). *Emerging concepts of alcohol dependence*, Springer, New York.

Patton, M. Q. (1980). *Qualitative evaluation methods*. Sage, Beverly Hills, Calif.

Paul, G. L. (1967). Strategy of outcome research in psychotherapy, *Journal of Consulting Psychology*, **31**, 109-18.

Pavlov, I. P. (1927). *Conditioned reflexes: An investigation of the physiological activity of the cerebral cortex*, trans. G. V. Anrep. Oxford University Press, London.

Peele, S. (1985). *The meaning of addiction: Compulsive experience and its interpretation*, Lexington Books, Lexington, Mass.

Peele, S. (1986). The implications and limitations of genetic models of alcoholism and other addictions, *Journal of Studies on Alcohol*, **47**, 63-73.

Peele, S. (1987). Why do controlled-drinking outcomes vary by investigator, by country and by era? Cultural conceptions of relapse and remission in alcoholism, *Drug and Alcohol Dependence*, **20**, 173-201.

Pemper, K. (1976). Dimensions of change in the improving alcoholic, *The International Journal of the Addictions*, **11**, 641–9.

Pendery, M. L., Maltzman, I. M., and West, L. J. (1982). Controlled drinking by alcoholics? New findings and a reevaluation of a major affirmative study, *Science*, **217**, 169–75.

Pervin, L. A. (1978). Definitions, measurements, and classifications of stimuli, situations, and environments, *Human Ecology*, **6**, 71–105.

Pettinati, H. M., Sugerman, A. A., DiDonato, N., and Maurer, H. S. (1982*a*). The natural history of alcoholism over four years after treatment, *Journal of Studies on Alcohol*, **43**, 201–15.

Pettinati, H. M., Sugerman, A. A., and Maurer, H. S. (1982*b*). Four year MMPI changes in abstinent and drinking alcoholics, *Alcoholism: Clinical and Experimental Research*, **6**, 487–94.

Pierce, R. M., Schanble, P. G., and Farkas, A. (1970). Teaching internalization behavior to clients, *Psychotherapy: Theory, Research, and Practice*, **7**, 217–20.

Pittel, S. M. and Hofer, R. (1974). A systematic approach to drug abuse treatment referral, *Journal of Psychedelic Drugs*, **6**, 253–8.

Pittman, D. J. and Tate, R. L. (1969). A comparison of two treatment programs for alcoholics, *Quarterly Journal of Studies on Alcohol*, **30**, 888–99.

Plant, M. A. (1977). Alcoholism and occupation: A review, *British Journal of Addiction*, **72**, 309–16.

Plant, M. A. (1979*a*). *Drinking careers: Occupations, drinking habits, and drinking problems*, Tavistock, London.

Plant, M. A. (1979*b*). Occupations, drinking patterns and alcohol-related problems: Conclusions from a follow-up study, *British Journal of Addiction*, **74**, 267–73.

Plato (1935). *The republic, Vol. 2*, trans. P. Shorey. William Heinemann, London.

Plotkin, W. R. (1985). A psychological approach to placebo: The role of faith in therapy and treatment. In *Placebo: Theory, research, and mechanisms* (ed. L. White, B. Tursky, and G. E. Schwartz) pp. 237–54. Guilford Press, New York.

Poldrugo, F. and Forti, B. (1988). Personality disorders and alcoholism treatment outcome, *Drug and Alcohol Dependence*, **21**, 171–6.

Polich, J. M. (1980). Patterns of remission in alcoholism. In *Alcoholism treatment in transition* (ed. G. Edwards and M. Grant) pp. 95–112. Croom Helm, London.

Polich, J. M., Armor, D. J., and Braiker, H. B. (1980). Patterns of alcoholism over four years, *Journal of Studies on Alcohol*, **41**, 397–416.

Polich, J. M., Armor, D. J., and Braiker, H. B. (1981). *The course of alcoholism: Four years after treatment*, Wiley, New York.

Pollack, I. W. and Kiev, A. (1963). Spatial orientation and psychotherapy: An experimental study of perception, *The Journal of Nervous and Mental Disease*, **137**, 93–7.

Pomerleau, O., Pertschuk, M., and Stinnet, J. (1976). A critical examination of some current assumptions in the treatment of alcoholism, *Journal of Studies on Alcohol*, **37**, 849–67.

Popper, K. R. (1959). *The logic of scientific discovery*, Hutchinson, London.

Porjesz, B. and Begleiter, H. (1983). Brain dysfunction and alcohol. In *The biology of alcoholism, Vol. 7: The pathogenesis of alcoholism—biological factors* (ed. B. Kissin and H. Begleiter) pp. 415–84. Plenum Press, New York.

Posthuma, A. B. and Carr, J. E. (1975). Differentiation matching in psychotherapy, *Canadian Psychological Review*, **16**, 35–43.

Powell, B. J., Penick, E. C., Read, M. R., and Ludwig, A. M. (1985). Comparison of three outpatient treatment interventions: A twelve-month follow-up of men alcoholics, *Journal of Studies on Alcohol*, **46**, 309–12.

Prioleau, L., Murdock, M., and Brody, N. (1983). An analysis of psychotherapy versus placebo studies, *The Behavioral and Brain Sciences*, **6**, 275–85.

Rachman, S. J. and Hodgson, R. J. (1980). *Obsessions and compulsions*, Prentice-Hall, Englewood Cliffs, NJ.

Rachman, S. J. and Wilson, G. T. (1980). *The effects of psychological therapy*, 2nd edn. Pergamon Press, Oxford.

Rankin, H. and Hodgson, R. (1977). Cue exposure: One approach to the extinction of addictive behaviors: In *Alcohol intoxication and withdrawal, Vol. 3b* (ed. M. M. Gross) pp. 621–30. Plenum Press, New York.

Rathod, R. (1977). Making treatment better. In *Alcoholism: New knowledge and new responses* (ed. G. Edwards and M. Grant) pp. 308–12. Croom Helm, London.

Reid, J. B. (1978). Study of drinking in natural settings. In *Behavioral approaches to alcoholism* (ed. G. A. Marlatt and P. E. Nathan) pp. 58–74. NIAAA–RUCAS Alcoholism Treatment Series, No. 2, Rutgers Center of Alcohol Studies, New Brunswick, NJ.

Renner, J. W., Stafford, D. G., Lawson, A. E., McKinnon, J. W., Friot, F. E., and Kellogg, D. N. (1976). *Research, teaching, and learning with the Piaget model*, University of Oklahoma Press, Norman, Okla.

Reynolds, C. M., Merry, J., and Coppen, A. (1977). Prophylactic treatment of alcoholism by lithium carbonate: An initial report, *Alcoholism: Clinical and Experimental Research*, **1**, 109–11.

Ridgely, M. S., ed. (1989). Special section on dual diagnosis, *Hospital and Community Psychiatry*, **40**, 1019–49.

Riley, D. M., Sobell, L. C., Leo, G. I., Sobell, M. B., and Klajner, F. (1987). Behavioral treatment of alcohol problems: A review and a comparison of behavioral and nonbehavioral studies. In *Treatment and prevention of alcohol problems: A resource manual* (ed. W. M. Cox) pp. 73–115. Academic Press, Orlando, Fla.

Robertson, L. (1973). Matching Instructional Method to Student Learning Style in Art Interpretation: A Replication. University of Toronto, Toronto. (Master's thesis)

Robins, L. N. (1966). *Deviant children grown up: A sociological and psychiatric study of sociopathic personality*, Williams and Wilkins, Baltimore.

Robinson, D. (1971). *The process of becoming ill*, Routledge and Kegan Paul, London.

Robinson, D. (1972). The alcohologist's addiction: Some implications of having lost control over the disease concept of alcoholism, *Quarterly Journal of Studies on Alcohol*, **33**, 1028–42.

Rogers, C. R. (1957). The necessary and sufficient conditions of therapeutic personality change, *Journal of Consulting Psychology*, **21**, 95–103.

Rohsenow, D. J. and O'Leary, M. R. (1978a). Locus of control research on alcoholic populations: A review. 1: Development, scales, and treatment, *The International Journal of the Addictions*, **13**, 55–78.

Rohsenow, D. J. and O'Leary, M. R. (1978b). Locus of control research on alcoholic populations: A review. 2: Relationship to other measures, *The International Journal of the Addictions*, **13**, 213–26.

Roizen, R., Cahalan, D., and Shanks, P. (1978). Spontaneous remission among untreated problem drinkers. In *Longitudinal research in drug use: Empirical findings and methodological issues* (ed. D. B. Kandel). Wiley, New York.

Roman, P. M. and Trice, H. M. (1968). The sick role, labelling theory, and the deviant drinker, *The International Journal of Social Psychiatry*, **14**, 245–51.

Rönnberg, S. (1979). Behavioral analysis of alcohol abuse. In *Trends in behavior therapy* (ed. P.-O. Sjödén, S. Bates, and W. S. Dockens III) pp. 181–97. Academic Press, New York.

Roodin, P. A., Broughton, A., and Vaught, G. M. (1974). Effects of birth order, sex, and family size on field dependence and locus of control, *Perceptual and Motor Skills*, **39**, 671–6.

Room, R. (1972). Comments on 'the alcohologist's addiction', *Quarterly Journal of Studies on Alcohol*, **33**, 1049–59.

Room, R. (1983). Sociology and the disease concept of alcoholism. In *Research advances in alcohol and drug problems, Vol. 7* (ed. R. G. Smart, F. B. Glaser, Y. Israel, H. Kalant, R. E. Popham, and W. Schmidt) pp. 47–91. Plenum Press, New York.

Room, R. (1984). A 'reverence for strong drink': The lost generation and the elevation of alcohol in American culture, *Journal of Studies on Alcohol*, **45**, 540–6.

Room, R. (1989). The U.S. general population's experiences of responding to alcohol problems, *British Journal of Addiction*, **84**, 1291–304.

Rose, G. S., Powell, B. J., and Penick, E. C. (1978). Determinants of locus of control orientation in male alcoholics, *Journal of Clinical Psychology*, **34**, 250–1.

Rosen, A. (1981). Psychotherapy and Alcoholics Anonymous: Can they be coordinated? *Bulletin of the Menninger Clinic*, **45**, 229–46.

Rosenbaum, M., Friedlander, J., and Kaplan, S. M. (1956). Evaluation of results of psychotherapy, *Psychosomatic Medicine*, **18**, 113–32.

Rosenbaum, P., Laverty, S. G., Ogurzsoff, S., and Bowman, M. (1977). *Development of an alcohol abuse treatment system: The Kingston treatment development research team, Third annual report*, Substudy No. 922, Addiction Research Foundation, Toronto.

Rosenthal, R. (1979). The 'file drawer problem' and tolerance for null results, *Psychological Bulletin*, **86**, 638–41.

Rosenzweig, S. (1936). Some implicit common factors in diverse methods of psychotherapy, *American Journal of Orthopsychiatry*, **6**, 412–15.

Ross, A. O. (1963). Deviant case analysis: Neglected approach to behavior research, *Perceptual and Motor Skills*, **16**, 337–49.

Ross, A. O. (1981). Of rigor and relevance, *Professional Psychology*, **12**, 318–27.

Rotter, J. B. (1954). *Social learning and clinical psychology*, Prentice-Hall, Englewood Cliffs, NJ.

Rotter, J. B. (1966). Generalized expectancies for internal versus external control of reinforcement, *Psychological Monographs*, **80** (1, Whole No. 609).

Rotter, J. B. (1975). Some problems and misconceptions related to the construct of Internal versus External control of reinforcement, *Journal of Consulting and Clinical Psychology*, **43**, 56–67.

Rounsaville, B. J., Dolinsky, Z. S., Babor, T. F., and Meyer, R. E. (1987). Psychopathology as a predictor of treatment outcome in alcoholics, *Archives of General Psychiatry*, **44**, 505–13.

Rush, B. (1785) *An inquiry into the effects of ardent spirits upon the human body and mind; with an account of the means of preventing and of the remedies for curing them.* (Reprinted in *Quarterly Journal of Alcohol Studies*, 1943, **4**, 324–41).

Rush, B. (1990). A systems approach to estimating the required capacity of alcohol treatment services, *British Journal of Addiction*, **85**, 49–59.

Rush, B., Brook, R., and Graham, K. (1982). Alcoholics in Ontario: Where do they go for help and what happens when they get there? *Canadian Journal of Community Mental Health*, **1**, 59-70.

Russakoff, L. M., Fontana, A. F., Dowds, B. N., and Harris, M. (1976). Psychological differentiation and psychotherapy, *The Journal of Nervous and Mental Disease*, **163**, 329-33.

Ryan, C. and Butters, N. (1983). Cognitive deficits in alcoholics. In *The biology of alcoholism, Vol. 7: The pathogenesis of alcoholism—biological factors* (ed. B. Kissin and H. Begleiter) pp. 485-538. Plenum Press, New York.

Rychtarik, R. G., Foy, D. W., Scott, T., Lokey, L., and Prue, D. M. (1987). Five-six-year follow-up of broad-spectrum behavioral treatment for alcoholism: Effects of training controlled drinking skills, *Journal of Consulting and Clinical Psychology*, **55**, 106-8.

Saliba, C. (1982). *La cure de désintoxication alcoolique et ses prolongements*, Presses Universitaires de Lyon, Lyon.

Samsonowitz, V. and Sjöberg, L. (1981). Volitional problems of socially adjusted alcoholics, *Addictive Behaviors*, **6**, 385-98.

Sanchez-Craig, M., Annis, H. M., Bornet, A. R., and MacDonald, K. R. (1984). Random assignment to abstinence and controlled drinking: Evaluation of a cognitive-behavioral program for problem drinkers, *Journal of Consulting and Clinical Psychology*, **52**, 390-403.

Sanchez-Craig, M. and Lei, H. (1986). Disadvantages to imposing the goal of abstinence on problem drinkers: An empirical study, *British Journal of Addiction*, **81**, 505-12.

Sandler, J. (1987). The concept of superego. In *From safety to superego* (ed. J. Sandler) pp. 17-44. Karnac, London.

Sarbin, T. R. (1943). A contribution to the study of actuarial and individual methods of prediction, *American Journal of Sociology*, **48**, 593-602.

Sarnecki, J. and Sollenhag, S. (1985). *Predicting social maladjustment*. Stockholm Boys Grown Up, Vol. 1, National Council for Crime Prevention (Report No. 17), Stockholm.

Saunders, W. M. and Kershaw, P. W. (1979). Spontaneous remission from alcoholism: A community study, *British Journal of Addiction*, **74**, 251-65.

Sawyer, J. (1966). Measurement *and* prediction, clinical *and* statistical, *Psychological Bulletin*, **66**, 178-200.

Schlesinger, H. J., Mumford, E., and Glass, G. V. (1980). Mental health services and medical utilization. In *Psychotherapy: Practice, research, policy* (ed. G. R. VandenBos) pp. 71-102. Sage, Beverly Hills, Calif.

Schmidt, W. and Popham, R. E. (1976). Impressions of Jewish alcoholics, *Journal of Studies on Alcohol*, **37**, 931-9.

Schmidt, W., Smart, R. G., and Moss, M. K. (1968). *Social class and the treatment of alcoholism*. Brookside Monograph of the Addiction Research Foundation No. 7, University of Toronto Press, Toronto.

Schroder, H. M. (1971). Conceptual complexity and personality organization. In *Personality theory and information processing* (ed. H. M. Schroder and P. Suedfeld) pp. 240-74. Ronald, New York.

Schroder, H. M., Driver, M. J., and Streufert, S. (1967). *Human information processing: Individuals and groups in complex social situations*, Holt, Rinehart and Winston, New York.

Schuckit, M. A. (1985). The clinical implications of primary diagnostic groups among alcoholics, *Archives of General Psychiatry*, **42**, 1043-9.

Schuckit, M. A. (1986). Genetic and clinical implications of alcoholism and affective disorder, *American Journal of Psychiatry*, **143**, 140–7.

Schuckit, M. A. and Cahalan, D. (1976). Evaluation of alcoholism treatment programs. In *Alcohol and alcohol problems: New thinking and new directions* (ed. W. J. Filstead, J. J. Rossi, and M. Keller) pp. 229–66. Ballinger, Cambridge, Mass.

Schuckit, M. A. and Winokur, G. (1972). A short term follow-up of women alcoholics, *Diseases of the Nervous System*, **33**, 672–8.

Searles, J. S. (1988). The role of genetics in the pathogenesis of alcoholism, *Journal of Abnormal Psychology*, **97**, 153–67.

Sechrest, L., White, S. O., and Brown, E. D., ed. (1979). *The rehabilitation of criminal offenders: Problems and prospects*. National Academy of Sciences, Washington, DC.

Seeley, J. R. (1962). Alcoholism is a disease: Implications for social policy. In *Society, culture, and drinking patterns* (ed. D. J. Pittman and C. R. Snyder) pp. 586–93. Wiley, New York.

Seeman, M. and Evans, J. W. (1962). Alienation and learning in a hospital setting, *American Sociological Review*, **27**, 772–82.

Seevers, M. H. (1969). Drugs, monkeys, and men, *Michigan Quarterly Review*, **8**, 3–14.

Seiden, R. H. (1960). The use of Alcoholics Anonymous members in research on alcoholism, *Quarterly Journal of Studies on Alcohol*, **21**, 506–9.

Seliger, R. V. (1938). The problem of the alcoholic in the community, *American Journal of Psychiatry*, **95**, 701–16.

Selzer, M. D. (1971). The Michigan Alcoholism Screening Test: The quest for a new diagnostic instrument, *American Journal of Psychiatry*, **127**, 1653–9.

Shadel, C. A. (1944). Aversion treatment of alcohol addiction, *Quarterly Journal of Studies on Alcohol*, **5**, 216–28.

Shapiro, D. A. and Shapiro, D. (1982). Meta-analysis of comparative therapy outcome studies: A replication and refinement, *Psychological Bulletin*, **92**, 581–604.

Shaw, S. (1980). A critique of the concept of the alcohol dependence syndrome, *British Journal of Addiction*, **74**, 339–48.

Shaw, S. (1985). The disease concept of dependence. In *The misuse of alcohol: Crucial issues in dependence, treatment and prevention* (ed. N. Heather, I. Robertson, and P. Davies) pp. 35–44. Croom Helm, Beckenham.

Shipman, S. and Shipman, V. C. (1985). Cognitive styles: Some conceptual, methodological, and applied issues. In *Review of research in education, Vol. 12* (ed. E. W. Gordon) pp. 229–91. American Educational Research Association, Washington, DC.

Short, J. F. and Nye, F. I. (1962). Reported behavior as a criterion of deviant behavior. In *The sociology of crime and delinquency* (ed. M. E. Wolfgang, L. Savitz, and N. Johnston) pp. 44–9. Wiley, New York.

Shows, W. D. and Carson, R. C. (1965). The A–B therapist 'type' distinction and spatial orientation: Replication and extension, *The Journal of Nervous and Mental Disease*, **141**, 456–62.

Shrauger, S. and Altrocchi, J. (1964). The personality of the perceiver as a factor in person perception, *Psychological Bulletin*, **62**, 289–308.

Siegler, M., Osmond, H., and Newell, S. (1968). Models of alcoholism, *Quarterly Journal of Studies on Alcohol*, **29**, 571–91.

Simmel, E. (1948). Alcoholism and addiction, *Psychoanalytic Quarterly*, **17**, 6–31.

Singer, M. (1984). Spiritual healing and family therapy: Common approaches to the treatment of alcoholism, *Family Therapy*, **11**, 155–62.

Sisson, R. W. and Azrin, N. H. (1986). Family-member involvement, to initiate and promote treatment of problem drinkers, *Journal of Behavior Therapy and Experimental Psychiatry*, **17**, 15–21.

Sjöberg, L. (1982). Aided and unaided decision making: Improving intuitive judgement, *Journal of Forecasting*, **1**, 349–63.

Sjöberg, L. and Samsonowitz, V. (1985). Coping strategies and relapse in alcohol abuse, *Drug and Alcohol Dependence*, **15**, 283–301.

Sjöberg, L., Samsonowitz, V., and Olsson, G. (1983). Volitional problems of Skid Row alcoholics, *Journal of Psychiatric Treatment and Evaluation*, **5**, 175–84.

Skinner, H. A. (1979). A model of psychopathology based on the MMPI. In *MMPI: Current clinical and research trends* (ed. C. S. Newmark) pp. 276–305. Praeger, New York.

Skinner, H. A. (1980*a*). Client–treatment matching and the anti-alcohol drugs. Paper presented at a symposium on the Anti-Alcohol Drugs: Current Status in Alcoholism Treatment, Toronto, Can., March 10–11.

Skinner, H. A. (1980*b*). Profiles of treatment-seeking populations. In *Alcoholism treatment in transition* (ed. G. Edwards and M. Grant) pp. 248–63. Croom Helm, London.

Skinner, H. A. (1981*a*). Assessment of alcohol problems: Basic principles, critical issues, and future trends. In *Research advances in alcohol and drug problems, Vol. 6* (ed. Y. Israel, F. B. Glaser, H. Kalant, R. E. Popham, W. Schmidt, and R. G. Smart) pp. 319–69. Plenum Press, New York.

Skinner, H. A. (1981*b*). Different strokes for different folks: Differential treatment for alcohol abuse. In *Evaluation of the alcoholic: Implications for research, theory and treatment* (ed. R. E. Meyer, B. C. Glueck, J. E. O'Brien, T. F. Babor, J. H. Jaffe, and J. R. Stabenau) pp. 349–67. Research Monograph No. 5, National Institute on Alcohol Abuse and Alcoholism, Rockville, Md.

Skinner, H. A. and Allen, B. A. (1982). Alcohol dependence syndrome: Measurement and validation, *Journal of Abnormal Psychology*, **91**, 199–209.

Skinner, H. A. and Allen, B. A. (1983). Does the computer make a difference? Computerized versus face-to-face versus self-report assessment of alcohol, drug, and tobacco use, *Journal of Consulting and Clinical Psychology*, **51**, 267–75.

Skog, O.-J. (1980). Social interaction and the distribution of alcohol consumption, *Journal of Drug Issues*, **10**, 71–92.

Skog, O.-J. (1985). The collectivity of drinking cultures: A theory of the distribution of alcohol consumption, *British Journal of Addiction*, **80**, 83–99.

Skog, O.-J. (1989). The socio-cultural foundation of drinking problems. In *Proceedings of the 35th International Congress on Alcoholism and Drug Dependence, Vol. 4.* (ed. R. B. Waahlberg) pp. 317–48. National Directorate for the Prevention of Alcohol and Drug Problems, Oslo.

Smart, R. G. (1975). Spontaneous recovery in alcoholics: A review and analysis of the available research, *Drug and Alcohol Dependence*, **1**, 277–85.

Smart, R. G. (1978*a*). Characteristics of alcoholics who drink socially after treatment, *Alcoholism: Clinical and Experimental Research*, **2**, 49–52.

Smart, R. G. (1978*b*). Do some alcoholics do better in some types of treatment than others? *Drug and Alcohol Dependence*, **3**, 65–75.

Smith, H. and Jackson, G. (1982). The Rand Reports reviewed: A critical analysis, *Advances in Alcohol and Substance Abuse*, **2** (2), 7–15.

Smith, M. L. (1980). Publication bias and meta-analysis, *Evaluation in Education*, **4**, 22–4.

Smith, M. L. and Glass, G. V. (1977). Meta-analysis of psychotherapy outcome studies, *American Psychologist*, **32**, 752-60.

Smith, M. L., Glass, G. V., and Miller, T. I. (1980). *The benefits of psychotherapy*. Johns Hopkins University Press, Baltimore, Md.

Smith, R. E. (1970). Changes in locus of control as a function of life crisis resolution, *Journal of Abnormal Psychology*, **75**, 328-32.

Snyder, C. R. (1958). *Alcohol and the Jews: A cultural study of drinking and sobriety*. Free Press, Glencoe, Ill.

Snyder, C. R. (1962). Culture and Jewish sobriety: The ingroup-outgroup factor. In *Society, culture, and drinking patterns* (ed. D. J. Pittman and C. R. Snyder) pp. 188-225. Wiley, New York.

Sobell, L. C. (1978). Critique of alcoholism treatment evaluation. In *Behavioral approaches to alcoholism* (ed. G. A. Marlatt and P. E. Nathan) pp. 166-82. NIAAA-RUCAS Alcoholism Treatment Series, No. 2, Rutgers Center of Alcohol Studies, New Brunswick, NJ.

Sobell, L. C. and Sobell, M. B. (1977). Alcohol problems. In *Behavioral approaches to medical treatment* (ed. R. B. Williams, Jr. and W. D. Gentry) pp. 183-201. Ballinger, Cambridge, Mass.

Sobell, L. C. and Sobell, M. B. (1982). Alcoholism treatment outcome evaluation methodology. In *Prevention, intervention and treatment: Concerns and models*. Alcohol and Health Monograph No. 3, National Institute on Alcohol Abuse and Alcoholism, Rockville, Md., pp. 293-321.

Sobell, M. B., Brochu, S., Sobell, L. C., Roy, J., and Stevens, J. A. (1987). Alcoholism treatment outcome evaluation methodology: State of the art 1980-1984, *Addictive Behaviors*, **12**, 113-28.

Sobell, M. B. and Sobell, L. C. (1973). Alcoholics treated by individualized behavior therapy: One year treatment outcome, *Behaviour Research and Therapy*, **11**, 599-618.

Sobell, M. B. and Sobell, L. C. (1976). Second year treatment outcome of alcoholics treated by individualized behavior therapy: Results, *Behavior Research and Therapy*, **14**, 195-215.

Sobell, M. B. and Sobell, L. C. (1978). *Behavioral treatment of alcohol problems: Individualized therapy and controlled drinking*. Plenum Press, New York.

Sobell, M. B. and Sobell, L. C. (1984). The aftermath of heresy: A response to Pendery *et al.*'s (1982) critique of 'Individualized behavior therapy for alcoholics', *Behaviour Research and Therapy*, **22**, 413-40.

Sobell, M. B. and Sobell, L. C. (1987). Conceptual issues regarding goals in the treatment of alcohol problems. In *Moderation as a goal or outcome of treatment for alcohol problems: A dialogue* (ed. M. B. Sobell and L. C. Sobell) pp. 1-37. Drugs and Society Series, Vol. 1, Nos. 2/3. Haworth Press, New York

Sobell, M. B., Sobell, L. C., and Sheahan, D. B. (1976). Functional analysis of drinking problems as an aid in developing individual treatment strategies, *Addictive Behaviors*, **1**, 127-32.

Sokolow, L., Welte, J. W., Hynes, G., and Lyons, J. P. (1980). Treatment-related differences between female and male alcoholics, *Focus on Women: Journal of Addictions and Health*, **1**, 43-56.

Solomon, D. and Kendall, A. J. (1976). Individual characteristics and children's performance in 'open' and 'traditional' classroom settings, *Journal of Educational Psychology*, **68**, 613-25.

Solomon, R. L. and Wynne, L. C. (1953). Traumatic avoidance learning: Acquisition in normal dogs, *Psychological Monographs*, **67** (Whole No. 354).

Sousa-Poza, J. F. and Rohrberg, R. (1976). Communicational and interactional aspects of self-disclosure in psychotherapy: Differences related to cognitive style, *Psychiatry*, **39**, 81–91.

Spoth, R. (1983). Differential stress reduction: Preliminary application to an alcohol-abusing population, *The International Journal of the Addictions*, **18**, 835–49.

Spradley, J. P. (1970). *You owe yourself a drunk: An ethnography of urban nomads*, Little, Brown and Company, Boston.

SPRI. See The Swedish Planning and Rationalization Institute for the Health and Social Services.

Stall, R. (1983). An examination of spontaneous remission from problem drinking in the Bluegrass region of Kentucky, *Journal of Drug Issues*, **13**, 191–206.

Stallings, D. L. and Oncken, G. R. (1977). A relative change index in evaluating alcoholism treatment outcome, *Journal of Studies on Alcohol*, **38**, 457–64.

Stanton, A. H. and Schwartz, M. S. (1954). *The mental hospital*. Basic Books, New York.

Stein, L. I., Newton, J. R., and Bowman, R. S. (1975). Duration of hospitalization for alcoholism, *Archives of General Psychiatry*, **32**, 247–52.

Stein, M. I., ed. (1961). *Contemporary psychotherapies*. Free Press of Glencoe, New York.

Stewart, M. J. (1989). Social support: Diverse theoretical perspectives, *Social Science and Medicine*, **28**, 1275–82.

Stiles, W. B., Shapiro, D. A., and Elliott, R. (1986). 'Are all psychotherapies equivalent?' *American Psychologist*, **41**, 165–80.

Stinson, D. J., Smith, W. G., Amidjaya, I., and Kaplan, J. M. (1979). Systems of care and treatment outcomes for alcoholic patients, *Archives of General Psychiatry*, **36**, 535–9.

Stockwell, T. (1986). Cracking an old chestnut: Is controlled drinking possible for the person who has been severely alcohol dependent? *British Journal of Addiction*, **81**, 455–6.

Stockwell, T. (1988). Can severely dependent drinkers learn controlled drinking? Summing up the debate, *British Journal of Addiction*, **83**, 149–52.

Stockwell, T., Hodgson, R. J., Rankin, H. J., and Taylor, C. (1982). Alcohol dependence, beliefs and the priming effect, *Behaviour Research and Therapy*, **20**, 513–22.

Stockwell, T., Smail, P., Hodgson, R., and Canter, S. (1984). Alcohol dependence and phobic anxiety states, 2: A retrospective study, *British Journal of Psychiatry*, **144**, 58–63.

Stoil, M. J. (1989). Problems in the evaluation of hypnosis in the treatment of alcoholism, *Journal of Substance Abuse Treatment*, **6**, 31–5.

Storm, T. and Cutler, R. E. (1970). Systematic desensitization in the treatment of alcoholics. University of British Columbia. (Unpublished manuscript)

Straus, R. (1974). *Escape from custody: A study of alcoholism and institutional dependency as reflected in the life record of a homeless man*, Harper and Row, New York.

Strupp, H. H. (1970). Specific versus nonspecific factors in psychotherapy and the problem of control, *Archives of General Psychiatry*, **23**, 393–401.

Strupp, H. H. (1973). *Psychotherapy: Clinical, research, and theoretical issues*, Jason Aronson, New York.

Strupp, H. H. (1977). A reformulation of the dynamics of the therapist's contribution. In *Effective psychotherapy: A handbook of research* (ed. A. S. Gurman and A. M. Razin) pp. 3–22. Pergamon Press, Oxford.

Strupp, H. H. (1978). Psychotherapy research and practice: An overview. In *Handbook of psychotherapy and behavior change: An empirical analysis*, 2nd edn. (ed. S. L. Garfield and A. E. Bergin) pp. 3–22. Wiley, New York.

Strupp, H. H. (1982). The outcome problem in psychotherapy: Contemporary perspectives. In *Psychotherapy research and behavior change* (ed. J. H. Harvey and M. M. Parks) pp. 39–71. Master Lecture Series, Vol. 1, American Psychological Association, Washington, DC.

Strupp, H. H. (1986). The nonspecific hypothesis of therapeutic effectiveness: A current assessment, *American Journal of Orthopsychiatry*, 56, 513–20.

Strupp, H. H. and Bergin, A. E. (1969). Some empirical and conceptual bases for coordinated research in psychotherapy: A critical review of issues, trends, and evidence, *International Journal of Psychiatry*, 7, 18–90.

Strupp, H. H. and Hadley, S. W. (1979). Specific vs. nonspecific factors in psychotherapy: A controlled study of outcome, *Archives of General Psychiatry*, 36, 1125–36.

Sugerman, A. A. and Schneider, D. U. (1976). Cognitive styles in alcoholism. In *Alcoholism: Interdisciplinary approaches to an enduring problem* (ed. R. E. Tarter and A. A. Sugerman) pp. 395–433. Addison-Wesley, Reading, Mass.

Sutherland, E. H., Schroeder, H. G., and Tordella, O. L. (1950). Personality traits and the alcoholic: A critique of existing studies, *Quarterly Journal of Studies on Alcohol*, 11, 547–61.

Sutker, P. B. and Allain, A. N., Jr. (1988). Issues in personality conceptualizations of addictive behaviors, *Journal of Consulting and Clinical Psychology*, 56, 172–82.

The Swedish Planning and Rationalization Institute for the Health and Social Services, SPRI (1983). *Dödsorsak? Dödsorsaksstatistik som underlag för planering* (Cause of death? Cause-of-death statistics as a basis for planning). SPRI Report No. 122, SPRI, Stockholm.

Syme, L. (1957). Personality characteristics and the alcoholic: A critique of current studies, *Quarterly Journal of Studies on Alcohol*, 18, 288–301.

Szasz, T. S. (1964). *The myth of mental illness: Foundations of a theory of personal conduct*. Hoeber/Harper, New York.

Szasz, T. S. (1970). *Ideology and insanity*. Doubleday, New York.

Szasz, T. S. (1972). Bad habits are not diseases: A refutation of the claim that alcoholism is a disease, *Lancet*, i, 83–4.

Talbott, J. A. and Gillen, C. (1978). Differences between nonprofessional recovering alcoholic counselors treating Bowery alcoholics: A study of therapist variables, *Psychiatric Quarterly*, 50, 333–42.

Tamerin, J. S., Weiner, S., and Mendelson, J. H. (1970). Alcoholics' expectancies and recall of experiences during intoxication, *American Journal of Psychiatry*, 126, 1697–1704.

Taylor, J. R., Helzer, J. E., and Robins, L. N. (1986). Moderate drinking in ex-alcoholics: Recent studies, *Journal of Studies on Alcohol*, 47, 115–21.

Telch, M. J. (1981). The present status of outcome studies: A reply to Frank, *Journal of Consulting and Clinical Psychology*, 49, 472–5.

Thoits, P. A. (1982). Conceptual, methodological, and theoretical problems in studying social support as a buffer against life stress, *Journal of Health and Social Behavior*, 23, 145–59.

Thornton, C. C., Gottheil, E. L., Skoloda, T. E., and Alterman, A. I. (1979). Alcoholics' drinking decision: Implications for treatment and outcome. In *Addiction research and treatment: Converging trends* (ed. E. L. Gottheil, A. T. McLellan, K. A. Druley, and A. I. Alterman) pp. 133-8. Pergamon Press, New York.

Throop, W. E. and Macdonald, A. P., Jr. (1971). Internal-external locus of control: A bibliography, *Psychological Reports*, Monograph Supplement No. 1-V28, 175-90.

Thurstin, A. H. and Alfano, A. M. (1988). The association of alcoholic subtype with treatment outcome: An 18-month follow-up, *The International Journal of the Addictions*, **23**, 321-30.

Tiebout, H. M. (1951). The role of psychiatry in the field of alcoholism, *Quarterly Journal of Studies on Alcohol*, **12**, 52-7.

Tiebout, H. M. (1961). Alcoholics Anonymous—an experiment of nature, *Quarterly Journal of Studies on Alcohol*, **22**, 52-68.

Tobacyk, J. J., Broughton, A., and Vaught, G. M. (1975). Effects of congruence-incongruence between locus of control and field dependence on personality functioning, *Journal of Consulting and Clinical Psychology*, **43**, 81-5.

Tolor, A. and LeBlanc, R. F. (1971). Personality correlates of alienation, *Journal of Consulting and Clinical Psychology*, **37**, 444.

Tomlinson, P. D. and Hunt, D. E. (1971). Differential effects of rule–example order as a function of conceptual level, *Canadian Journal of Behavioural Science*, **3**, 237-45.

Tomsovic, M. and Edwards, R. V. (1970). Lysergide treatment of schizophrenic and nonschizophrenic alcoholics: A controlled evaluation, *Quarterly Journal of Studies on Alcohol*, **31**, 932-49.

Tourney, G. (1970). Psychiatric therapies: 1800-1968. In *Changing patterns in psychiatric care: An anthology of evolving scientific psychiatry in medicine* (ed. T. Rothman) pp. 3-42. Crown Publishers, New York.

Treffert, D. Specific Treatment in Two Sub-Groups of Alcoholics. Final report to research grant MH18441-02, US Department of Health, Education, and Welfare, Public Health Service, Health Service and Mental Health Administration. National Institute of Mental Health, US Government Printing Office, Washington, DC. N.d.

Trice, H. M. and Beyer, J. M. (1981). A data-based examination of selection-bias in the evaluation of a job-based alcoholism program, *Alcoholism: Clinical and Experimental Research*, **5**, 489-96.

Trice, H. M. and Beyer, J. M. (1982). Social control in worksettings: Using the constructive confrontation strategy with problem-drinking employees, *Journal of Drug Issues*, **12**, 21-49.

Trice, H. M. and Beyer, J. M. (1984). Work related outcomes of constructive confrontation strategies in a job-based alcoholism program, *Journal of Studies on Alcohol*, **45**, 393-404.

Trice, H. M., Roman, P. M., and Belasco, J. A. (1969). Selection for treatment: A predictive evaluation of an alcoholism treatment regimen, *The International Journal of the Addictions*, **4**, 303-17.

Trice, H. M. and Sonnenstuhl, W. J. (1988). Constructive confrontation and other referral processes. In *Recent developments in alcoholism, Vol. 6* (ed. M. Galanter) pp. 159-70. Plenum Press, New York.

Trotter, T. (1804). *An essay, medical, philosophical, and chemical on drunkenness and its effects on the human body.* London. (Reprinted 1988 by Routledge, London. Tavistock Classics in the History of Psychiatry Series.)

Tuchfeld, B. S. (1981). Spontaneous remission in alcoholics: Empirical observations and theoretical implications, *Journal of Studies on Alcohol*, **42**, 626-41.

Tuchfeld, B. S. and Marcus, S. H. (1982). Methodological issues in evaluating alcoholism treatment effectiveness, *Advances in Alcoholism*, **2** (Whole No. 23).

Ullman, L. P. and Krasner, L. (1969). *A psychological approach to abnormal behavior*. Prentice-Hall, Englewood Cliffs, NJ.

Vaillant, G. E. (1980*a*). Natural history of male psychological health, 8: Antecedents of alcoholism and 'orality', *American Journal of Psychiatry*, **137**, 181-6.

Vaillant, G. E. (1980*b*). The doctor's dilemma. In *Alcoholism treatment in transition* (ed. G. Edwards and M. Grant) pp. 13-31. Croom Helm, London.

Vaillant, G. E. (1981). Dangers of psychotherapy in the treatment of alcoholism. In *Dynamic approaches to the understanding and treatment of alcoholism* (ed. M. H. Bean and N. E. Zinberg) pp. 36-54. Free Press/Macmillan, New York.

Vaillant, G. E. (1983*a*). Natural history of male alcoholism, 5: Is alcoholism the cart or the horse to sociopathy? *British Journal of Addiction*, **78**, 317-26.

Vaillant, G. E. (1983*b*) *The natural history of alcoholism: Causes, patterns, and paths to recovery*. Harvard University Press, Cambridge, Mass.

Vaillant, G. E. (1984). The contribution of prospective studies to the understanding of etiologic factors in alcoholism. In *Research advances in alcohol and drug problems, Vol. 8* (ed. R. G. Smart, H. D. Cappell, F. B. Glaser, Y. Israel, H. Kalant, R. E. Popham, W. Schmidt, and E. M. Selles) pp. 265-89. Plenum Press, New York.

Vaillant, G. E. (1986). Cultural factors in the etiology of alcoholism: A prospective study, *Annals of the New York Academy of Sciences*, **472**, 142-8.

Vaillant, G. E. (1988). What can long-term follow-up teach us about relapse and prevention of relapse in addiction? *British Journal of Addiction*, **83**, 1147-57.

Vaillant, G. E., Clark, W., Cyrus, C., Milofsky, E. S., Kopp, J., Wulsin, V. W., and Mogielnicki, N. P. (1983). Prospective study of alcoholism treatment: Eight-year follow-up, *The American Journal of Medicine*, **75**, 455-63.

Vaillant, G. E. and Milofsky, E. S. (1982*a*). Natural history of male alcoholism, 4: Paths to recovery, *Archives of General Psychiatry*, **39**, 127-33.

Vaillant, G. E. and Milofsky, E. S. (1982*b*). The etiology of alcoholism: A prospective viewpoint, *American Psychologist*, **37**, 494-503.

van Dijk, W. K. (1972). Where are we, what is permitted, what is the impact? Plenary lecture given at the 30th International Congress on Alcoholism and Addictions, Amsterdam, September.

van Dijk, W. K. (1977). Vicious circles in alcoholism and drug dependence. In *Drug dependence: Current problems and issues* (ed. M. M. Glatt) pp. 97-104. MTP Press, Lancaster, England.

Van Hasselt, V. B., Hersen, M., and Milliones, J. (1978). Social skills training for alcoholics and drug addicts: A review, *Addictive Behaviors*, **3**, 221-33.

Vannicelli, M. (1984). Treatment outcome of alcoholic women: The state of the art in relation to sex bias and expectancy effects. In *Alcohol problems in women: Antecedents, consequences, and intervention* (ed. S. C. Wilsnack and L. J. Beckman) pp. 369-412. Guilford Press, New York.

Vannicelli, M. and Nash, L. (1984). Effect of sex bias on women's studies on alcoholism, *Alcoholism: Clinical and Experimental Research*, **8**, 334-6.

Verden, P. and Shatterly, D. (1971). Alcoholism research and resistance to understanding the compulsive drinker, *Mental Hygiene*, **55**, 331-6.

Voegtlin, W. L. and Lemere, F. (1942). The treatment of alcohol addiction: A review of the literature, *Quarterly Journal of Studies on Alcohol*, **2**, 717-803.

Vogler, R. E., Lunde, S. E., Johnson, G. R., and Martin, P. L. (1970). Electrical aversion conditioning with chronic alcoholics, *Journal of Consulting and Clinical Psychology*, **34**, 302-7.

Vogler, R. E., Lunde, S. E., and Martin, P. L. (1971). Electrical aversion conditioning with chronic alcoholics: Follow-up and suggestions for research, *Journal of Consulting and Clinical Psychology*, **36**, 450.

von Knorring, A.-L., Bohman, M., von Knorring, L., and Oreland, L. (1985*a*). Platelet MAO-activity as a biological marker in subgroups of alcoholism, *Acta Psychiatrica Scandinavica*, **72**, 51-8.

von Knorring, L., Palm, U., and Andersson, H.-E. (1985*b*). Relationship between treatment outcome and subtype of alcoholism in men, *Journal of Studies on Alcohol*, **46**, 388-91.

Vuchinich, R. E. and Tucker, J. A. (1988). Contributions from behavioral theories of choice to an analysis of alcohol abuse, *Journal of Abnormal Psychology*, **97**, 181-95.

Wagman, A. M. I. and Allen, R. P. (1975). Effects of alcohol ingestion and abstinence in slow wave sleep of alcoholics. In *Alcohol intoxication and withdrawal: Experimental studies 2* (ed. M. M. Gross) pp. 453-66. Plenum Press, New York.

Walker, R. D., Donovan, D. M., Kivlahan, D. R., and O'Leary, M. R. (1983). Length of stay, neuropsychological performance, and aftercare: Influences on alcohol treatment outcome, *Journal of Consulting and Clinical Psychology*, **51**, 900-11.

Wallerstein, R. S. (1956). Comparative study of treatment methods for chronic alcoholism: The alcoholism research project at Winter VA Hospital, *American Journal of Psychiatry*, **113**, 228-33.

Wallerstein, R. S. (1957). *Hospital treatment of alcoholism: A comparative experimental study*, Basic Books, New York.

Ward, D. A., Bendel, R. B., and Lange, D. (1982). A reconsideration of environmental resources and the posttreatment functioning of alcoholic patients, *Journal of Health and Social Behavior*, **23**, 310-17.

Ward, R. F. and Faillace, L. A. (1970). The alcoholic and his helpers: A systems view, *Quarterly Journal of Studies on Alcohol*, **27**, 620-35.

Warren, M. Q. (1969). The case for differential treatment of delinquents, *Annals of the American Academy of Politics and Social Science*, **381**, 47-59.

Watson, C. G. and Pucel, J. (1985). Consistency of posttreatment alcoholics' drinking patterns, *Journal of Consulting and Clinical Psychology*, **53**, 679-83.

Weiner, M. F. and Crowder, J. D. (1986). Psychotherapy and cognitive style, *American Journal of Psychotherapy*, **40**, 17-25.

Welte, J. W., Hynes, G., Sokolow, L., and Lyons, J. P. (1979). Outcome study of alcoholism rehabilitation units: An outcome study of New York State operated alcoholism rehabilitation units. Research Institute on Alcoholism, New York State Division of Alcoholism and Alcohol Abuse, Albany, NY.

Welte, J. W., Hynes, G., Sokolow, L., and Lyons, J. P. (1981). Effect of length of stay in inpatient alcoholism treatment on outcome, *Journal of Studies on Alcohol*, **42**, 483-91.

Welte, J. W., Lyons, J. P., and Sokolow, L. (1983). Relapse rates for former clients of alcoholism rehabilitation units who are drinking without symptoms, *Drug and Alcohol Dependence*, **12**, 25-9.

Whitehead, P. C. and Simpkins, J. (1983). Occupational factors in alcoholism: In *The biology of alcoholism, Vol. 6: The pathogenesis of alcoholism—psychosocial factors* (ed. B. Kissin and H. Begleiter) pp. 405-553. Plenum Press, New York.

WHO. *See* World Health Organization.

Wiens, A. N. and Menustik, C. E. (1983). Treatment outcome and patient characteristics in an aversion therapy program for alcoholism, *American Psychologist*, **38**, 1089–96.

Wiggins, J. S. (1973). *Personality and prediction: Principles of personality assessment*. Addison-Wesley, Reading, Mass.

Wiggins, N. and Hoffman, P. J. (1968). Three models of clinical judgement, *Journal of Abnormal Psychology*, **73**, 70–7.

Wilbur, B. M., Salkin, D., and Birnbaum, H. (1966). The response of tuberculous alcoholics to a therapeutic community, *Quarterly Journal of Studies on Alcohol*, **27**, 620–35.

Wilkins, W. (1979). Expectancies in therapy research: Discriminating among heterogeneous nonspecifics, *Journal of Consulting and Clinical Psychology*, **47**, 837–45.

Wilkins, W. (1984). Psychotherapy: The powerful placebo, *Journal of Consulting and Clinical Psychology*, **52**, 570–3.

Wilkinson, D. A. and Carlen, P. L. (1981). Chronic organic brain syndromes associated with alcoholism: Neuropsychological and other aspects. In *Research advances in alcohol and drug problems, Vol. 6* (ed. Y. Israel, F. B. Glaser, H. Kalant, R. E. Popham, W. Schmidt, and R. G. Smart) pp. 107–45. Plenum Press, New York.

Wilkinson, D. A. and Sanchez-Craig, M. (1981). Relevance of brain dysfunction to treatment objectives: Should alcohol-related cognitive deficits influence the way we think about treatment? *Addictive Behaviors*, **6**, 253–60.

Willems, P. J. A., Letemendia, F. J. J., and Arroyave, F. (1973). A two-year follow-up study comparing short with long stay in-patient treatment of alcoholics, *British Journal of Psychiatry*, **122**, 637–48.

Wilson, G. T. and Rachman, S. J. (1983). Meta-analysis and the evaluation of psychotherapy outcome: Limitations and liabilities, *Journal of Consulting and Clinical Psychology*, **51**, 54–64.

Wilson, G. T. (1988). Alcohol use and abuse: A social learning analysis. In *Theories on alcoholism* (ed. C. D. Chaudron and D. A. Wilkinson) pp. 239–87. Addiction Research Foundation, Toronto.

Winokur, G., Clayton, D. J., and Reich, T. (1969). *Manic depressive illness*. C. V. Mosby, St. Louis.

Wise, R. A. (1988). The neurobiology of craving: Implications for the understanding and treatment of addiction, *Journal of Abnormal Psychology*, **97**, 118–32.

Wise, R. A. and Bozarth, M. A. (1987). A psychomotor stimulant theory of addiction, *Psychological Review*, **94**, 469–92.

Witkin, H. A. (1950). Individual differences in ease of perception of embedded figures, *Journal of Personality*, **19**, 1–15.

Witkin, H. A. (1965). Psychological differentiation and forms of pathology, *Journal of Abnormal Psychology*, **70**, 317–36.

Witkin, H. A., Dyk, R. B., Faterson, H. F., Goodenough, D. R., and Karp, S. A. (1962). *Psychological differentiation: Studies of development*, Wiley, New York.

Witkin, H. A. and Goodenough, D. R. (1977). Field dependence and interpersonal behavior, *Psychological Bulletin*, **84**, 661–89.

Witkin, H. A. and Goodenough, D. R. (1981). *Cognitive styles, essence and origins: Field dependence and field independence*. Psychological Issues, Monograph No. 51, International Universities Press, New York.

Witkin, H. A., Goodenough, D. R., and Oltman, P. K. (1979). Psychological differentiation: Current status, *Journal of Personality and Social Psychology*, **37**, 1127–45.

Witkin, H. A., Lewis, H. B., Hertzman, M., Machover, K., Meissner, P. B., and Wapner, S. (1954). *Personality through perception: An experimental and clinical study*. Harper and Brothers, New York.

Witkin, H. A., Lewis, H. B., and Weil, E. (1968). Affective reactions and patient–therapist interactions among more differentiated and less differentiated patients early in therapy, *The Journal of Nervous and Mental Disease*, **146**, 193–208.

Witkin, H. A., Moore, C. A., Goodenough, D. R., and Cox, P. W. (1977). Field-dependent and field-independent cognitive styles and their educational implications, *Review of Educational Research*, **47**, 1–64.

Witkin, H. A. and Oltman, P. K. (1967). Cognitive style, *International Journal of Neurology*, **6**, 119–37.

Witkin, H. A., Oltman, P., Raskin, E., and Karp, S. A. (1971). *A manual for the Embedded Figures Tests*. Consulting Psychologists Press, Palo Alto, Calif.

Wolberg, L. R. (1967). *The technique of psychotherapy*, 2nd edn., 2 vols. Grune and Stratton, New York.

Wolfe, B. E. and Goldfried, M. R. (1988). Research on psychotherapy integration: Recommendations and conclusions from an NIMH workshop, *Journal of Consulting and Clinical Psychology*, **56**, 448–51.

Woody, G. E., Luborsky, L., McLellan, A. T., O'Brien, C. P., Beck, A. T., Blaine, J., Herman, I., and Hole, A. (1983). Psychotherapy for opiate addiction: Does it help? *Archives of General Psychiatry*, **40**, 639–45.

Woody, G. E., McLellan, A. T., Luborsky, L., O'Brien, C. P., Blaine, J., Fox, S., Herman, I., and Beck, A. T. (1984). Severity of psychiatric symptoms as a predictor of benefits from psychotherapy: The Veterans Administration-Penn Study, *American Journal of Psychiatry*, **141**, 1172–7.

World Health Organization, WHO (1952). Expert Committee on Mental Health, Alcoholism Subcommittee, Second Report. Technical Report Series, No. 48, WHO, Geneva.

World Health Organization, WHO (1977). *International classification of diseases: Manual of the international statistical classification of diseases, injuries, and causes of death, Vol. 1*, 9th edn. WHO, Geneva.

World Health Organization, WHO (1986). Regional Office for Europe, Health Education Unit. Life-styles and health, *Social Science and Medicine*, **22**, 117–24.

World Health Organization, WHO (1989*a*). *International classification of diseases*, 10th edn. Draft of Chapter 5. WHO, Geneva.

World Health Organization, WHO (1989*b*). *Lexicon of psychiatric and mental health terms, Vol. 1*. WHO, Geneva.

Wright, C. and Moore, R. D. (1990). Disulfiram treatment of alcoholism, *The American Journal of Medicine*, **88**, 647–55.

Yeaton, W. H. and Sechrest, L. (1981). Critical dimensions in the choice and maintenance of successful treatments: Strength, integrity, and effectiveness, *Journal of Consulting and Clinical Psychology*, **49**, 156–67.

Yersin, B. and Paccaud, F. (1989). Alcoholism in hospitalized patients in Switzerland, *The Journal of the American Medical Association*, **262**, 772.

Yohman, J. R. and Parsons, O. A. (1987). Verbal reasoning deficits in alcoholics, *The Journal of Nervous and Mental Disease*, **175**, 219–23.

Young, R. McD., Oei, T. P. S., and Knight, R. G. (1990). The tension reduction hypothesis revisited: An alcohol expectancy perspective, *British Journal of Addiction*, **85**, 31–40.

Zola, I. K. (1972). Medicine as an institution of social control, *The Sociological Review*, **20**, 487–504.

Zucker, R. A. (1987). The four alcoholisms: A developmental account of the etiologic process. In *Alcohol and addictive behaviors* (ed. P. C. Rivers) pp. 27–83. University of Nebraska Press, Lincoln, Nebraska.

Zucker, R. A. and Gomberg, E. S. L. (1986). Etiology of alcoholism reconsidered: The case for a biopsychosocial process, *American Psychologist*, **41**, 783–93.

Zucker, R. A. and Noll, R. B. (1987). The interaction of child and environment in the early development of drug involvement: A far ranging review and a planned very early intervention, *Drugs and Society*, **2** (1), 57–97.

Zweben, A., Pearlman, S., and Li, S. (1988). A comparison of brief advice and conjoint therapy in the treatment of alcohol abuse: The results of the Marital Systems Study, *British Journal of Addiction*, **83**, 899–916.

Name index

Abbott, M. 221
Abramowitz, C. V. 223
Abrams, D. B. 83
Adamson, J. D. 295
Adler, A. 35
Adler, M. J. 16
Ågren, G. 90
Aiken, M. 150
Albert, B. M. 223
Albrecht, G. L. 82
Alfano, A. M. 194
Alfie, S. 290
Allain, A. N., Jr. 68
Allen, B. A. 61, 147
Allen, R. P. 78
Allen, V. L. 299
Allman, L. R. 74
Almond, R. 36, 231
Alterman, A. I. 194
Altrocchi, J. 212
Åmark, C. 117
Amidjaya, I. 181
Anastasi, A. 189
Anderson, J. G. 82
Andersson, H. E. 195
Andrews, G. 32
Annis, H. M. 5, 6, 26, 27, 85–7, 120, 124,
    189–93, 246, 258–60, 266, 270, 272,
    281–2, 299
Aristotle 2–3
Armor, D. J. 52, 154–5, 162–3, 173, 177,
    178–9, 183, 237–40, 242–3, 258–9, 267,
    268, 270
Armstrong, J. D. 68
Arroyave, F. 26
Ashem, B. 23
Atthowe, J. M. 294
Attia, P. R. 78
Austrian, R. W. 217, 275
Ausubel, D. P. 50
Azrin, N. H. 23, 30–1, 85, 99–101, 102, 118,
    258–60, 279, 287

Babor, T. F. 23, 31, 45, 194, 238, 293
Babow, I. 124
Bacon, F. 28–9
Bacon, S. D. 56
Baekeland, F. 21, 98, 186, 270, 295
Bakan, D. 156, 193

Balch, P. 223
Bandura, A. 120, 223, 298
Barlow, D. H. 36, 136, 174
Barnes, G. E. 68, 219, 275
Barry, H. III, 68
Bateson, G. 47, 96
Bean-Bayog, M. 77
Beardslee, W. R. 70, 73
Beattie, M. 102, 281
Beaubrun, M. H. 39
Beauchamp, D. E. 95
Begleiter, H. 75, 220
Beigel, A. 88
Bejerot, N. 63, 108, 110
Bellak, A. S. 84
Bem, D. J. 274
Bendel, R. B. 96
Bentler, P. M. 81
Beresford, T. P. 45
Berg, B. 104
Bergin, A. E. 31, 32–3, 35, 191, 266, 294
Berglund, M. 67, 94, 117, 195, 248, 293–4
Bergman, H. 75, 220, 275
Berman, J. S. 31
Berzins, J. I. 36
Best, J. A. 223, 225, 276
Beutler, L. E. 36, 226, 276, 278
Beyer, J. M. 56, 238
Billings, A. G. 96
Birnbaum, H. 192
Bittner, E. 55
Bjerver, K. 118
Björnstad, S. 30
Blaine, G. B. 300
Blanchard, E. B. 298
Blane, H. T. 20, 21, 22, 68
Blashfield, R. K. 66, 71
Bloch, S. 188–9
Blose, J. O. 269
Blow, F. C. 45
Blumberg, L. 145
Blume, S. B. 193
Bohman, M. 71, 190
Bond, C. F. 83
Bootzin, R. B. 120
Bornet, A. R. 246
Bowlby, J. 302
Bowman, K. M. 3, 67
Bowman, R. S. 27, 272
Bozarth, M. A. 63

Braiker, H. B. (Stambul) 52, 238–9, 240, 242–3, 267, 270
Bratt, I. 10, 51
Brewer, C. 101
Brickman, B. 67, 76, 77, 291
Brill, R. 208
Brody, N. 25
Bromet, E. 97, 98, 141, 156, 179
Brook, R. 150, 211
Brooks, M. 212
Brophy, J. E. 205
Broughton, A. 277
Brower, K. J. 45, 47, 78
Brown, E. D. 190
Brown, Sandra A. 78, 82, 96
Brown, Stephanie 77
Brownell, K. D. 84, 294
Bruun, K. 54, 70, 93, 95, 103, 106
Buchanan, T. K. 269
Butcher, J. N. 32
Butler, S. F. 120
Butters, N. 220

Caddy, G. R. 22, 45, 81
Cadogan, D. A. 23
Cadoret, R. J. 70, 71
Cahalan, D. 22, 50, 91, 117
Campbell, D. T. 22, 117, 135, 148, 173
Campbell, P. 23
Cappell, H. 80
Carey, K. B. 29
Carlen, P. L. 220
Carr, J. E. 212–14, 274–5
Carson, R. C. 218
Castaneda, R. 27
Caudill, B. D. 102
Chafetz, M. E. 118
Chalupsky, A. B. 9, 21
Chan, Darrow A. 72, 294
Chan, David 124, 189–92, 266, 282, 299
Chan, R. M. 188, 281–2
Chebib, F. S. 295
Chen, H.-T. 288
Chertok, L. 120
Chick, J. 25, 238, 247
Childress, A. R. 30
Chipperfield, B. 103
Christiansen, B. A. 82
Clancy, J. 23
Clark, D. C. 123
Clark, S. 39
Clark, W. B. 111, 117
Clarkin, J. 36
Clayton, D. J. 68
Cloninger, C. R. 66, 71, 194–5
Clopton, J. R. 193
Coe, R. 126, 138, 139, 180
Cohen, M. 52
Cohen, S. 75

Cole, S. G. 270
Collins, C. 81
Collins, J. L. 191, 266
Collins, R. L. 102
Colón, I. 93, 106
Conger, J. J. 80
Conrad, P. 58
Conradsson, C. 20, 295
Cook, C. C. H. 30
Cook, T. D. 22, 173
Cooney, N. 195, 196
Cooper, H. M. 7
Cooper, M. L. 84
Coppen, A. 123
Corrigan, B. 134
Cosper, R. 90
Costello, R. M. 29, 115, 125
Cox, W. M. 68
Crawford, A. 90
Crawford, J. J. 9, 21
Crawford, J. R. 57
Cristoph, P. 168
Critchlow Leigh, B. 82, 85
Cronbach, L. J. 34, 124, 208, 211, 261–2, 263–4, 265, 282
Cronkite, R. C. 22, 96, 97, 156, 180–1
Cross, D. G. 300
Cross, G. M. 98
Crowder, J. D. 212
Crowe, L. C. 83
Cunningham, W. G. 124
Curtin, M. E. 180
Cushing, H. 40
Cutler, R. E. 23
Cutter, H. S. G. 93

Dahlgren, L. 193, 260, 263, 281, 299
Davies, D. L. 51, 52, 237
Davies, J. B. 91
Davis, C. S. 85, 86–7, 120, 258, 259, 260, 282
Davis, D. I. 82
Dawes, R. M. 31, 134
Deever, S. G. 277
Demming, B. 82
DeSisto, M. 35
Dewey, M. E. 250, 268
Diagoras 28–9
Dickerson, M. 53
Dies, R. R. 223
Dinardo, P. A. 36
Dobson, K. S. 37
Dodes, L. M. 77
Doerr, H. O. 126, 138, 139, 180
Donner, L. 23
Donovan, D. M. 83, 84, 196, 220, 221, 225
Dougherty, F. E. 283
Dowds, B. N. 217, 275
Drake, R. E. 70
Drew, L. R. H. 117

Driver, M. J. 204
Druley, K. A. 152, 173
Dua, P. S. 221
Dukta, C. 149
Dunham, R. G. 47
Dunn, R. 124, 212
Durlak, J. A. 32, 301
Dwyer, D. 150-1

Eddy, N. B. 59, 62
Edgerton, R. B. 82
Edwards, G. 24-7 *passim*, 37-8, 52-4, 57-8,
    60-2, 65-6, 87, 94-5, 98, 102, 104, 110-11,
    118-19, 122-3, 142, 145-6, 163, 180, 233-8,
    247, 257, 260, 263, 267, 269, 271-2, 294
Edwards, R. V. 23
Einstein, A. 18
Einstein, S. 124
Eisler, R. M. 81
Elal-Lawrence, G. 250, 260, 268-9
Elliott, R. 32, 34
Elliott, W. A. 220
Ellsworth, R. B. 26
Empedocles 14
Emrick, C. D. 1, 5, 20, 22-3, 25, 31, 37, 48,
    96, 117, 119, 139, 160, 173, 270
Ends, E. J. 23
English, G. E. 180
Eriksen, L. 26, 30
Erlebacher, A. 135
Erwin, J. E. 219, 220, 275, 285, 302
Evans, G. D. 149-50
Evans, J. W. 221, 223
Evans, K. 78
Ewing, J. A. 77, 291
Eysenck, H. J. 25, 120

Fabrega, H. 108
Fagan, R. W. 56
Faillace, L. A. 52, 126
Fairbairn, W. R. D. 301
Farkas, A. 221
Farrington, B. 13
Faulkner, W. 91
Fawcett, J. 123
Feuerlein, W. 178
Fillmore, K. M. 69, 71
Fingarette, H. 47, 51
Fink, E. B. 23, 26, 160
Finney, J. W. 5, 22, 72, 96-7, 118, 141, 160,
    173, 179-81, 197, 212, 248, 259, 263, 265,
    294
Flanagan, J. 175, 201-2
Flores, P. J. 47, 96
Foon, A. E. 223
Forti, B. 195
Fostakowsky, R. T. 295
Foy, D. W. 24, 245-7, 249, 258, 260, 267-8,
    285, 292

Frances, A. 36
Frances, R. 67
Frank, A. F. 36, 228-32, 278
Frank, J. D. 37-9, 42-3, 120, 222, 224, 228,
    295, 298-9, 301, 302
Frederiksen, N. 274
Freed, E. X. 68
Freud, S. 17, 34, 35, 75, 299
Friedlander, J. 139
Friedman, M. L. 223
Fries, J. F. 124
Fromm, E. 35
Funder, D. C. 274
Fusco, E. 212

Galanter, M. 27, 67, 98, 126
Gallant, D. M. 23
Gallo, P. S. 32, 191
Garfield, S. L. 32, 33, 136
Gaston, L. 300
Gazda, P. 147
Gecht, D. 124
Gelso, C. J. 32
George, W. H. 79, 83, 84
Gerard, D. L. 74, 291, 293
Gergen, K. J. 263
Gerstein, D. R. 106
Getter, H. 195
Ghertner, S. 88
Gibbs, L. E. 5, 141, 175, 201-3
Giesbrecht, N. A. 56, 94
Giffen, P. J. 56
Gilbert, F. S. 82
Gillen, C. 116
Gillespie, D. G. 20
Gillis, J. S. 223
Gitlow, S. E. 49
Glad, D. D. 104
Glaser, F. B. 3, 4, 5, 115, 123, 126-7, 142-9,
    179, 236, 260, 279, 283
Glass, G. V. 23, 32, 174, 265, 301
Glassner, B. 104
Glatt, M. 49
Glueck, E. 69
Glueck, S. 69
Goldberg, L. R. 131, 134, 136
Goldbergèr, L. 217, 275
Goldfried, M. R. 36, 120, 289, 301
Goldman, M. S. 75, 82, 220
Goldman, R. D. 45
Goldstein, M. S. 22
Goldstein, S. G. 194
Gomberg, E. S. L. 69
Gomes-Schwartz, B. 36
Good, T. L. 205
Goodenough, D. R. 216, 218, 274-8
Goodwin, D. W. 66, 71, 74, 91, 106, 123
Gordis, E. 20
Gordon, J. R. 83-4, 87

Götestam, K. G. 30
Gottheil, E. 173
Gottlieb, B. H. 98
Gow, J. 136
Graham, J. R. 193–4
Graham, K. 150
Greeley, J. 80
Greenberg, L. S. 36
Greenwald, A. G. 174, 175
Grennon, J. 212
Gripp, R. 17–18, 38
Gross, H. W. 193
Gross, M. M. 53–4, 65, 87, 238
Gunderson, J. G. 35–6, 228–32, 278
Guntrip, H. 301
Guthrie, A. 220
Guthrie, S. 27, 269, 272
Guze, S. B. 66

Hadley, S. W. 36, 299
Halikas, J. A. 201
Hall, J. J. 196
Halleck, S. L. 47
Hansen, J. 20, 22
Hanson, M. 108
Harding, G. T. 75
Hare, F. 39
Hartman, L. M. 30, 225–6, 258, 260, 277, 302
Harvey, O. J. 204, 211, 273
Harvey, R. 32
Hattie, J. A. 32, 301
Hayes, S. C. 136
Hayman, M. 67
Heather, N. 51, 57, 64, 101, 250–1, 269
Hegel, G. W. F. 110
Helzer, J. E. 247, 248, 260
Hemingway, E. 91
Hendriks, V. M. 160
Herman, C. P. 80
Hersen, M. 84, 174
Hershon, H. 51
Hesselbrock, M. N. 193, 194
Hester, R. K. 5, 26, 27, 29, 30, 74, 80, 98, 101, 117, 146, 270
Hiatt, H. H. 147
Hill, M. J. 20, 21
Hill, S. Y. 51
Hingson, R. 61
Hinrichsen, J. J. 225
Hippocrates 13–16, 18–19, 256, 296
Hodgson, R. J. 31, 53, 62, 64–6, 86, 239
Hofer, R. 149
Hoffman, P. J. 136
Hoffmann, H. 48, 68
Holder, H. D. 126, 269
Holmgren, S. 20, 295
Holt, R. R. 132
Holt, S. 61
Hopkins, T. K. 20

Howard, K. I. 120
Howden Chapman, P. L. 26
Howell, R. J. 223
Hubbard, R. N. 144, 148
Huebner, R. 45
Hulbert, R. J. 220
Hull, J. G. 83
Hume, W. I. 300
Hunt, D. D. 213, 274
Hunt, D. E. 124, 136, 204–9, 211, 221, 226, 227, 273–4
Hunt, G. H. 23, 30, 85, 99–100, 279
Hunter, J. J. 219, 220, 275, 285, 302
Huss, M. 49
Hustmyer, F. E. 218
Huygens, I. 25
Hyman, H. 20

Ingram, J. A. 82, 84
Intagliata, J. C. 219
Irwin, M. 78
Isaiah 48
Ito, J. R. 196
Iversen, L. 90

Jackson, G. 241
Jeffrey, D. B. 22
Jellinek, E. M. 3, 49–50, 51, 52, 54–6, 57, 64, 65, 67, 82–3, 86, 105–6, 236, 256
Jessor, R. 221
Joe, V. C. 221
Johnson, D. H. 32
Johnson, R. K. 223
Jones, B. A. 120, 302
Jones, E. 299
Jones, W. C. 93
Jones, W. H. S. 13, 18
Joyce, B. R. 209
Jung, C. G. 35, 299
Jyrkämä, J. 90

Kadden, R. 195–7, 258, 259, 260, 278, 281–2, 299, 302
Kahneman, D. 135
Kammeier, M. L. 48
Kaplan, J. M. 181
Kaplan, S. M. 139
Karasu, T. B. 120, 279
Karp, S. A. 218, 275, 302
Kazdin, A. E. 32, 34, 120, 174
Keddie, A. 249–51, 260, 268–9
Keller, M. 1, 49, 63, 68
Kelly, G. A. 212
Kendall, A. J. 124
Kendall, P. C. 32
Kendell, R. E. 54, 57, 90, 117
Kernberg, O. F. 299
Kershaw, P. W. 94, 117–18, 294
Keso, L. 30

Khan, J. A. 300
Khantzian, E. J. 95–6, 101, 290
Kiesler, D. J. 34–5, 120
Kiev, A. 218
Kilmann, P. R. 223
King, L. S. 296
Kish, G. B. 26
Kissin, B. 21, 23, 25, 104–5, 106, 108, 110, 113, 115, 125, 152, 186, 198–201, 203, 218, 233, 258, 260–2, 264, 270–1, 272, 275, 303
Kivlahan, D. R. 220
Klajner, F. 30
Klausen, H. 90
Kline, N. S. 123
Knight, R. G. 80
Knight, R. P. 67, 179
Knupfer, G. 92–3, 293
Koester, H. 5
Kohut, H. 301
Kornreich, M. 32
Koss, M. P. 32
Kraepelin, E. 48, 49
Krasner, L. 51
Kratochwill, T. R. 174
Kristenson, H. 238, 267–8, 293, 298
Krywonis, M. 225, 277
Küfner, H. 178
Kuller, L. H. 22
Kurosawa, K. 174
Kurtz, N. R. 57
Kyle, E. 180

Laberg, J. C. 85
Lambert, M. J. 31, 32–3, 191, 266, 294
Lambert, S. 56
Landfield, A. W. 213, 274
Landman, J. T. 31
Lange, D. 96
Lansky, D. 22, 98
LaPorte, D. J. 161, 200
Laufer, M. W. 290
Laundergan, J. C. 187
Lazarus, A. A. 36
Leach, J. 218, 273, 287
Leber, W. R. 220
LeBlanc, R. F. 221
Lefcourt, H. M. 221, 276, 277
Lei, H. 246
Leidner, B. 5
Leigh, H. 108
Leitner, L. M. 120
Lemere, F. 20, 39, 263
Lens, W. 220
Lesyk, J. J. 221
Letemendia, F. J. J. 26
Lettieri, D. J. 22
Levinson, T. 23, 75, 125, 235, 292
Levy, M. 76–7, 291
Lewin, K. 204, 211, 273

Lewinsohn, P. M. 68
Lewis, H. B. 217
Lewis, S. 91
Li, S. 26
Liban, C. B. 193
Liberman, B. L. 221–2, 223, 225, 228, 276, 294
Lick, J. R. 120
Liebson, I. A. 52
Light, R. J. 175
Lindberg, S. 90
Linden, J. D. 194
Lindman, R. 80
Liskow, B. I. 123
Lisman, S. A. 80
Litman, G. K. 300
Litt, M. 195, 196
Llewelyn, S. P. 300
Logue, P. E. 74
Lomp, K. G. E. 28, 97
London, P. 120
Longabaugh, R. 6, 26, 101, 102, 260, 261, 264, 266, 281, 299
Loper, R. G. 48
Lovibond, S. H. 82
Luborsky, Lester 32, 152, 168, 214, 265, 295, 300
Luborsky, Lise 32
Ludwig, A. M. 74, 79–80, 94, 200
Lunde, S. E. 23
Lundwall, L. 21
Lyons, J. P. 192–3, 244, 260, 263, 266, 281

MacAndrew, C. 82
McArthur, C. C. 300
McCabe, R. J. R. 248
McCance, C. 23
McCance, P. F. 23
McCord, J. 72
McCord, W. 72
McCrady, B. S. 26, 30, 220, 269
MacDonald, A. P., Jr. 221
MacDonald, K. R. 246
MacDowell, D. J. 17–18, 38
McGahan, P. L. 161
Machover, S. 25
Mack, J. E. 95–6, 101, 290
McLachlan, J. F. C. 26, 192, 204–12, 229, 258–9, 260, 261, 263, 273–4, 275, 278, 302
McLatchie, B. H. 28, 97
McLean, P. D. 35
McLellan, A. T. 5, 30, 127–8, 152–69, 173, 192, 203, 255, 259–65 passim, 271–2, 278, 281–2, 283–4, 295, 302, 303
McNamee, H. B. 74
Magaro, P. A. 17–18, 20, 35, 36, 38, 127
Magnusson, D. 71, 299
Maher, B. A. 183
Maier, S. F. 221

Maisto, S. A. 29, 83
Mäkelä, K. 56, 57, 93, 95, 106
Malikin, D. 50
Mallams, J. H. 30, 99
Maltzman, I. M. 24
Mandell, W. 22
Mann, M. 49
Marcus, S. H. 22
Marlatt, G. A. 6, 79, 80, 82–3, 84, 85–6, 87, 102
Marmar, C. 36
Martin, P. L. 23
Maskin, M. 35
Matakas, F. 5
Maurer, H. S. 72
Mauss, A. L. 47, 56
May, S. J. 22
Mayer, J. 227, 260, 278
Meehl, P. E. 130–1, 134
Megargee, E. I. 196
Mello, N. K. 51, 74, 80
Meltzoff, J. 32
Mendelson, J. H. 51, 74
Menustik, C. E. 280
Merry, J. 123
Meyer, R. E. 45, 194
Meyer, R. G. 223
Miller, A. 124, 204–5
Miller, B. A. 10, 20
Miller, P. M. 30, 81–2, 85, 99
Miller, S. I. 67, 126
Miller, T. I. 32
Miller, William R. 5, 26, 27, 29, 30, 51, 67, 74, 80, 98, 101, 104, 117, 146, 244, 270
Milliones, J. 84
Milofsky, E. S. 48, 69, 72, 106, 111, 118, 247, 260
Mintz, J. 168
Mirkin, P. M. 194
Mischel, W. 42
Moll, J. K. 1
Moore, M. H. 106
Moore, R. A. 269
Moore, R. D. 61, 101
Moos, R. H. 6, 22, 72, 96–8, 118, 141, 156, 173, 179–81, 197, 212, 248, 259, 263, 265, 274, 294
Morey, L. C. 66, 71, 193, 194
Morgan, R. 300
Morrison, E. 225, 277
Mosher, V. 26
Moskowitz, J. M. 93, 106
Moss, M. K. 180
Mumford, E. 23
Murdock, M. 25
Murray, R. M. 91
Muuronen, A. 75, 220
Myers, J. L. 175
Myerson, D. J. 227, 260, 278

Nace, E. P. 28
Narin, F. 1
Naroll, R. 1, 16
Nash, L. 193
Nathan, P. E. 22, 68, 74, 80, 98, 108, 126
Nelson, R. O. 136
Nerviano, V. J. 193
Neuringer, C. 68
Newcomb, M. D. 81
Newell, S. 45
Newton, J. R. 23, 27, 272
Niaura, R. S. 83
Nicholls, P. 180
Nicholson, R. A. 31
Nisbett, R. 135
Noll, R. B. 71
Norcross, J. C. 36
Nordström, G. 94, 117, 195, 248, 251, 286, 293–4
Norman, J. 116, 192, 278, 302
Norton, G. R. 36
Norton-Ford, J. D. 32
Nunn, L. B. 24, 245, 267
Nye, F. I. 68

Obitz, F. W. 227, 276, 302
O'Brien, C. P. 152, 168
Ockham, W. of, 72
O'Doherty, F. 91
Oei, T. P. S. 80
Ogborne, A. C. 5, 48, 93, 148, 149–51, 152, 176, 199, 204, 279
Öjehagen, A. 67
Öjesjö, L. 117
Okpaku, S. O. 67
O'Leary, D. E. 84
O'Leary, M. R. 84, 221, 224, 225
Olson, R. P. 75, 266, 292
Olsson, G. 278
Oltman, P. K. 205, 215, 216, 274
Omer, H. 120
Oncken, G. R. 140
O'Neill, E. 91
Oppenheimer, E. 52, 122, 237, 263, 267
Orford, J. 25, 37–8, 52, 98, 118, 122–3, 142, 145–6, 163, 233–8, 249–51, 258, 260, 263, 267–9
Orlinsky, D. E. 120
Osler, W. 40, 296
Osmond, H. 45
Öst, L.-G. 35

Paccaud, F. 61
Padawer, W. 120
Page, C. W. 23
Page, R. D. 26
Palm, U. 195
Papernik, D. S. 217
Paracelsus 296

Pardes, H. 217, 275
Paré, A. 119
Park, P. 92
Parloff, M. B. 38, 189
Parsons, O. A. 75, 220
Parsons, T. 55, 58
Pattison, E. M. 2, 5, 37, 50, 51, 82, 104,
    107–9, 111, 115, 124, 126–7, 137–41, 152,
    157, 180, 200, 201, 203, 266
Patton, M. Q. 189
Paul, G. L. 35–6, 42, 123
Pavlov, I. P. 79
Pearlman, S. 26
Peele, S. 51, 71, 247, 248
Pemper, K. 125
Pendery, M. L. 24
Penick, E. C. 227
Pertschuk, M. 51
Pervin, L. A. 274
Pettinati, H. M. 23, 72, 98, 160, 248
Piaget, J. 218–19, 221, 275
Pierce, R. M. 221
Pittel, S. M. 149
Pittman, D. J. 23, 26
Plant, M. A. 90, 91, 92
Plato 296–7
Platz, A. 23, 218, 262, 270, 272
Plotkin, W. R. 295
Poldrugo, F. 195
Polich, J. M. 52, 61, 154, 177, 178, 238–9,
    240, 242–3, 244, 258, 260, 262–4, 267–8,
    270
Pollack, I. W. 218
Pomerleau, O. 51
Popham, R. E. 105
Popper, K. R. 4, 18
Porjesz, B. 75, 220
Posthuma, A. B. 212
Powell, B. J. 27, 227
Prioleau, L. 25
Pucel, J. 117

Rachman, S. J. 32, 53, 62, 124
Rank, O. 35
Rankin, H. 53
Rathod, R. 125
Regier, M. 57
Reich, T. 68
Reid, J. B. 82, 102
Reiser, M. F. 108
Renner, J. W. 275
Reynolds, C. M. 123, 260
Rhodes, R. J. 126
Ridgely, M. S. 78
Riley, D. M. 29
Ritson, E. B. 25, 31, 54, 90
Robertson, I. 51, 64, 250, 269
Robertson, L. 208
Robins, L. N. 68, 247

Robinson, D. 51, 55
Rogers, C. R. 34, 35, 211, 301
Rogers, H. J. 32, 301
Rohrberg, R. 217
Rohsenow, D. J. 85–6, 224, 225
Roizen, R. 117
Roman, P. M. 56
Rönnberg, S. 82
Roodin, P. A. 277
Room, R. 50, 51, 88, 91, 97, 293
Rose, G. S. 227
Rosen, A. 77
Rosenbaum, Michael 68
Rosenbaum, Milton 139
Rosenbaum, P. 149
Rosenblatt, S. M. 25
Rosenthal, R. 174
Rosenzweig, S. 37
Ross, A. O. 136
Ross, A. W. 223
Ross, L. 135
Rossi, P. H. 288
Rotter, J. B. 221, 226, 276, 277
Roumanie, M. de, 54, 90
Rounsaville, B. J. 78
Rush, Benjamin 49
Rush, Brian R. 150–1, 283
Russakoff, L. M. 217, 275
Russell, M. 84
Ryan, C. 220
Rychtarik, R. G. 24, 245, 248–9, 251, 267

Saenger, G. 74, 291, 293
Sakel, M. 17
Salamon, I. 27
Salaspuro, M. 30
Saliba, C. 75, 119, 291
Salkin, D. 192
Salzberg, H. C. 82, 84
Samsonowitz, V. 85, 278
Sanchez-Craig, M. 220, 245–7, 267–8, 293
Sandler, J. 290
Sarbin, T. R. 130
Sarnecki, J. 106
Saunders, W. M. 94, 117–18, 294
Sawyer, J. 131–4
Schanble, P. G. 221
Schaub, K. H. 26
Schefft, B. K. 83
Schlesinger, H. J. 23
Schmidt, W. 105, 180, 200
Schneider, D. U. 219, 275
Schneider, J. W. 58
Schroder, H. M. 204–5, 211, 273
Schroeder, H. G. 68
Schuckit, M. A. 22, 66, 77–8, 81
Schulze, R. 192, 278, 302
Schwartz, M. S. 232
Searles, J. S. 71, 194

Sechrest, L. B. 190, 196, 278
Seeley, J. R. 58
Seeman, M. 221, 223, 276
Seevers, M. H. 63
Seiden, R. H. 51
Seliger, R. V. 270
Seligman, M. E. P. 221
Selzer, M. D. 156
Sereny, G. 23, 75, 125, 235, 292
Shadel, C. A. 39–40
Shanks, P. 117
Shapiro, David A. 32–3, 34, 175, 301
Shapiro, Diana 32, 175, 301
Sharpley, C. F. 32, 301
Shatterly, D. 51
Shaw, S. 64
Sheahan, D. B. 82
Sheehan, P. W. 300
Shipman, S. 212
Shipman, V. C. 212
Short, J. F. 68
Shows, W. D. 218
Shrauger, S. 212
Siegler, M. 45
Sigvardsson, S. 71
Simmel, E. 68
Simpkins, J. 91
Singer, B. 32
Singer, M. 38
Sisson, R. W. 30, 99, 101, 102
Sjöberg, L. 85, 135, 278
Skinner, H. A. 4, 5, 61, 66, 71, 135, 147, 173, 193–4, 226–8, 276
Skinstad, A. H. 22
Skog, O.-J. 88, 102, 105
Slade, P. D. 250, 268
Slovic, P. 135
Smart, R. G. 117, 173, 178–9, 180, 183, 198, 248, 259, 270, 288
Smith, D. E. 220
Smith, H. 241
Smith, M. L. 32, 174, 301
Smith, P. V. 175
Smith, R. E. 221
Smith, W. G. 181
Snow, R. E. 124, 208, 265
Snyder, C. R. 104
Sobell, L. C. 21, 23–5, 29, 39–40, 50, 82, 93, 104, 107, 109, 111, 243, 247–8
Sobell, M. B. 21–30 passim, 39–40, 50, 82, 93, 104, 107, 109, 111, 243, 247, 248
Socrates 295, 296–7
Sokolow, L. 192–3, 244, 260, 263, 264, 266, 281, 299
Sollenhag, S. 106
Solomon, D. 124
Solomon, R. L. 53
Son, L. 70
Sonnenstuhl, W. J. 56, 115

Sotile, W. M. 223
Sousa-Poza, J. F. 217
Sperber, J. 126
Spoth, R. 225, 226, 258, 260, 277, 302
Spradley, J. P. 145
Stall, R. 94
Stallings, D. L. 140
Stambul, H. B., see Braiker, H. B
Stanley, J. C. 117, 173
Stanton, A. H. 232
Stark, L. H. 74, 79–80
Staton, M. C. 117
Steffy, R. A. 223, 225, 276
Stein, L. I. 23, 27, 273
Stein, M. I. 34
Stein, R. L. 26
Steinbeck, J. 91
Stengers, I. 120
Stewart, M. J. 97
Stiles, W. B. 32, 34, 36
Stinnet, J. 51
Stinson, D. J. 27, 173, 181–3, 258, 292, 301
Stockwell, T. R. 53, 65–6, 80, 85, 247, 258
Stoil, M. J. 187
Storm, T. 23
Stratas, N. E. 126
Straus, R. 145
Strenger, V. E. 193–4
Streufert, S. 204
Strupp, H. H. 35, 36, 120, 295, 296, 299, 301
Su, W. H. 23, 218, 262, 270, 272
Sugerman, A. A. 72, 219, 275
Sullivan, H. S. 35
Sullivan, J. M. 78
Surber, M. 22
Sutherland, E. H. 68
Sutker, P. B. 68
Syme, L. 68
Szasz, T. S. 51

Talbott, J. A. 116
Tamerin, J. S. 74
Tarter, R. E. 194
Tate, R. L. 23, 26
Taylor, H. A. 74
Taylor, J. R. 247
Telch, M. J. 42
Telegdi, M. 277
Thoits, P. A. 97
Thornton, C. C. 161
Throop, W. E. 221
Thurstin, A. H. 194
Tiebout, H. M. 47, 67, 96
Tobacyk, J. J. 277
Tolor, A. 221
Tomlinson, P. D. 207
Tomosovic, M. 23
Tordella, O. L. 68
Tourney, G. 17

Treffert, D. 203
Trice, H. M. 56, 115, 200, 238
Trotter, T. 3, 49, 63, 300-1
Tuchfeld, B. S. 22, 94
Tucker, J. A. 93
Tversky, A. 135

Ullman, L. P. 51

Vaillant, G. E. 20, 22, 25, 28, 38-40, 47-8,
    68-73, 76-8, 94-5, 97-8, 102, 106, 111,
    117, 118, 186, 247, 260, 264, 291-4, 295
Valverius, S. 8
Vanderhoof, E. 23
van Dijk, W. K. 108, 110
Van Hasselt, V. B. 84
Vannicelli, M. 193
Vaught, G. M. 277
Verden, P. 51
Voegtlin, W. L. 20, 39, 263
Vogel-Sprott, M. 103
Vogler, R. E. 23
von Knorring, A.-L. 195
von Knorring, L. 195
Vuchinich, R. E. 93

Wagman, A. M. I. 78
Walker, R. D. 26, 220
Wallerstein, R. S. 39, 184-9, 197, 258,
    259-61, 280-1, 299
Ward, D. A. 96
Ward, R. F. 126
Warren, M. Q. 124
Watson, C. G. 117
Webb, N. 211, 263
Weil, E. 217
Weiner, M. F. 212
Weiner, S. 74
Welte, J. W. 182, 244, 266, 268, 271-2, 292,
    301, 303

West, L. J. 24
White, S. O. 190
Whitehead, P. C. 91
Whitton, B. 250, 269
Wiens, A. N. 280
Wiggins, J. S. 135
Wiggins, N. 136
Wikler, A. 74, 79-80
Wilbur, B. M. 191, 278, 281, 302
Wile, R. 293
Wilkins, W. 119-20
Wilkinson, D. A. 220
Willander, A. 193, 260, 263, 281, 299
Willems, P. J. A. 26
Wilner, D. M. 22
Wilson, G. T. 32, 34, 83, 124
Wing, J. 218, 273, 287
Winnicott, D. 301
Winokur, G. 68, 78
Winston, A. 217
Wise, R. A. 63
Witkin, H. A. 205, 214-19, 274-5, 279
Wolberg, L. R. 75, 291
Wolfe, B. E. 301
Wolfson, E. 124
Woody, G. E. 152, 168, 186
Woody, M. M. 26
Wright, Charles R. 20
Wright, Curtis 101
Wynne, L. C. 53

Yeaton, W. H. 196, 278
Yersin, B. 61
Yohman, J. R. 75
Young, L. D. 298
Young, R. McD. 80

Zola, I. K. 58
Zucker, R. A. 69, 71, 78
Zweben, A. 26

Subject index

abstinence
  controlled drinking *versus* 233–51, 266–9,
    285–6, 292
  dependence and 51–2, 59, 63, 65, 111–12
  environmental resources 96–8, 242–3
addiction (alcohol), *see* alcohol dependence
Addiction Research Foundation 26, 127,
  142–3, 145–6, 148–51, 189, 226, 236
Addiction Research Unit 108, 233
Addiction Severity Index (ASI) 127, 153,
  156–66, 169, 196, 259, 261
  psychiatric severity 161–9, 196, 260, 271–3,
    284–7
advice *versus* treatment 25–6, 233–6
  see also brief counselling
aftercare 181–3, 195–7, 210–11, 218–19, 273,
  278–9
age
  age factor 182–3, 192, 220, 227, 237, 240–3,
    244, 259, 262, 266, 267
  age of onset 71, 194–5
agency level (regional system) 150–1
aggression (aversion therapy) 186–7, 280
Al-Anon 98, 102, 292
alcohol availability 70, 84–5, 93, 101–3, 106,
  293
alcohol consumption (quantity) 61–2, 82–3,
  103, 242, 258, 267
alcohol dependence 52–4, 59, 86
  definition 59, 63–4, 65, 109
  dependence as syndrome 63–6, 109–10
  disabilities 60–1, *see also* alcohol-related
    disabilities
  multivariant conception 107–12
  persuasion and 249–51
  physical dependence 62–3
  quantity of consumption 61–2
  severity, *see* alcohol dependence (degree of)
  see also alcohol dependence (degree of);
    alcohol-dependence syndrome; Gamma
    alcoholics
alcohol dependence (degree of) 65–6, 266–9,
  278, 285–7, 292
  Annis–Davis study 86–7, 282
  Edwards–Orford study 233–8, 267–8
  Foy–Sanchez-Craig studies 245–7, 267–8,
    285, 292–3
  long-term outcome 247–9
  persuasion *versus* 249–51, 268–9
  Rand Report II 238–43, 267–8
  Welte study 244, 266, 268

alcohol-dependence syndrome 59–66, 107,
  109–10, 111, 257, 258
alcohol expectancies 51, 79, 80, 82–3, 84, 85–6
alcohol industry 50, 92
alcohol-related disabilities 59, 60–2, 66, 70,
  109, 111, 257
alcohol tolerance 52–3, 59, 64, 65, 236, 248–9
alcoholics
  'affiliative'/'schizoid' 71
  Delta 49
  'developmentally cumulative'/'antisocial' 71
  differences 115–16, 120–2, 256–8
  Epsilon 49, 248
  'essential'/'reactive' 179
  Gamma 24–5, 49–50, 94–5, 122, 236–7,
    248, 267
  'hidden' 70, 138, 139
  'milieu-limited'/'male-limited' 66, 194
  personality typologies 193–5
  primary/secondary 66, 78
  type 1/type 2 194–5
Alcoholics Anonymous 39–40, 82, 125, 161,
  200, 211, 292, 298
  persuasion and 250
  disease model 49–51, 55, 57
  effectiveness 97–8
  moral model 47–8
  self governance and 95–6, 290–1
  social model 94–9 *passim*, 102
  superego support and 291
  symptomatic model 76, 77
  see also Al-Anon
alcoholism (conceptions) 45, 256–8
  biopsychosocial perspective 104–12
  dependence 59–66
  disease model 49–58
  learning model 79–87
  moral model 47–8
  social model 88–103
  symptomatic model 67–78
  see also specific conceptions
alcoholism treatment, *see* treatment; treatment
  effectiveness; treatment in perspective;
  treatment strategies
American College of Physicians 101
American Medical Association 30, 49
American Psychiatric Association 49, 59, 67, 70
analogue studies 35, 82–3, 85
Ancient Medicine 13–15, 17, 19
Antabuse 39–40, 99–101, 184–8, 226–8,
  276–80, 286, 291, 297–8

anti-alcohol drugs 226-8
  see also Antabuse; Temposil
antisocial behaviour 48, 71, 73, 106, 194-5, 256
  see also sociopathy
ASIST 150
assessment (individual) 128, 143-4, 146-8,
  150-1, 283
attachment factor 187-8, 280-1
attachment theory 302
attenuated drinking 237, 266
attribution orientation
  active/responsive 94
  self-/external 223-4
  see also locus of control
Attributions Inventory 94
aversion therapy 30, 39-40, 276, 280
  personality traits 184, 186-7, 188, 280
  treatment profile 138-41, 180

basic assumptions 40-3, 117-24, 261-4
behaviour therapy 18, 32, 34, 36, 39-40, 75,
  291, 292
  cognitive 36-7, 83-6, 291
  learning model 79-87
  see also relapse prevention; self-control
    training
behavioural analysis 82, 86
biofeedback 222, 238, 267, 286, 297-8
biopsychosocial approach 58, 66, 85, 104-12,
  242-3, 257-8, 269
boys 71-2, 73, 106, 208
brain damage 75, 220, 285
brief counselling 25-6, 122-3, 145, 233-8
Brookfield Clinics 128, 148
buffer hypothesis 97

California Psychological Inventory Socialization Scale 196
career (social model) 52, 101-3
case studies 35, 136, 174
childhood environment 68-9, 70-3
chronicity, see problem chronicity
classical disease model 49-51, 54, 57-8, 81,
  108, 236, 256-7
client-centred therapy 32, 34, 210
client–treatment interaction, see interaction;
  interaction studies; interaction studies
  (negative results)
Client Profile
  generalized/differentiated 87, 202
clinical
  assessment 134, 188-9
  composite (prediction) 131-4
  interview (ASI) 156-60
  prediction 130-6, 147
  replication 174
  strategies 289-90, 291, 295
co-operative arts 16, 38, 145, 280
Coatesville and Philadelphia Veterans Administration Medical Centers 153, 161-9

cognitive-behavioural therapy 36-7, 83-5,
  196, 291
  see also relapse prevention
cognitive ability 75, 218-20, 274-6, 277, 279,
  285, 302
  see also intelligence/intellect; restructuring
    ability
cognitive matching 212
cognitive personality theories 204, 212, 215-16,
  273-5
cognitive styles 273, 275, 277, 279
  conceptual differentiation 212-14, 274
  definition 205
  field dependence/restructuring 214-20,
    274-6, 285, 302
  locus of control 221-8, 276-7, 285, 302
  McLachlan study 204-12, 273-4, 285, 302
  Skinner's hypothesis 226-8
  therapist–milieu interaction 228-32, 278
community/specialist collaboration 128
community reinforcement approach 30-1,
  99-101, 118-19, 279, 287
community support networks 97, 98
competitive monolithic approach 124-5
compulsive behaviour
  drinking as 50, 59, 62-6 passim
  personality trait 185-6, 280
conceptual complexity 204-5, 207, 274
conceptual differentiation 212-14, 274
  see also conceptual level; psychological
    differentiation
conceptual level 204-12, 273-4, 275, 277-9,
  285, 302
conceptual systems theory 204-5, 273-4
concrete operational level 218-19, 275
conditioning theories 53-4, 74, 79-82, 85
conjoint therapy, see marital therapy
constructive confrontation 238
consumption levels, see alcohol consumption
  (quantity)
contemporaneous matching models 205-7,
  221, 226-7
continuity of care 108, 113, 128, 143, 144, 283-4
contra-indications 77, 78, 139, 164, 282, 291
control
  concept 95-6
  locus of 221-8, 276-7, 279, 285, 302
  see also powerlessness; self-control; social
    control
control (loss of)
  Gamma alcoholics 24-5, 49-50, 94-5, 122,
    236-7, 248, 267
  hypothesis 51-3, 65, 79-80, 82-3, 85, 95-6,
    257
  powerlessness 47-8, 290-1, 292
  recovery patterns 93-6
control policies 54, 56, 62, 93, 103, 257
controlled drinking
  abstinence versus 233-51, 266-9, 285-6, 292

controlled drinking (*cont*)
  definitions 237, 239, 244, 246, 248, 266, 268
  dependence and 52, 111
controlled studies 6, 22, 25, 148, 173–4, 258, 260
coping skills
  availability of 84, 96, 278
  training 82, 86, 196–7, 225, 269, 277, 282
  see also relapse prevention; social skills training
Core City study 69–72, 94–5, 247
core–shell system 128, 179
  background 142–3
  core and shell 143–4
  implementation 148–9, 283–7
  individual assessment 146–7
  primary care 144–6
  regional systems 149–51
  treatment research 147–8
counselling 27, 28, 138, 180
  brief 25–6, 122–3, 145, 233–8
  group 99, 100
couples
  marital status 88–90, 96–8, 100, 240–3, 267, 272, 279
  Maudsley Hospital study 25, 94, 122–3, 233–8, 267–8
  therapy 26, 30, 101
craving 50, 53, 54, 63, 79–80, 110
culture
  -based interaction 17–18, 39–40, 263–4
  socio-cultural factors 82, 104–6, 257
  subcultures 70–1, 90–1, 104–5, 106, 145
  therapy as cultural phenomenon 16–19
  transcultural model 38–9, 295
  values and expectations 93, 101–2, 293

degree of structure 164, 205–11, 272
  directiveness and 196–7, 209–11, 217, 219, 225–6, 273–9, 284–7, 301–2
demoralization 38, 298
dependence, *see* alcohol-dependence syndrome;
  alcohol dependence; alcohol dependence
  (degree of); Gamma alcoholics
depression 63, 68–9, 72–4, 78, 81, 123, 158, 162, 186–7, 280, 284, 286
developmental matching models 207–8, 221, 227–8
deviant case analysis 136
differential assessment of disability 139–40, 156–60
differential treatment 3–4, 113, 115, 138, 142, 265, 283–7, 289
  see also matching; matching clients to treat-
    ments; systems of alcoholism treatment
directiveness 209–11, 217, 219, 225–6, 273–9, 284–7, 301–2
disabilities, alcohol-related 59, 60–2, 66, 70, 109, 111, 257
disease model 47, 63, 64–5, 67, 86
  classical model 49–51, 54, 57–8, 81, 108, 236

interpretations and trends 57–8, 256–7
multivariant model 107–12, 113, 115, 116, 142, 201
scientific critique 51–4
social consequences 55–7
divorce 63, 88–9, 93, 271, 284
drink-seeking behaviour 54, 65, 109
drink centredness 64
  see also drink-seeking behaviour
Drinking-Related Locus of Control Scale 221, 278
drinking behaviour (and improvement) 22–3, 116–17, 159–60, 256
drinking pattern
  prognostic indicators 115–16, 202–3, 258–61, 283–7
  see also abstinence; controlled drinking
drinking repertoire 53, 65, 87, 109
dropout (selective) 153, 154, 164, 173, 177–8, 200
drug addicts 161, 168, 189–92, 281
drug therapy 198–200, 218, 270–1, 272, 279
  see also Antabuse; lithium therapy; Temposil
DSM-III 59, 70, 247, 248
dual diagnosis 78
dynamic psychotherapy 67–8, 74–8, 266, 291–2
  see also insight-oriented therapy

early intervention, *see* secondary prevention
educational research 188, 205–9, 211, 212, 273, 281
effectiveness, *see* treatment effectiveness
Embedded Figures Test 198, 215–16, 217–19, 220, 274–5
employment 90–2, 93, 96–7, 98, 271, 284
environment 51, 70–2, 106
  degree of structure 164, 205–11, 225, 273–9, 285, 301–2
  resources 93–103 *passim*, 256, 259, 272, 281, 294
ethnicity 70–1, 104–5, 106
expectancy effect 82–3, 85–6
  see also alcohol expectancies
experimental studies 6, 22, 25, 148, 173–4, 258, 260
external control 221, 223–8, 276–7, 279, 285, 302

family
  alcoholism in relatives 70–2, 103, 106
  -related problems 271, 284, 287
  therapy 30
  see also couples; divorce; marital status;
    marital therapy
female alcoholics 78, 90, 192–3, 263, 281
field dependence–independence 214–16
  cognitive style 214–18, 219, 274–5, 279, 285
  restructuring ability 198–200, 214–20, 270–1, 272, 274–6, 279, 285
'file drawer problem' 174, 175

'fishing expedition' 3, 183, 288
follow-up 148, 283
    change scores 139–40, 158, 159–60
    intervals 21, 23–4, 28, 29, 155–6
    spontaneous remission 117–19
formal operational level 218–20, 275–7

Gamma alcoholics 24–5, 49–50, 94–5, 122,
    236–7, 248, 267
Gamma GT tests 238, 267, 286, 297–8
gender differences 78, 90, 92–3, 192–3, 263, 281
    see also men; women
genetic factors 70–1, 106, 194–5
group effects 192–3, 197, 211–12, 263
group hypnotherapy 184, 187
group therapy 32, 39, 125, 179, 192–3, 263,
    281
    confrontational 190–2, 266, 281
    counselling 99, 100
    interactional 196–7, 281–2
    psychological meaning 280–1
    see also milieu therapy

halfway house 28, 138–41, 180, 182
heavy drinking, see alcohol consumption
    (quantity)
helping alliance 295, 297–303
heredity, see genetic factors
'hidden' alcoholics 70, 138, 139
higher-order interaction 262–4, 265, 288
high-risk situations 84, 86–7, 269, 282
Hippocratic tradition 13–19, 36, 38–40, 43,
    113, 119, 145, 266, 279–80, 296
    craftsmen and philosophers 13–16
    therapy as cultural phenomenon 16–19
homelessness 27, 115–17, 138, 139, 141,
    200–1, 218, 273, 287
hope 25, 32–33, 39, 40, 47, 50, 224, 229
hospitalization 177–8, 220, 269, 272, 273
    see also inpatient treatment
hypnotherapy, see group hypnotherapy

iatrogenic effects 24, 25, 75, 76, 145, 191–2,
    265–6, 281, 292, 299
indirect effects (interaction) 180–1
individual
    assessment 128, 143–4, 146–8, 150–1, 283
    therapy 32, 179
inpatient treatment 125
    intensive/peer-oriented 181–3
    Kissin study 198–200, 270–2, 303
    need for structure 284–7
    outpatient treatment versus 26, 27, 269–73,
        284–7, 302–3
    Penn-VA Project 161–9, 271–2, 284, 303
insight-oriented therapy
    alcoholism treatment 67, 74–5, 78, 218,
        291–2
    psychiatry 229–31, 278
Institute of Medicine (US) 3–4, 6, 30, 116,

    119, 128–9, 143, 149, 173, 269
integrative review 6–10
intelligence/intellect 198–9, 202–3, 206, 215,
    220, 270, 275
intensive treatment 26–8, 122–3, 145–6,
    181–3, 255–6
    group therapy 189–92, 281
interaction 41–3, 121–3, 136
    higher-order 262–4, 265, 288
    therapist–milieu 228–32, 278
interaction studies 35–6, 171, 258–64, 282–3,
    285–6, 288, 297, 299, 301–2, 303
    cognitive styles 204–32
    degree of dependence 233–51
    negative results 177–183
    personality traits 184–97
    research methodology 173–6
    social and psychological resources 198–203
    see also matching clients to treatments
interaction studies (other)
    Annis–Davis study 86–7, 282
    Azrin study 100, 279
    Glaser reanalysis 123
    Orford study 122–3
    Longabaugh study 102, 266, 281, 299
    Penn-VA Project 161–4, 262, 271–2, 278,
        284, 295, 302, 303
interdisciplinary approach 85–7, 108, 112,
    257–8
Internal–External Locus of Control Scale 221,
    276
    see also locus of control
International Classification of Diseases 59,
    109, 258
Interpersonal Discrimination Task 212, 213, 274
interpersonal relationships 189, 216, 276, 277
    attachment 187–8, 280–1
    helping alliance 295, 297–303
    maturity 204–5, 274
    therapeutic 38–9, 120, 289, 290, 299–302
    see also social investment; sociopathy
intervention, see treatment

learning model 79
    alcohol expectancies 51, 79, 80, 82–3, 84,
        85–6
    cognitive-behavioural model 83–5, 86
    conditioning approaches 79–82
    interdisciplinary approach 85–7, 257
legal model 47
life health 137–40
locus of control 221–8, 276–7, 279, 285, 302
lithium therapy 123
long-term
    outcome 28, 29–30, 31, 94–5, 97–8, 160,
        239–43, 247–9, 261, 267, 293–4
    prospective studies 48, 69–74, 94–5, 247
    treatment 26–7, 32, 154–6, 177–8, 256
loss of control, see control (loss of)

marital status 88–90, 96–8, 100, 240–3, 267, 272, 279
marital therapy 26, 30, 101
mastery 36, 86, 222–4, 282
matching
  definition 4
  hypothesis 2–6, 37, 40–3, 120–4, 147, 152, 173, 236, 255, 265, 283
  fruitfulness of hypothesis 4–5, 261–4
  prospective study 164–9
  systems approach 3–6, 126–9
matching clients to treatments 265–6
  abstinence/controlled drinking 266–9, 285, 292–3
  degree of structure 273–9, 285, 301–2
  inpatient/outpatient treatment 269–73, 284, 303
  systems approach 282–7
  treatment task 279–82, 299
Maudsley Hospital 25, 233–8, 300
mechanical composite (prediction) 131–4
men 78, 88–90, 192–3, 194–5, 281
  boys 71–2, 73, 106, 208
  married (study) 25, 94, 122–3, 233–8, 267–8
Menninger Foundation 39–40, 184, 299
meta-analysis 8, 23, 31–32
Michigan Alcoholism Screening Test (MAST) 156
milieu therapy 18, 99, 184, 187–8, 197, 280–1, 286, 292
Minnesota Model 30
Minnesota Multiphasic Personality Inventory (MMPI) 132, 193–4
mismatched/matched patients 164–9, 210–11, 213–14, 230
moderation-oriented approaches 24–5, 243, 244, 245–7, 249–51, 266–9, 286, 292
monolithic approach 124–5
mood states (impact) 68–9
Moral Maturity Scale 205
moral model 47–8
morning drinking 62, 64, 236, 239, 246
mortality (alcohol-related) 70, 88–90, 93
motivation 124, 146, 150
multifactorial relationships 239, 240
  see also higher-order interaction
multivariant approach
  to alcoholism 107–12, 113, 115, 116, 142, 201
  to treatment 35, 37, 137, 142, 152, 198–201, 203
multivariate analysis 174, 257

National Collaborative Matching Project 3
National Institute on Alcohol Abuse and Alcoholism (NIAAA) 3, 20, 239
natural healing processes 16, 38, 40–3, 117–19, 279–81, 293–7
  see also recovery patterns; self-healing; spontaneous remission

neuropsychological dysfunction 75, 220, 275
no treatment 22–31 passim, 154, 169, 174, 198
non-directive therapy 209–11, 225, 273, 277, 278
  see also directiveness
non-problem drinking 239–44 passim, 247, 248, 266–8
  see also controlled drinking
non-specific hypothesis 37, 38, 40–2, 117, 119–20
'normal' drinking 239, 240, 268
Northern Addiction Centre 149

occupational factors 56, 90–2, 93, 97, 98
offenders (self-image) 189–91, 281
operant conditioning 79, 81–2
operative arts 16
'oral' traits 73
outcome research (review)
  alcoholism treatment 20–31, 255–6
  psychotherapy 31–33
outpatient treatment
  detoxification 272
  inpatient treatment versus 26, 27, 269–73, 284–7, 302–3
  Kissin study 198–200, 270–2, 303
  need for structure 284–6
  network/informal 181–3
  Penn-VA Project 161–9, 271–2, 284, 303
  see also aftercare

Paragraph Completion Method 204, 274
paraprofessionals 32, 144, 192, 292, 301
  see also peer-oriented programmes
parental relations 69, 71–3, 76
Patton State Hospital 39–40
peer-oriented programmes 27, 138, 181–3, 192–3, 281, 291, 292, 301
  see also self-help
pendulum problem 218–19, 220, 275
Penn-VA Project 127–8, 152
  Addiction Severity Index 156–60, 259, 261
  effectiveness of treatment 152–6
  matching (prospective study) 164–9, 261, 271–2, 303
  psychiatric severity 161–4, 271–2, 284, 303
Penn Psychotherapy Project 152, 265
personality disorder 48, 67–74, 77–8
personality traits 256
  Annis–Chan study 189–92, 266, 281, 299
  Kadden study 195–7, 278, 281–2, 299, 302
  Longabaugh study 102, 266, 281, 299
  Lyons–Sokolow study 192–3, 281, 299
  personality typologies 193–5
  Wallerstein study 184–9, 280–1, 299
persuasion hypothesis 249–51
physical dependence 62–3, 236

placebo effects
  alcohol 82–3, 85–6
  treatment 39, 119–20, 222–5, 295
  see also non-specific hypothesis
plant problem 218–19, 220, 275
powerlessness
  over alcohol 47–8, 290–1, 292
  component of alienation 221, 223, 276
  see also control (loss of)
prealcoholic personality 68–74, 77–8, 105
prediction 127, 130–6, 147
preoperational level 218–19, 275
prescriptive treatment model 18
prevention
  policies (primary) 54, 56, 62, 93, 103, 257
  programmes (secondary) 31, 246–7, 256,
    267–8, 293
  relapse 84, 86–7, 120, 144, 145, 196, 282,
    284–6
primary care 143–9 passim
problem (matching hypothesis) 2–6
problem chronicity 237, 258, 288
profile interpretation 131–4
profiles
  client 87, 282
  treatment 137–41, 157
prognostic indicators 115–16, 121–2, 135,
    202–3, 258–61, 295–6
projective test (Szondi Test) 185, 189
prospective studies
  matching 164–9, 261
  symptomatic model 48, 68–74, 256
protracted abstinence 78
psychiatric severity 158, 161–4, 196–7, 260,
    262, 271, 281, 284–7, 295, 203
psychic dependence, see psychological de-
    pendence
psychoanalysis 34, 68, 76–7, 291, 299
  see also insight-oriented therapy
psychobiological processes 64, 86, 242, 257
psychodrama 210
psychological
  dependence 59, 62, 63, 65, 288
  differentiation 216
  meanings 185, 280, 281, 282
  and social resources 198–203, 270–3, 284, 303
  variables 288–9
psychology (and predictions) 130–6
psychopathology 34, 68, 73, 77, 104–5, 194,
    196–7
  see also psychiatric severity
psychosocial equation 104
psychosocial treatment 50, 120, 279–80
  clinical strategies 288–303
  dynamics of 288–90
  effectiveness 17–18, 20–33, 39–40, 255–6
  research strategies 4, 11, 13, 17–19, 34–7,
    40–3, 117–24, 261–4, 283
  transcultural model 38–40, 295

see also psychotherapy; treatment; treatment
    effectiveness; treatment in perspective
psychotherapy
  dynamic 67–8, 74–8, 266, 291–2
  Penn Project 152, 265
  research findings 17–18, 31–3, 184, 187–8,
    198–200, 213–14, 218, 220, 221, 222–4,
    265, 271–6 passim, 279, 299, 300
  therapist–milieu interaction 228–32
  see also psychosocial treatment; treatment

qualitative approach 8
quasi-experimental approach 173–4, 178, 182,
    292

Rand Report I 154, 163, 173, 177–8, 183,
    239–40, 258, 268, 270
Rand Report II 154, 177–8, 238–43, 244, 262,
    267–8
reaction-formation 187
recovery patterns 93–6, 117–19, 195, 247–9,
    293–4
referral system 128, 150–1
regional systems (core–shell) 149–51
regional variations (alcohol problems) 70,
    93
regression artefact 117, 153–4
rehabilitation
  criteria 22–3, 116–17, 159–60, 256
  potential 115–16, 120–1, 136, 141
reinforcement
  of drinking 52–3, 81–2, 194, 257
  of sobriety 97, 98
  training 30–1, 99–101, 118–19, 279, 287
relapse 79–80, 82–4
  accepting 292
  controlled drinking and 24, 239–43, 244,
    246, 250, 266–8, 285, 292
  prevention 84, 86–7, 120, 144, 145, 196,
    282, 284–6
relatives, alcoholism in 70–2, 103, 106, 194–5
relaxation training 147, 225, 277
  see also stress management
remission 117, 239, 243
  environmental resources 96–8
  natural healing processes 38, 40–3, 117–19,
    279–81, 293–7
  spontaneous 37, 40–3, 94, 117–19
  see also recovery patterns
research 11
  basic assumptions 40–3, 117–24, 261–4
  core–shell system 143–4, 147–8, 283–4
  integrative review 6–10
  methodology (interaction studies) 173–6,
    258–61
  new directions 34–43
  outcome research 20–33, 255–6
  overview 1–2
  problem 2–6

research (*cont*)
  see also Hippocratic tradition; psychosocial
    treatment (research strategies)
restructuring ability 198–200, 214–20, 270–1,
    274–6, 277, 279
retrospective illusion 73, 77, 256
retrospective studies 68–9, 71, 94, 96
rod-and-frame test 214–18, 274–5
Role Construct Repertory Test 212
role modelling 84, 93, 102–3

Salvation Army 141, 180
schizophrenia 186, 228–32, 280
scientific critique (disease model) 51–4
secondary prevention 31, 246–7, 256, 267–8, 293
secure base 302–3
self-control training 29–30, 86–7, 282
self-efficacy 120, 223–4, 282, 298
self-esteem 74, 95–6, 192–3, 298–9
  superego 290–3
self-governance 95–6, 101, 290–1
self-healing 280, 295, 298–9, 302
self-help 27, 97, 98, 251, 295–7
  see also Alcoholics Anonymous; Al Anon
self-image 189–92, 215, 266, 281
self-medication 74, 77–8
self-reliance 207, 223, 276, 277
self-responsibility 204–5, 274
sentence-completion test 204, 209
Shadel Clinic 39–40
sheltered environment 273, 284–5, 287
short-term treatment 26–7, 32, 154–6, 177–8
shotgun approach 124, 125–6
sick role 55, 57, 257
skid-row alcoholics 115, 116, 201
  see also homelessness
smokers 73, 225, 276
social class 92–3, 205, 272, 288
'social competence' 200
social consequences (disease model) 55–7
social control 52, 55, 58, 88, 94–5, 97, 103,
    104, 119, 291
social drinking 83, 94–5, 163, 195, 248–9, 286
social investment 102, 281
social model 88, 258
  career 52, 101–3
  environmental resources 93–103 *passim*, 256,
    259, 272, 281, 294
  recovery patterns 93–6, 117–19, 195, 247–9,
    293–4
  social treatment approach 98–101
  symptomatic conception 88–93
social network 88, 97–8, 195, 272
  see also support
social and psychological resources
  Azrin study 100, 279
  Gibbs study 201–3
  Kissin study 198–201, 270–2, 303
  Penn-VA Project 161–9, 271–2, 284, 303

social skills training 30, 82, 245, 286
social stability/instability 199, 202–3, 227,
    270–2, 278, 284–6, 303
social treatment approach 98–101
  see also community reinforcement approach
socialization 115, 139, 196, 197
Society for the Exploration of Psychotherapy
    Integration (SEPI) 36
socio-cultural factors 82, 104–6, 257
  see also subcultures
socioeconomic status 200, 203, 270, 272
  see also social class
sociopathy 68, 70–1, 164, 196–7, 272, 278,
    282, 285, 302
spiritual model 47, 139, 297
spontaneous remission 37, 40–3, 94, 117–19
  see also natural healing processes; recovery
    patterns; self-healing
statistical prediction 130–6, 147
statistical significance 175
stereotyping of behaviour 53–4
stimulus generalization 74
stress management 30, 80–1
  see also relaxation training
stress theories 90–2
structure (degree of) 164, 196–7, 205–11, 217,
    219, 225–6, 272, 273–9, 284–7, 301–2
strychnine injections 39, 263
subcultures 70–1, 90–1, 104–5, 106, 145
superego support 290–3, 295
support (environmental resources) 57, 94, 96–8,
    102
  see also social network
supportive therapy 67, 227–8, 286, 291, 297–8
Swedish Planning and Rationalization Institute
    for the Health and Social Services (SPRI)
    88, 93
symptomatic conceptions (social model) 88–93
symptomatic model 67–8, 105, 289, 294
  dynamic psychotherapy 67–8, 74–8, 266,
    291–2
  evaluation and trends 77–8, 256
  prospective studies 48, 68–74
systems of alcoholism treatment 3, 126–9, 152
  clinical/statistical prediction 130–6, 147
  core–shell system 128, 142–51
  implementation 282–7
  monolithic and shotgun approaches 124–6
  Penn-VA Project 128, 152–69, 271–2
  treatment profiles 137–41

technique hypothesis 40–3
Temposil 226–8, 276, 286
tension-reduction theory 79, 80–1
therapeutic
  community 161, 180, 192, 281
  relationship 36, 38–9, 289–90, 297–302
therapist–milieu interaction 228–32, 278
therapy

as cultural phenomenon 16–19
  see also specific therapies
tolerance, see alcohol tolerance
trait ratings 131–34
transactional analysis 75
transcultural model 38–9, 295
treatment
  advice versus 25–6, 233–6
  approach 279–82, 289–90, 297–9
  changing notions 37–40
  definition 6
  duration 26–7, 32, 154–6, 177–8, 255–6,
    271–2, 281
  dynamics 288–90
  environment, see environment
  goal 116–17, 137–9, 146, 266–9, 285, 289–93
  intensity 26–8, 122–3, 145–6, 181–3, 255–6
  milieu 228–32, 278
  negative effects, see iatrogenic effects
  profiles 137–41, 157
  research, see research
  setting 269–73, 289–90, 302–3
  task 279–82, 289, 299
  see also matching clients to treatment;
    psychosocial treatment; rehabilitation;
    systems of alcoholism treatment; treat-
    ment effectiveness, etc.
treatment effectiveness
  review 20–33, 255–6
  project 152–6

test of time 17–18, 39–40, 263–4
treatment in perspective
  alcoholics (differences) 256–8
  interaction effects 258–61
  matching (conclusion) 261–4
  superiority of method 255–6
treatment strategies
  dynamics of 288–90
  helping alliance 297–303
  natural healing processes 293–7
  supporting the superego 290–3

unemployment 90, 93, 271, 284
uniformity assumption myth 35

verbal psychotherapy 275–6, 302
vulnerability 69, 105–6

will-power 95, 296
Winter Veterans Administration Hospital 184
withdrawal symptoms 52–3, 62–5 passim, 81,
    86, 234, 236, 249
  see also protracted abstinence
women
  alcoholics 78, 90, 192–3, 263, 281
  wives of alcoholics 233–7, 242–3
World Health Organization 56–66 passim,
    109, 160, 257
writers (alcoholism rate) 91